OXFORD MEDICAL PUBLICATIONS

Infectious Disease Epidemiology

Oxford Specialist Handbooks published and forthcoming

General Oxford Specialist Handbooks
A Resuscitation Room Guide
Addiction Medicine
Day Case Surgery
Perioperative Medicine, 2e
Pharmaceutical Medicine
Postoperative Complications, 2e
Renal Transplantation

Oxford Specialist Handbooks in Anaesthesia
Anaesthesia for Medical and Surgical Emergencies
Cardiac Anaesthesia
Neuroanaethesia
Obstetric Anaesthesia
Ophthalmic Anaesthesia
Paediatric Anaesthesia
Regional Anaesthesia, Stimulation and Ultrasound Techniques
Thoracic Anaesthesia

Oxford Specialist Handbooks in Cardiology
Adult Congenital Heart Disease
Cardiac Catheterization and Coronary Intervention
Cardiac Electrophysiology and Catheter Ablation
Cardiovascular Computed Tomography
Cardiovascular Magnetic Resonance
Echocardiography, 2e
Fetal Cardiology
Heart Failure, 2e
Hypertension
Inherited Cardiac Disease
Nuclear Cardiology
Pacemakers and ICDs
Pulmonary Hypertension
Valvular Heart Disease

Oxford Specialist Handbooks in Critical Care
Advanced Respiratory Critical Care
Cardiothoracic Critical Care

Oxford Specialist Handbooks in End of Life Care
End of Life Care in Cardiology
End of Life Care in Dementia
End of Life Care in Nephrology
End of Life Care in Respiratory Disease
End of Life in the Intensive Care Unit

Oxford Specialist Handbooks in Infectious Diseases
Infectious Disease Epidemiology

Oxford Specialist Handbooks in Neurology
Epilepsy
Parkinson's Disease and Other Movement Disorders, 2e
Stroke Medicine

Oxford Specialist Handbooks in Oncology
Practical Management of Complex Cancer Pain

Oxford Specialist Handbooks in Paediatrics
Paediatric Dermatology
Paediatric Endocrinology and Diabetes
Paediatric Gastroenterology, Hepatology, and Nutrition
Paediatric Haematology and Oncology
Paediatric Intensive Care
Paediatric Nephrology, 2e
Paediatric Neurology, 2e
Paediatric Radiology
Paediatric Respiratory Medicine
Paediatric Rheumatology

Oxford Specialist Handbooks in Pain Medicine
Spinal Interventions in Pain Management

Oxford Specialist Handbooks in Psychiatry
Child and Adolescent Psychiatry
Forensic Psychiatry
Old Age Psychiatry

Oxford Specialist Handbooks in Radiology
Interventional Radiology
Musculoskeletal Imaging
Pulmonary Imaging
Thoracic Imaging

Oxford Specialist Handbooks in Surgery
Cardiothoracic Surgery, 2e
Colorectal Surgery
Gastric and Oesophageal Surgery
Hand Surgery
Hepatopancreatobiliary Surgery
Neurosurgery
Operative Surgery, 2e
Oral and Maxillofacial Surgery, 2e
Otolaryngology and Head and Neck Surgery
Paediatric Surgery
Plastic and Reconstructive Surgery
Surgical Oncology
Urological Surgery
Vascular Surgery, 2e

Oxford Specialist Handbook of Infectious Disease Epidemiology

Edited by

Ibrahim Abubakar
Professor of Infectious Disease Epidemiology and Director,
Centre for Infectious Disease Epidemiology,
University College London,
London, UK

Helen R. Stagg
Senior Research Fellow,
Centre for Infectious Disease Epidemiology,
University College London,
London, UK

Ted Cohen
Associate Professor in Epidemiology of Microbial Diseases,
Yale School of Public Health,
New Haven, USA

Laura C. Rodrigues
Professor of Infectious Disease Epidemiology,
Faculty of Epidemiology and Population Health,
London School of Hygiene and Tropical Medicine,
London, UK

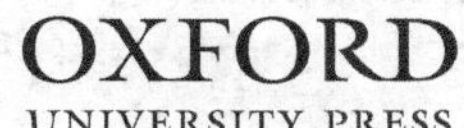

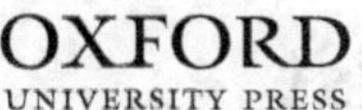

Great Clarendon Street, Oxford, OX2 6DP,
United Kingdom

Oxford University Press is a department of the University of Oxford. It furthers the University's objective of excellence in research, scholarship, and education by publishing worldwide. Oxford is a registered trade mark of Oxford University Press in the UK and in certain other countries

First Edition published in 2016

Published in the United States of America by Oxford University Press
198 Madison Avenue, New York, NY 10016, United States of America

British Library Cataloguing in Publication Data

Data available

Library of Congress Control Number: 2015947355

ISBN 978–0–19–871983–0

Printed in Great Britain by
Ashford Colour Press Ltd, Gosport, Hampshire

Preface

The discipline of epidemiology has undergone remarkable advances over the last two decades as a result of progress in computing, statistics, molecular biology, genomics, and immunology. These changes have allowed previously unimagined approaches that range from simple molecular-level outbreak investigations to the more complex analysis of routinely collected data needed for selection of vaccine viral strains, or for predicting resistance to antimicrobial agents. Such advances are powerful, often automated, and a great addition to 21st-century epidemiology. But their use, often through clear and proven protocols, could result in neglect in first developing a solid foundation in the basic epidemiological and data analysis principles that underpin them.

While many courses allow students and practitioners to gain a full understanding of epidemiology and biostatistics during their time of study, a quick reference text that comprehensively covers this discipline for use was lacking. The *Oxford Specialist Handbook of Infectious Disease Epidemiology* fills this gap.

Section 1 of the handbook covers a comprehensive list of methods relevant to the study of infectious disease epidemiology, from a general introduction to topics such as mathematical modelling and sero-epidemiology.

Section 2 addresses major infectious diseases that are of global significance, either due to their current burden or their potential for causing morbidity and mortality. This concise handbook for the pocket/electronic pocket of practising infectious disease epidemiologists is a welcome addition to the medical literature.

David L. Heymann, MD
Professor, Infectious Disease Epidemiology
London School of Hygiene and Tropical Medicine

Acknowledgements

Our sincere gratitude goes to several individuals who helped to make this book a reality. We gratefully acknowledge the colleagues who contributed chapters and put up with our repeated requests for changes over the last year. The following helped bring the book to life through their invaluable thoughts and contributions: Adrian A. Root, Joanna Lewis, Vanessa Hack, and Joanne R. Winter. Technical editing prior to submission was performed by Jemma Lough, Independent Medical Editor.

To David Pencheon, many thanks for the helpful insight and for sharing your experience of what to do and, more importantly, what not to do when editing a handbook.

We would also like to acknowledge the support of colleagues, family, and friends. IA would like to thank Sani, Amita, and Ginnie; HRS would like to thank all the individuals who have made her the scientist and person she is today (*sapere aude*—Horace), as well as acknowledge the invaluable editing support provided by some wonderful symphonic power metal bands; TC would like to thank Alexandra, Jack, and Poppy; and LCR would like to thank Chris Yara and George, and friends and colleagues at the LSHTM.

Although the book is written with a primary focus on tackling infections in wealthy and middle-income countries, it is the hope of the authors that it would prove to be a useful reference for emerging economies and low-income/high disease-burden countries. Responsibility for the final version and any errors rests with us.

Finally, this book is dedicated to you, the reader, in the hope that you will find it useful in your quest to understand and apply the many aspects of infectious disease epidemiology that underpin the prevention, control, and elimination of disease.

IA
HRS
TC
LCR
2016

Contents

Contributors

Ibrahim Abubakar (editor)
Professor of Infectious Disease Epidemiology and Director,
Centre for Infectious Disease Epidemiology,
University College London;
MRC Clinical Trials Unit at University College London,
London, UK
(Chapters 1, 6, and 11)

Robert Aldridge
Academic Clinical Lecturer
Institute of Health Informatics,
The Farr Institute of Health Informatics Research,
University College London,
London, UK
(Chapter 7)

Sani H. Aliyu
Consultant in Infectious Diseases and Microbiology
Cambridge University Hospital NHS Trust,
Cambridge, UK
(Chapter 9)

Koye Balogun
Senior Scientist
Department of Immunisation, Hepatitis and Blood Safety,
Public Health England,
Colindale,
London, UK
(Chapter 22)

Mauricio L. Barreto
Professor
Instituto de Saude Coletiva,
Federal University of Bahia,
Salvador,
Brazil and Fundacao Oswaldo Cruz, Brazil
(Chapter 26)

Alexandre Blake
Medical Epidemiologist
Epicentre,
Paris, France
(Chapter 14)

Andrew Boulle
Associate Professor
School of Public Health and Family Medicine,
Centre for Infectious Disease Epidemiology and Research,
University of Cape Town,
Cape Town, South Africa
(Chapter 25)

Mike Catchpole
Chief Scientific Officer
European Centre for Disease Prevention and Control,
Stockholm, Sweden
(Chapter 2)

Ted Cohen (editor)
Associate Professor in Epidemiology of Microbial Diseases
Yale School of Public Health,
New Haven, USA
(Chapter 16)

Mary Cooke
Research Associate
Department of Infection and Population Health,
Centre for Infectious Disease Epidemiology,
University College London,
London, UK
(Chapter 18)

Barry Cookson
Professor
Centre for Clinical Microbiology,
University College London,
London, UK
(Chapter 7)

Phil J. Cooper
Professor
St George's University of London,
London, UK
(Chapter 26)

Ken Eames
Lecturer
Centre for the Mathematical
Modelling of Infectious Diseases,
Department of Infectious Disease
Epidemiology,
London School of Hygiene and
Tropical Medicine,
London, UK
(Chapter 15)

Nigel M. Field
Academic Clinical Lecturer
Research Department of
Infection and Population Health,
University College London,
London, UK
(Chapters 9 and 10)

Lakshmi Ganapathi
Clinical Fellow
Division of Infectious Diseases,
Boston Children's Hospital and
Harvard Medical School,
Boston, USA
(Chapter 27)

Walter Haas
Head of Respiratory Diseases
Robert Koch Institute,
Berlin, Germany
(Chapter 3)

Paul Hunter
Professor of Health Protection
Norwich Medical School,
University of East Anglia,
Norwich, UK
(Chapter 19)

Charlotte Jackson
Research Associate
Research Department of
Infection and Population Health,
Centre for Infectious Disease
Epidemiology,
University College London,
London, UK
(Chapter 15)

Mark Jit
Senior Lecturer in Vaccine
Epidemiology
Department of Infectious Disease
Epidemiology,
London School of Hygiene and
Tropical Medicine,
London, UK;
Senior Scientist
Modelling and Economics Unit,
Public Health England,
London, UK
(Chapter 17)

Anne Johnson
Professor of Infectious Disease
Epidemiology
Research Department of
Infection and Population Health,
University College London,
London, UK
(Chapter 23)

Leigh Johnson
Epidemiologist
Centre for Infectious Disease
Epidemiology and Research,
University of Cape Town,
Cape Town, South Africa
(Chapter 25)

Marc Lipman
Clinical Senior Lecturer
and Consultant Physician in
Respiratory and HIV Medicine,
Division of Medicine,
University College London,
London, UK
(Chapter 6)

Duncan MacCannell
Senior Advisor for Bioinformatics
Centers for Disease Control and Prevention,
Atlanta, USA
(Chapter 10)

Sema Mandal
Consultant Epidemiologist
Department of Immunisation, Hepatitis and Blood Safety,
Public Health England,
Colindale, London, UK
(Chapter 22)

Punam Mangtani
Senior Lecturer
Faculty of Epidemiology and Population Health,
London School of Hygiene and Tropical Medicine,
London, UK
(Chapter 4)

Noel McCarthy
Professor and Honorary Consultant Epidemiologist
Division of Health Sciences,
Warwick Medical School,
University of Warwick, UK;
Field Epidemiology Service,
Public Health England, UK
(Chapter 8)

Emma Meader
Clinical Scientist
Norfolk and Norwich University Hospital NHS Trust,
Norwich, UK
(Chapter 19)

Andrew J. Nunn
Professor of Epidemiology
MRC Clinical Trials Unit,
University College London,
London, UK
(Chapter 5)

Patrick P.J. Phillips
Senior Statistician
MRC Clinical Trials Unit,
University College London,
London, UK
(Chapter 5)

Molebogeng X. Rangaka
UCL Excellence Fellow and Clinical Lecturer
Centre for Infectious Disease Epidemiology,
University College London,
London, UK
(Chapter 6)

Laura C. Rodrigues (editor)
Professor of Infectious Disease Epidemiology
Faculty of Epidemiology and Population Health,
London School of Hygiene and Tropical Medicine,
London, UK
(Chapter 12)

Katherine Russell
Specialist Registrar in Public Health
Centre for Infectious Disease Surveillance and Control,
Public Health England,
Colindale, London, UK
(Chapter 2)

William A. Rutala
Director/Professor
Division of Infectious Diseases,
University of North Carolina School of Medicine;
Department of Hospital Epidemiology,
University of North Carolina Health Care,
Chapel Hill, USA
(Chapter 21)

Tanvi Sharma
Assistant Professor of Paediatrics and Director of Fellowship Programme
Pediatric Infectious Diseases,
Boston Children's Hospital and Harvard Medical School,
Boston, USA
(Chapter 27)

Emily E. Sickbert-Bennett
Division of Infectious Diseases,
University of North Carolina School of Medicine;
Department of Hospital Epidemiology,
University of North Carolina Health Care,
Chapel Hill, USA
(Chapter 21)

Adrian Smith
Associate Professor
Nuffield Department of Population Health,
University of Oxford,
Oxford, UK
(Chapter 8)

Peter G. Smith
Professor of Tropical Epidemiology
Department of Infectious Disease Epidemiology,
London School of Hygiene and Tropical Medicine,
London, UK
(Chapter 24)

Pam Sonnenberg
Reader in Infectious Disease Epidemiology
Research Department of Infection and Population Health,
University College London,
London, UK
(Chapter 23)

Saranya Sridhar
Clinical Research Fellow
Jenner Institute,
University of Oxford,
Oxford, UK
(Chapter 11)

Helen R. Stagg (editor)
Senior Research Fellow
Research Department of Infection and Population Health,
Centre for Infectious Disease Epidemiology,
University College London,
London, UK
(Chapters 9 and 10)

Clarence Tam
Assistant Professor
Saw Swee Hock School of Public Health,
National University of Singapore,
Singapore
(Chapter 3)

Frank Tanser
Professor
School of Nursing and Public Health,
University of KwaZulu-Natal,
Durban, South Africa
(Chapter 14)

Maria Gloria Teixeira
Professor
Instituto de Saude Coletiva,
Federal University of Bahia,
Salvador, Brazil
(Chapter 20)

John M. Watson
Deputy Chief Medical Officer for England
Department of Health,
London, UK
(Chapter 18)

David J. Weber
Professor of Medicine and Pediatrics, School of Medicine, Professor of Epidemiology, Gillings School of Public Health, University of North Carolina, Chapel Hill, USA
(Chapter 21)

Laura F. White
Associate Professor in Biostatistics
Boston University School of Public Health, Boston, USA; Adjunct Associate Professor, Harvard School of Public Health, Boston, USA
(Chapter 13)

Peter White
Reader in Public Health Modelling
MRC Centre for Outbreak Analysis and Modelling, and NIHR Health Protection Research Unit in Modelling Methodology, Imperial College, London, UK; Head of Modelling and Economics Unit
Public Health England, London, UK
(Chapters 16 and 17)

Tom A. Yates
PhD student
Centre for Infectious Disease Epidemiology,
University College London, London, UK
(Chapter 14)

Symbols and abbreviations

~	approximately
β	beta
©	copyright
°C	degree Celsius
$	dollar
γ	gamma
>	greater than
<	less than
μ	mu
φ	omega
%	percent
±	plus or minus
£	pound sterling
σ	sigma
θ	theta
➲	cross-reference
ACDP	Advisory Committee on Dangerous Pathogens
AIDS	acquired immune deficiency syndrome
ART	antiretroviral therapy
AR	attack rate *or* attributable risk
ARI	acute respiratory illness
ARR	attack rate ratio
AUROC	area under the receiver operating characteristic
BCG	bacille Calmette–Guérin
BSE	bovine spongiform encephalopathy
BSI	bloodstream infection
CA-UTI	catheter-associated urinary tract infection
CAPI	computer-assisted personal interviews
CAR	clinical attack rate
CDC	Centers for Disease Control and Prevention
CDI	*Clostridium difficile* infection
CFR	case fatality ratio/rate

CFU	colony-forming unit
CHF	congestive heart failure
CJD	Creutzfeldt–Jakob disease
CLA-BSI	central-line bloodstream infection
CMV	cytomegalovirus
CONSORT	Consolidated Standards of Reporting Trials
CPE	carbapenemase-producing *Enterobacteriaceae*
CRP	C-reactive protein
CRS	congenital rubella syndrome
CSR	complete spatial randomness
DAA	direct-acting antiviral
DALY	disability-adjusted life-year
DENV	dengue virus
DF	dengue fever
DFA	direct immunofluorescence assay
DHF	dengue haemorrhagic fever
DNA	deoxyribonucleic acid
DSS	dengue shock syndrome
EBA	early bactericidal activity
EBS	event-based surveillance
ECDC	European Centre for Disease Prevention and Control
EIA	enzyme immunoassay
ELDSNet	European Legionnaires' Disease Surveillance Network
ELISA	enzyme-linked immunosorbent assay
ELISpot	enzyme-linked immunospot
EOC	emergency operations centre
ES	electrospray
ESEN2	European Sero-Epidemiology Network
ETEC	enterotoxigenic *Escherichia coli*
EU	European Union
EWRS	Early Warning and Response System
FN	false negative
FP	false positive
ft	foot/feet

GAM	generalized additive model
GAVI Alliance	Global Alliance for Vaccines and Immunisation
GBD	global burden of disease
GCP	*Good Clinical Practice*
GDP	gross domestic product
GEE	generalized estimating equation
GISRS	Global Influenza Surveillance and Response System
GIS	geographical information systems
GOARN	Global Outbreak Alert and Response Network
GP	general practitioner
GPHIN	Global Public Health Intelligence Network
GPS	global positioning system
GPW	Gridded Population of the World
HAART	highly active antiretroviral therapy
HAI	healthcare-associated infection
HBc	hepatitis B core
HBeAg	hepatitis B e antigen
HBIG	hepatitis B immunoglobulin
HBsAg	surface antigen of the hepatitis B virus
HBV	hepatitis B virus
HCC	hepatocellular carcinoma
HCP	healthcare personnel
HCT	HIV counselling and testing
HCV	hepatitis C virus
hGH	human growth hormone
Hib	*Haemophilus influenzae* type b
HIV	human immunodeficiency virus
HPV	human papillomavirus
HSV	herpes simplex virus
HTLV-1	human T-lymphocytic virus 1
HUS	haemolytic–uraemic syndrome
IBM	individual-based model
ICER	incremental cost-effectiveness ratio
ICH	International Conference on Harmonisation of Technical Requirements for Registration of Pharmaceuticals for Human Use

ICT	infection control team
IDMC	independent data monitoring committee
IFN	interferon
IFN-γ	interferon gamma
Ig	immunoglobulin
IHR	International Health Regulations
IL	interleukin
ILI	influenza-like illness
INICC	International Nosocomial Infection Control Consortium
IPP	inhomogeneous Poisson process
ISRCTN	International Standard Randomised Controlled Trial Number Register
ISTM	International Society of Travel Medicine
IT	information technology
IU	international unit
JCVI	Joint Committee on Vaccination and Immunisation
kg	kilogram
LGV	lymphogranuloma venereum
LR	likelihood ratio
LR–	negative likelihood ratio
LR+	positive likelihood ratio
LRTI	lower respiratory tract infection
m	metre
MAC-ELISA	M antibody capture enzyme-linked immunosorbent assay
MALDI-TOF MS	matrix-assisted laser desorption/time of flight mass spectrometry
MAMS	multi-arm multi-stage
MBM	meat and bone meal
MCID	minimum clinically important difference
MDR-TB	multidrug-resistant tuberculosis
MERS	Middle East respiratory syndrome
MERS-CoV	Middle East respiratory syndrome coronavirus
MHRA	Medicines and Healthcare products Regulatory Agency

MIRU-VNTR	mycobaterial interspersed repetitive units–variable number tandem repeat
mIU	milli international unit
mL	millilitre
MLST	multilocus sequence typing
MLVA	multilocus variable-number tandem repeat analysis
mm	millimetre
MMR	measles–mumps–rubella
MOOSE	meta-analysis of observational studies
MRC	Medical Research Council
MRSA	methicillin-resistant *Staphylococcus aureus*
MS	mass spectrometry
MSM	men who have sex with men
NAAT	nucleic acid amplification test
NATSAL	National Survey of Sexual Attitudes and Lifestyle
ng	nanogram
NGS	next-generation sequencing
NHSN	National Healthcare Safety Network
NICE	National Institute for Health and Care Excellence
NPV	predictive value of a negative test
NS1	non-structural protein 1
OCT	outbreak control team
OI	opportunistic infection
OR	odds ratio
PCR	polymerase chain reaction
PCR-ESI MS	polymerase chain reaction-electrospray ionization mass spectrometry
PCT	procalcitonin
PCV	proportion of cases vaccinated
PEP	post-exposure prophylaxis
PFGE	pulse field gel electrophoresis
PHEIC	Public Health Event of International Concern
PHL	public health laboratory
PKDL	post-kala-azar dermal leishmaniasis
PMTCT	prevention of mother-to-child transmission
PN	partner notification

POC	point-of-care
PPV	predictive value of a positive test or proportion of population vaccinated
PrEP	pre-exposure prophylaxis
Pro-Med	Programme for Monitoring Emerging Diseases
PrP	prion protein
PWID	people who inject drugs
QALY	quality-adjusted life-year
R_0	basic reproductive number
$R_{effective}$	effective reproductive number
RCT	randomized controlled trial
RDT	rapid diagnostic/detection test
RFLP	restriction fragment length polymorphism
RNA	ribonucleic acid
ROC	receiver operating characteristic
RR	relative risk *or* risk ratio
rRNA	ribosomal ribonucleic acid
RSV	respiratory syncytial virus
RT-PCR	reverse transcription polymerase chain reaction
SAE	serious adverse event
SAR	secondary attack rate
SARS	severe acute respiratory syndrome
sCFR	symptomatic case fatality ratio or rate
SD	standard deviation
SEIR	susceptible–exposed–infectious–recovered
SFC	spot-forming count
SI	susceptible–infectious
SIR	susceptible–infectious–recovered
SIS	susceptible–infectious–susceptible
SLTEC	Shiga-like toxin-producing *Escherichia coli*
SMART	sequential multiple assignment randomized trial
SMR	standardized morbidity ratio
SNP	single nucleotide polymorphism
SSI	surgical site infection
STD	sexually transmitted disease

STEC	Shiga toxin-producing *Escherichia coli*
STH	soil-transmitted helminth
STI	sexually transmitted infection
SUSAR	suspected unexpected serious adverse reaction
SVR	sustained virological response
TB	tuberculosis
TN	true negative
TNF	tumour necrosis factor
TP	true positive
TSC	Trial Steering Committee
TSE	transmissible spongiform encephalopathy
UK	United Kingdom
URTI	upper respiratory tract infection
USA	United States of America
USD	United States dollar
UTI	urinary tract infection
VAERS	Vaccine Adverse Event Reporting System
VAP	ventilator-associated pneumonia
VBD	vector-borne disease
vCJD	variant Creutzfeldt–Jakob disease
VE	vaccine efficacy
VHF	viral haemorrhagic fever
VL	visceral leishmaniasis
VRE	vancomycin-resistant *Enterococcus* species
VTEC	verocytotoxin-producing *Escherichia coli*
WASH	water, sanitation, and hygiene
WGS	whole-genome sequencing
WHO	World Health Organization
ZIKV	Zika virus

Section 1

Epidemiologic Methods

Chapter 1

Introduction

Ibrahim Abubakar

What is infectious disease epidemiology?

Epidemiology provides the tools to understand why and how infections spread and how they might be prevented or contained. For example, when a new infection emerges or there is an outbreak of a known disease, infectious disease epidemiologists are the scientists that collect, analyse, and interpret data to inform interventions to halt further spread. Many infectious diseases do not respect national boundaries, and some that initially affect only one part of the globe can rapidly spread to other populations. The dramatic rise in commercial air travel has ensured that the time between the appearance of a new pathogen and its global spread is much shorter than ever before. Outbreaks of viral haemorrhagic fevers (VHFs), such as Ebola and Lassa fever, and respiratory viruses, such as influenza, typically attract media and political interest due to the potentially high morbidity and mortality. An infectious disease epidemiologist is concerned with a range of pathogens—from viruses through fungi to infestation with parasites. Infectious agents are also important underlying causes of subsequent disease. For example, some infections, such as hepatitis C virus (HCV) and human papillomavirus (HPV), cause cancers, while others increase the risk of subsequent autoimmune disease.

More formally, infectious disease epidemiology is the application of methods and approaches used to understand the distribution and determinants of health and disease to the study of infections. This definition provides a framework to help our understanding of infectious disease epidemiology, and the ability to prevent, treat, and control morbidity and mortality from infectious causes. Very broadly, the discipline of epidemiology allows us to take information from individuals and to aggregate it into logical groups (defined by the characteristics of the person, the environment, or time) to understand from where the infection has arisen, how it might be spreading, and thereby the potential means for prevention and containment. This simple analysis is usually referred to as 'descriptive epidemiology' and is mainly useful for the generation of hypotheses. To formally test a hypothesis that aims to explain these observations, we require more sophisticated approaches that use a variety of study designs to minimize bias and statistical methods to quantify the role of chance, which is referred to as 'analytical epidemiology'. Such techniques are explored in Section 1 of this book, with general overviews in ➔ Chapter 4, which outlines study designs and issues specific to infections, and ➔ Chapter 13, which describes statistical approaches for analysis. The second half of the book describes the epidemiology of common infections and is organized mainly into chapters covering particular body systems such as respiratory or gastrointestinal infections. Hospital-acquired infections are addressed in two chapters: a methods chapter covering hospital outbreak investigation (➔ Chapter 7) and a descriptive epidemiology chapter with a US perspective (➔ Chapter 21).

The objectives of infectious disease epidemiology include:

- assessing the extent of the disease in a given population in terms of transmission, new 'incident' cases, and existing 'prevalent' cases
- understanding the prognosis and natural history of infections, including links to diseases not previously considered to be of infectious origin

- determining the infection causing a particular disease and the risk factors that increase the frequency of infection acquisition and progression from infection to disease, sequelae, and different clinical outcomes
- assessing the efficacy and effectiveness of preventive and curative measures
- informing the development of policies that would aid the prevention, control, and eventual elimination of the infection.

An understanding of the host response to pathogen exposure is a prerequisite for the study of the epidemiology of infections. Similarly, the development of vaccines, antibiotics, and antiviral agents continues to play a central role in epidemiology and control of infectious disease:

- The development of some vaccines, which educate the immune system by pre-exposure to infectious agents or subunits of such agents, occurred prior to the discovery of the microbial origin of the particular infectious disease. Vaccines have remained central to the prevention and control of infectious disease.
- The discovery of antibiotics has changed the natural history of bacterial infections. Unfortunately, antimicrobial resistance emerged almost immediately and has now reached alarming levels globally.
- Although antivirals historically have had modest effectiveness, recent advances have been made in the treatment of viral infections such as human immunodeficiency virus (HIV) and hepatitis C.

More recently, newer treatments, such as immunomodulatory therapies, have been investigated in infections, such as monoclonal antibodies, which have shown promise in chronic diseases.[1] For example, a Cochrane review concluded that prophylaxis with palivizumab is effective in reducing the frequency of hospitalizations due to respiratory syncytial virus (RSV).[2] A recent trial in multidrug-resistant tuberculosis (MDR-TB) confirmed the safety of autologous mesenchymal stromal cell infusion as adjunctive treatment.[3] Further research capitalizing on improved knowledge of the immunological response to pathogens might lead to alternative therapies.

Infectious disease epidemiology has also been influenced by the emergence of new areas of biological research (including genomics and other 'omics'—metagenomics, transcriptomics, proteomics, and metabolomics), as well as advances in disciplines, such as immunology, which have extended our understanding of the biology and natural history of infections and opportunities for interventions. For example, stratified therapy, where the choice of treatment regimen takes into account the genetic make-up of the patient, has become possible with faster and cheaper genomic sequencing. However, this is accompanied by added complexity in terms of analysing the data generated and the tools required to undertake such analyses, given the sheer volume of data generated. The implications of these issues are addressed in ➲ Chapters 9 and 11.

How is infectious disease epidemiology different from non-infectious disease epidemiology?

The key concepts developed and used in epidemiology are applicable to the study of infections; indeed, several of these were developed originally to study infections, as they were major causes of morbidity and mortality globally at the time. Classically, the approach John Snow used to describe the cholera outbreak of 1854 in London is one of the earliest uses of epidemiology. An even earlier example is Daniel Bernoulli's study of the benefits of variolation on smallpox mortality, which demonstrated limited gains.[4]

As the incidence of major infectious diseases declined in industrialized nations over the past century, chronic conditions, such as cancer and cardiovascular disease, have become the predominant focus of epidemiological studies in these settings. Nevertheless, infectious disease epidemiology continues to play an important role in the control of morbidity and mortality globally, with a disproportionate impact in the developing world.

The discipline of infectious disease epidemiology does, however, differ from non-infectious disease epidemiology in several ways.

Agent, host, and the environment

Unlike in non-infectious diseases, which are not transmitted from host to host, mixing patterns with other people, as well as with animals, influence the frequency of infectious diseases. The transmission dynamics of infections must be taken into account when investigating the spread of infections and measures required for disease control. Figure 1.1 shows a widely used model to account for the role of the infectious agent, host, and environment. This model assumes that the three elements have attributes that influence each other in a complex way and contribute to the spread of infections.

Transmission and transmission dynamics

A second largely unique feature of infectious diseases is that their causative agents can be transmitted from person to person (or between animals and people, or animals and animals), leading to sustained transmission and often to outbreaks that may require prompt public health action.

Another unique characteristic of infections is that some animals, typically insects, may serve as vectors to transmit the infection to humans. Examples include mosquitoes that can carry the dengue virus or the parasite that causes malaria, and the *Triatominae* that carry the parasite that causes Chagas' disease. Non-infectious diseases, such as those caused by environmental contamination, may arise from exposure through a vehicle, but, unlike the vectors for infectious diseases, these vehicles are non-living and the causative agent within them may not evolve.

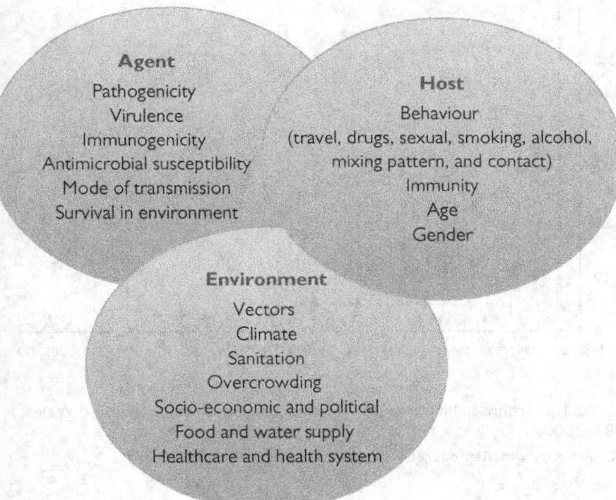

Figure 1.1 The interplay between the agent, host, and environment.

Transmission is the cause of the recurrent patterns often observed with infectious disease, which may vary in their predictability. For example, Figure 1.2 shows the yearly fluctuations in rates of influenza disease between 1989 and 2000 in England and Wales. It is logical to imagine that such a pattern may be described by a simple mathematical equation. If essential determinants of the observed pattern can be described, such a model might provide a mechanism to assess the impact of interventions and to inform planning of disease control. Mathematical modelling is discussed further in ➲ Chapter 16.

The transmissible nature of infections also means that, for most infectious diseases, the impact of any single case and its public health and economic consequences may go beyond those attributable to the loss of quality of life and risk of death to that individual. Cancer may result in a substantial loss of healthy life-years among those directly affected, while a single infection could spread and eventually affect many individuals. Assessment of the public health impact of interventions against infections therefore will usually use models that account for the non-static nature of infectious disease spread. Such models are presented in ➲ Chapter 16, and approaches to economic evaluation that consider the impact of transmission are presented in ➲ Chapter 17.

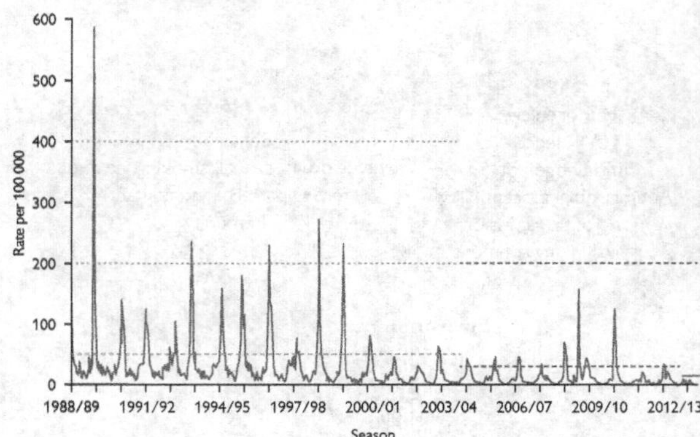

Figure 1.2 Trends in influenza per 100 000 population in England and Wales, 1989–2000.

Subclinical infections

Another unique feature of infections is the observation that subclinical infections in individuals who are asymptomatic carriers or who are in the preclinical or convalescent phase of illness may still transmit infection to others. This means that knowledge of the observed number of symptomatic cases of a particular infection alone may not be sufficient to fully understand trends or to assess the effects of interventions.

Immunity

Infections also differ from non-infectious diseases because the natural history of an infection in the human host is altered by previous levels of exposure to the organism or by active or passive immunization. For some infectious diseases, immunity can be conferred for life, while repeat episodes due to recurrence or reinfection are possible for other infections.

Host and causative organism genomes

The genomes of microorganisms determine the behaviour, drug susceptibility, pathogenicity, and virulence of the infecting agent, and thus the characteristics of the disease; to varying degrees, the human genome also influences the susceptibility of the host, as well as its reaction to specific treatments. Although older genetic typing methods allowed the identification of some resistance mutations and typing of strains, whole-genome sequencing (WGS) has facilitated the investigation of the entire genes of pathogens, leading to a fuller understanding of their evolution (phylogenetics), transmission patterns, and resistance, which is further discussed in ➔ Chapter 10. The interactions between humans and microorganisms are complicated; in certain parts of the body, such as the gut, an abundant pool of usually harmless and beneficial bacteria—the microbiome—may alter the behaviour of pathogenic organisms. The discipline of metagenomics aims to investigate the full genomic material of host organisms and coexisting microorganisms.

Concepts in infectious diseases epidemiology

Comprehensive dictionaries of epidemiological terms are available online and as published books;[5] an overview of basic concepts is provided here.

The temporal stages after exposure to an infectious agent are illustrated in Figure 1.3. After a person is exposed to a pathogen, they may become infected. The time between exposure and the onset of symptoms is referred to as the incubation period, and the time between exposure and the onset of infectiousness is called the latent period. The average period between two equivalent stages of consecutive infected cases is the serial interval, which is most frequently measured at symptom onset, due to the clinical ease of defining this time point. Often, some individuals are asymptomatic and yet transmit the organism to others, which is known as a carrier state (see ➜ Chapters 13 and 16).

One of the most widely used concepts in infectious disease epidemiology is the idea of a reproductive number (R), which is used to denote the number of secondary cases attributable to a single infectious individual (see ➜ Chapters 13 and 16). The basic reproductive number (R_0) for a pathogen is R when the infection is introduced into a fully susceptible population, and the effective reproductive number ($R_{effective}$) is R in a population where some individuals may be immune.

Herd immunity refers to the indirect protection of individuals in a population who are not vaccinated or otherwise immune; this indirect protection arises as a consequence of the immunity of others in their community.

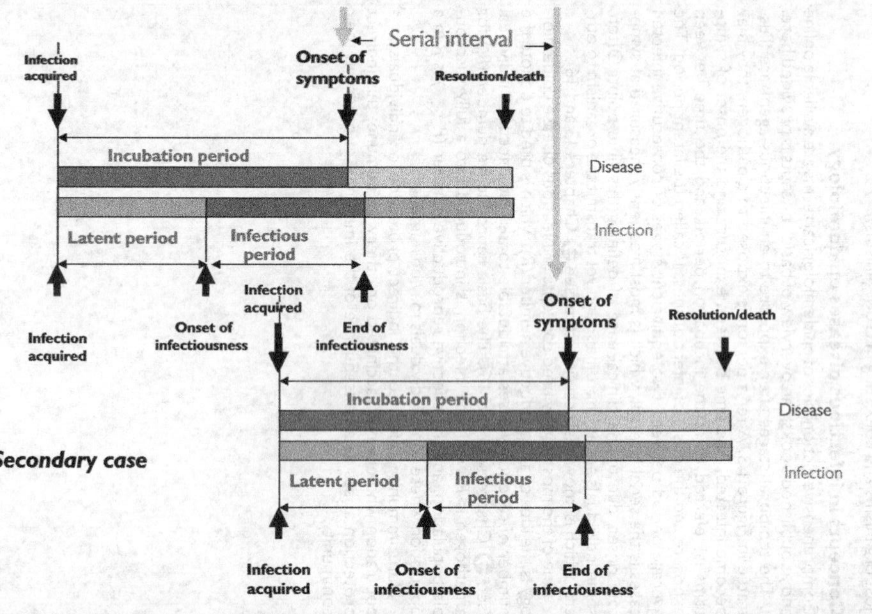

Figure 1.3 Temporal stages of an infection.

Source/reservoir, mode of transmission, and host response

Source/reservoir

Sources of infections include symptomatic human cases, animals, and the environment. For example, respiratory viruses may be spread by coughing and aerosolization of organisms that are then inhaled, causing infections in susceptible people. Some infections, such as typhoid fever, may be transmitted by asymptomatic or convalescent human carriers, while others are acquired from animals (e.g. zoonotic infections such as salmonella) or the environment (e.g. legionnaires' disease).

Mode of transmission

An infection can be transmitted:

- directly, e.g. sexually (HIV), by touching (scabies), by biting (rabies), or vertically from mother to child (rubella and cytomegalovirus (CMV))
- indirectly via a vector or vehicle (food- and water-borne pathogens, healthcare-associated infections (HAIs), e.g. an infected catheter). Infections can also be spread by droplets over very short distances (Ebola) and by droplet nuclei, which are smaller and can travel longer distances (airborne transmission, e.g. influenza and tuberculosis (TB)).

Host response

Normally, the host's immune response is a key determinant of susceptibility to an infection. Broadly, this includes both innate and adaptive immunity.

Innate defence mechanisms include barriers like the skin and secretions, as well as immunological cells such as macrophages; their effectiveness varies with age and underlying illness. Adaptive immunity may be acquired through previous exposure to the pathogen, as well as through active and passive immunization. The implications of immunity on infectious disease epidemiology are discussed in more detail in ➲ Chapter 11.

Global burden of infections

Studies of the global burden of disease synthesize data from a variety of sources to highlight the changing pattern of infectious diseases. Remarkable declines in mortality from many infections have been observed, with the largest mortality decreases over the past three decades from diarrhoeal diseases, lower respiratory infections, TB, and measles.[6] Many countries experiencing these declines are going through a demographic transition. However, mortality data from the Global Burden of Disease (GBD) study also showed an increase in the age-standardized death rate from HIV/acquired immune deficiency syndrome (AIDS) in 2013, compared to 1990.[6]

More detailed analysis of global trends in the incidence of major infections, such as TB, HIV, and malaria, showed substantial variation by world region.[7] The incidence of all three infections has declined since 2000, with recent major reductions in TB, suggesting that global action may be working in many settings.

Management and control of infectious diseases: general principles

Traditional approaches to manage and control infections have been effective in tackling many pathogens. Although these approaches are being extended with modern technology, the basic principles of infectious disease control remain important.

Underpinning any infectious disease control or elimination plan is the need for a robust surveillance system. A strategic plan to control infectious disease must rely on sound knowledge of infectious disease epidemiology, evidence-based public health, and effective implementation, including appropriate and clear communication. Elements of a strategic plan for infectious disease control would include:

- assessing health needs and required resources
- setting objectives, identifying evidence-based interventions, and planning their implementation
- implementing the strategic plan, which includes:
  - an action plan covering containment and treatment
  - preventative interventions, including addressing wider social determinants and vaccination
  - prompt detection and management of outbreaks
- monitoring, evaluation, and lessons learned
- communication.

The continuing emergence of new pathogens, such as Middle East Respiratory Syndrome coronavirus (MERS-CoV), and new forms of known pathogens, such as Ebola virus and avian influenza, changing patterns of some infections, such as dengue fever (DF) and Chikungunya, re-emergence of previously endemic infections, and the development of antimicrobial resistance, such as methicillin-resistant *Staphylococcus aureus* (MRSA), all pose serious threats to the control of infections (see ➲ Chapter 6). For the foreseeable future, infections are likely to remain a challenge due to the movement of pathogenic species between animals and humans and the ability of microorganisms to evolve via mutations and the exchange of plasmids. The importance of infectious disease epidemiology is therefore here to stay for many decades to come.

References

1. Beck A, Wurch T, Bailly C, Corvaia N (2010). Strategies and challenges for the next generation of therapeutic antibodies. *Nat Rev Immunol*, **10**, 345–52.
2. Andabaka T, Nickerson JW, Rojas-Reyes MX, Rueda JD, Bacic Vrca V, Barsic B (2013). Monoclonal antibody for reducing the risk of respiratory syncytial virus infection in children. *Cochrane Database Syst Rev*, **4**, CD006602.
3. Skrahin A, Ahmed RK, Ferrara G, *et al.* (2014). Autologous mesenchymal stromal cell infusion as adjunct treatment in patients with multidrug and extensively drug-resistant tuberculosis: an open-label phase 1 safety trial. *Lancet Respir Med*, **2**, 108–22.
4. Bernoulli D (1971). An attempt at a new analysis of the mortality caused by smallpox and of the advantages of inoculation to prevent it. In: Bradley L, *Smallpox inoculation: an eighteenth century mathematical controversy*, Adult Education Department, Nottingham, p. 21, reprinted in Haberman S, Sibbett TA (eds) (1995). *History of actuarial science, volume VIII, multiple decrement and multiple state models*. William Pickering, London, p. 1.
5. Porta M, Last JM (2008). *Dictionary of epidemiology*. Oxford University Press, New York.

6. Murray CJL (2015). Global, regional, and national age-specific all-cause and cause-specific mortality and 240 causes of death, 1990–2013: a systematic analysis for the Global Burden of Disease Study 2013. *Lancet*, **385**, 117–71.
7. Murray CJL (2014). Global, regional, and national incidence and mortality for HIV, tuberculosis, and malaria 1990–2013: a systematic analysis for the Global Burden of Disease Study 2013. *Lancet*, **384**, 1005–70.

Chapter 2

Surveillance

Katherine Russell and Mike Catchpole

Definition of surveillance

Surveillance was defined within the 2005 International Health Regulations (IHR) as the 'systematic ongoing collection, collation and analysis of data for public health purposes and the timely dissemination of public health information for assessment and public health response as necessary'.[1] This definition highlights the three integral parts of any surveillance system—collection of data, analysis, and interpretation, and dissemination of results—and the underlying principle that surveillance outputs should be linked directly to implementation of public health actions.

Surveillance is an essential component of all public health practice. Although surveillance is most commonly used to guide the control and prevention of infectious disease, particularly through the detection of outbreaks, the principles and practice of surveillance are relevant to all domains of public health and ultimately can be considered as providing the evidence or information that should inform most public health actions.

Purpose of surveillance

Surveillance systems for infectious diseases may serve as a general 'safety net' to identify incidents and untoward trends or may be designed to deliver more specific detailed epidemic intelligence on the frequency, distribution, and determinants of infectious diseases with particular public health significance, thus providing information that can inform actions and decisions about programmes of public health interventions. The key aims of surveillance include:

- informing immediate public health actions, including providing reassurance that new or further action is not required
- guiding policy decisions and allocation of resources
- evaluating the delivery and outcomes of public health programmes
- generating hypotheses and stimulating research.

These aims are achieved by ascertaining information about cases of infectious diseases, the distribution of determinants of diseases, the outcomes of diseases, and performance of intervention programmes (e.g. coverage of vaccination programmes). The commonest aim is to measure disease occurrence. At its most basic, this may begin with initial recording of numbers of incident and/or prevalent cases, although demographic information is also collected in most instances, which allows analysis of risk by, for example, age and sex. With the addition of supplementary descriptive information on physical, behavioural, and environmental characteristics of cases, more specific risk factors can be elicited. The axiom that infectious disease surveillance is continuous and systematic enables trends in the incidence and distribution of disease to be observed.

Design of surveillance systems

Surveillance programmes vary according to the specific public health issues surrounding each disease and often also the type of healthcare systems from which case-based data are collected. Not every surveillance system will need to be, nor can be, set up in the same way. An initial assessment should be made of the feasibility of data collection for a new disease. If possible, data collection should be integrated with other data collection systems to reduce the burden on healthcare workers. The most effective and efficient surveillance systems are usually those that have the best fit with the local healthcare system infrastructure in terms of data collection and collation.

An effective surveillance system should have a documented protocol, with clearly defined aims and objectives to guide the process. Case definitions to be used in the surveillance system should be clearly laid out, which may include definitions for possible, probable, and confirmed cases. Desired sensitivity and specificity of case definitions will depend on the public health consequences of failing to detect true cases, the resources available to confirm a diagnosis, and the consequences of initiating public health actions in response to false-positive cases. Case definitions for a surveillance system may change over time, as more information is learned about a disease and new diagnostic tests are introduced.

Many factors will affect the design and scope of a surveillance system, including:

- disease characteristics such as the natural history of the disease and current understanding of its epidemiology
- opportunities for data capture and reporting
- public health impact of the disease
- political interest in the disease
- information needs of public health decision-makers
- available funding sources
- availability of relevant diagnostic technology, effective treatment, and preventive measures.

Plans for the analysis, interpretation, and dissemination of results should be considered in advance to ensure they are appropriate for the needs of the stakeholders.

Ensuring quality of surveillance systems

Good surveillance systems have several common attributes, but the importance of each factor will vary according to the disease itself and the ultimate outputs required from the surveillance data.[2] A surveillance system should be:

- simple—a simple system requires fewer resources and is more likely to be acceptable and timely
- relevant—the system should be useful and deliver outputs with content and a format that meet the needs of the public health system
- flexible—the system should be able to adapt to changing demands and be integrated with other surveillance systems, where appropriate
- acceptable—patients and healthcare workers should be willing to participate in the system
- sensitive—the system should be capable of detecting reliably any changes in disease frequency or distribution and/or detecting a high proportion of cases with a high positive predictive value
- complete—this is particularly important for diseases that require immediate public health actions or have significant health implications and for rare diseases that are either severe in nature or the subject of an elimination programme
- timely—the system should process the information within a useful time frame
- representative—the system should be able to describe the disease distribution accurately in terms of time, place, and person, without any obvious evidence of bias within the population under surveillance (which may be different from the general population)
- stable—the system should be reliable and not prone to changing levels of ascertainment.

Types of surveillance systems

Surveillance systems may be described as 'active' or 'passive' (Table 2.1); these labels are often used to distinguish whether the system operator (receiver of reports) or the data provider initiates the process of reporting and therefore will reflect the degree of effort put in to ensuring that cases under surveillance are identified to the system by the system operator. In an active surveillance system, the organization running the surveillance programme actively solicits reports of cases, often including null reports if no cases have been seen. In a passive surveillance system, information on cases is sent to the health agency without prompting.

Passive surveillance is commonly used for conditions with a high incidence and when high levels of ascertainment are not essential, such as *Campylobacter* infections, whereas active surveillance is generally reserved for conditions with a lower incidence for which complete ascertainment is important such as verocytotoxin-producing *Escherichia coli*. The impact of different types of surveillance may be seen in the level of case ascertainment achieved from each type; passive systems may be prone to more under-reporting than active systems, but this must be balanced by the additional resources required for an active system.

Table 2.1 Comparison of active and passive surveillance systems

Comparator	Type of system	
	Active	Passive
Benefits	• Increased completeness of data • Can improve timeliness of reporting • More reflective of true changes in disease activity	• Require fewer resources for a given level of coverage (number of potential data providers) • Generally easier to set up and operate • More feasible approach for diseases with high incidence
Drawbacks	• More resources required to obtain information • Timeliness limited by frequency of reporting prompts (capacity and acceptability constraints) • Can be difficult to sustain for long periods	• Under-reporting may be common • Bias in case reporting (according to case age, severity, etc.) • Lack of motivation and/or awareness to report among health professionals

Sources of data

Many different sources of data are employed in surveillance systems, each of which has its benefits and drawbacks. For some infectious diseases—HIV, for example—combining numerous sources of surveillance data may produce a richer picture of the disease, so that public health actions can be targeted appropriately.

With many disease surveillance systems, only a small proportion of the total number of cases will present to health services and so be identified. These clinically apparent cases represent the tip of the 'prevalent disease iceberg' and can be picked up through a surveillance system based on healthcare system reporting (the commonest form of reporting). A further proportion of clinically apparent cases—the bulk of the iceberg below the surface—may not be identified through the surveillance system due to lack of awareness of the need to report or due to lack of clinicians' time or resources for reporting; these represent clinical cases not presenting to the health services, preclinical, subclinical, latent, or chronic cases.

Statutory notifications of infectious diseases

Many countries have a defined list of diseases that all physicians are required to notify to the relevant public health authority (Box 2.1). Submission of these reports is a legal obligation and may be based on clinical suspicion of the disease, as well as reporting of confirmed cases.

Benefits

- A legal requirement to report is usually applicable to all clinical services, so offering potentially comprehensive coverage.
- A legal requirement will often specify the need for rapid reporting, which allows early detection of outbreaks and interventions.
- Once established, the data can be used to monitor trends in endemic diseases.

Drawbacks

- Despite a legal requirement for reporting, notification rates often vary for different diseases (reflecting variations in clinician awareness and motivation to report), and this can result in substantial under-reporting for some diseases, although effective surveillance can still occur with some degree of under-reporting.
- Surveillance is limited to the diseases, and often the level of data, specified in the legislation and so lacks flexibility, particularly for surveillance of new or emerging diseases.

Laboratory reports

Laboratory reports are based on laboratory-confirmed diagnoses of infectious diseases. Laboratories are often provided with lists of diseases for which they must provide information.

Benefits

- High specificity (high diagnostic validity).
- Particularly relevant for diseases that require laboratory results to distinguish the cause of disease, e.g. different forms of hepatitis.

Box 2.1 Notifiable diseases in the United Kingdom (UK), based on Health Protection (Notification) Regulations, 2010

- Acute encephalitis
- Acute infectious hepatitis
- Acute meningitis
- Acute poliomyelitis
- Anthrax
- Botulism
- Brucellosis
- Cholera
- Diphtheria
- Enteric fever (typhoid or paratyphoid fever)
- Food poisoning
- Haemolytic uraemic syndrome (HUS)
- Infectious bloody diarrhoea
- Invasive group A streptococcal disease
- Legionnaires' disease
- Leprosy
- Malaria
- Measles
- Meningococcal septicaemia
- Mumps
- Plague
- Rabies
- Rubella
- Severe acute respiratory syndrome (SARS)
- Scarlet fever
- Smallpox
- Tetanus
- Tuberculosis
- Typhus
- Viral haemorrhagic fever (VHF)
- Whooping cough
- Yellow fever

- May provide additional information on typing and antimicrobial resistance of the pathogen.
- Can be automatically extracted.
- Can monitor long-terms trends in diagnoses.

Drawbacks

- Still a voluntary system in many countries and so will be affected by participation bias.
- Only captures cases for which laboratory investigations are undertaken (e.g. severe cases, very young patients, and very old patients); laboratories may not receive, and hence be able to report, demographic or risk factor data.

Death notifications

Registration of all deaths is a legal requirement in most countries, and a death certificate, including a cause of death and contributing factors, must be completed by a doctor.

Benefits

- Usually very complete data.
- Can be used to compare trends over long periods.

Drawbacks

- Not useful to monitor mild diseases.
- Relies on accurate recording of contributing diagnoses by the doctor completing the death certificate.
- Can be affected by coding issues.

Hospital admission data

Most healthcare systems keep accurate records of all hospital admissions or attendances, which may include demographic data, the reasons for admission, diagnoses made, and patient-reported outcome measures for certain interventions. These records enable trends in hospital activity to be monitored, planning of future services, setting of targets, performance management, and monitoring of the effective delivery of healthcare.

Benefits

- Cover all hospitals.
- May be possible to link to other sources of data.
- Provides a measure of the severity/impact of a disease (e.g. seasonal or pandemic influenza).

Drawbacks

- Can be affected by inaccurate diagnoses or coding problems.
- Often a significant time delay in the coding process.
- Not suitable for diseases that rarely result in hospitalization.

Syndromic surveillance

Syndromic surveillance is based on reporting of clinical symptoms or signs by clinicians, providers of telephone-based health advice lines, or self-reports by members of the public, including Internet-based surveillance like Flunet. It typically looks specifically at common syndromes such as cold/flu, fever, cough, shortness of breath, vomiting, diarrhoea, and eye problems.

Benefits

- Can avoid delays related to laboratory confirmation of diagnosis or obtaining an appointment with healthcare providers and so provides an early-warning system.
- Provides an opportunity to monitor population groups not seen by clinical services.
- Can be used to monitor for emerging disease.

Drawbacks

- Lack of diagnostic certainty.

Other sources of data

- Sexually transmitted infection (STI) reporting: in the United Kingdom (UK), genitourinary medicine clinics are required to report anonymized data on a range of STIs.
- Primary care sentinel reporting systems: these use sentinel sites in general practice to monitor consultations in order to assess acute illness in the community; the Royal College of General Practitioners' weekly returns service[3] is a well-established system in the UK.
- Vaccine uptake: this can be monitored through child health information systems.
- Vaccine adverse incident reports: most countries have a specific mechanism for reporting side effects or incidents relating to the administration of vaccines. In the UK, this is known as the Yellow Card system and relies on clinicians filling in and returning cards following any incidents.
- Rare infections: these can be monitored through an active surveillance system that requires clinicians to submit a monthly return reporting, whether or not they have seen specific conditions. The British Paediatric Surveillance Unit,[4] in which paediatricians are asked to complete a card each month to document whether or not they have treated any specified childhood diseases, is an example of this type of system.
- International alerts and surveillance systems: a range of international systems provide alerts or surveillance information between countries. The IHR[5] require countries to build capacity for disease surveillance and share reports on specific diseases (Box 2.2). PulseNet[6] is a network of laboratories that detect food-borne infections worldwide using standardized typing methods and sharing real-time data. The European Legionnaires' Disease Surveillance Network (ELDSNet)[7] is coordinated by the European Centre for Disease Prevention and Control (ECDC) to monitor cases of legionnaires' disease across Europe.
- Event information: information about public health events can be collected on an ad hoc basis or via more structured methods. Global Public Health Intelligence Network (GPHIN) is an electronic public health early-warning system, developed by Canada's Public Health Agency in collaboration with the World Health Organization (WHO), which searches global media for information about events of public health concern. ProMed[8] is an international open-access source of public health alerts.
- Big data: more recently, evidence is appearing that monitoring use of keywords in search engines, Twitter, and other open digital content may be a useful contribution to surveillance.

Box 2.2 International Health Regulations (IHR) (2005)

The IHR is an international law that requires participating countries to prevent and respond to acute public health risks that have the potential to cross borders and threaten populations worldwide. The key requirements of the 2005 IHR include:

- Notification:
  - All events that may contribute to a public health emergency of international concern should be notified to the WHO, and countries must respond to requests for information about such events.
- National IHR focal point:
  - All countries must report through a national focal point that is accessible 24 hours a day, 7 days a week.
- Requirements for national core capabilities:
  - Each state must develop, strengthen, and maintain core public health capabilities for surveillance and response; sanitary and health services should be put in place at international airports, ports, and border crossings.
- Recommended measures:
  - Each state must abide by recommendations from the WHO in response to public health emergencies of international concern.

Source: data from World Health Organization, *International Health Regulations*, Copyright © WHO 2005, available from http://www.who.int/topics/international_health_regulations/en/.

Analysis and interpretation of surveillance data

All too often, the main focus of the design and running of a surveillance system is the process of collecting and collating data, with insufficient thought put into the analysis, and particularly the interpretation and dissemination. If these crucial steps are not well planned, surveillance signals may not lead to relevant public health actions.

Analysis

The type of analysis required for a surveillance system will depend on the data available and how it is used. The overall aim for analysis is to provide information of a content and format that allows stakeholders to use it directly to inform decisions and guide actions.

Simple descriptive statistics based on person, place, and time are the most basic form of analyses for surveillance data. This information can be presented using graphs showing trends over times or using geographical information systems (GIS) to produce maps of disease distribution. If denominator data are available, rates for specific diseases can be calculated and compared with those for previous time periods.

To detect outbreaks or determine if a change in frequency is significant, a range of different statistical techniques may be employed. For example, scan statistics may identify locations of disease clusters in space and time (➔ Chapter 14). More complex model-based approaches can be used to take additional variables into account, e.g. the exceedance score approach used by Public Health England.[9,10]

Interpretation

Surveillance systems for infectious diseases are often designed to provide rapid insight into the changing frequency or distribution of disease, rather than provide complete and fully validated information on cases. Careful interpretation of surveillance data is therefore important to ensure that real or potential limitations in data quality and representativeness are taken into account before public health actions are taken. Apparent increases or decreases in cases reported through surveillance systems may be the result of true changes in disease frequency or artefacts related to the surveillance system itself or to clinical or diagnostic practice. Potential causes of a 'signal' in surveillance outputs include the following.

True changes

- Changes in disease incidence, e.g. an increase in influenza cases at the start of a new pandemic.
- Seasonality of the disease, e.g. increases in norovirus infections during autumn and winter.
- Periodicity of the disease, e.g. the incidence of pertussis seems to increase every 3–4 years.
- Effects of an intervention, e.g. the introduction of a new vaccination programme.

Artefacts

- Introduction of a new, more sensitive laboratory diagnostic test.
- Changes in clinical practice that lead to more cases being diagnosed e.g. after the introduction of a new screening programme.
- Changes in clinical coding systems.
- Reporting delays.

Analysis and interpretation challenges

- Some of the problems faced in the analysis of surveillance data include:
    - lack of clear case definitions
    - under-reporting of cases
    - delays in reporting
    - lack of denominator data.

Dissemination of surveillance data and evaluation of the surveillance system

Dissemination

Dissemination of surveillance data in a form that is useful to the stakeholders is a vital part of the surveillance process. The manner and format of the output needs to be appropriate for the type of surveillance and for the audience requiring the information. The potential target audience for surveillance outputs may include the public; doctors, nurses, and other healthcare workers; health service managers; public health professionals; health promotion practitioners; environmental health professionals; government (local or national); and international organizations.

Sometimes it will be sufficient to disseminate data on a quarterly, or even yearly, basis; in other circumstances, such as when the prime purpose is to detect outbreaks or during epidemics, data may be required on a weekly, or even daily, basis. Some stakeholders may require short summaries with the key messages in order to influence their public health actions, whereas others may require extensive analysis of the results or the ability to download the results and manipulate the data themselves.

A clear understanding of the purpose of the surveillance system and who will require the information will allow it to be produced in an appropriate format.

Evaluation

All surveillance systems should be evaluated on a regular basis to determine whether they are fit for purpose. Guidelines for evaluating public health surveillance systems have been published by Centers for Diseases Control and Prevention (CDC) in the United States of America (USA).[2] This process will identify changes in the disease, difficulties in the reporting systems, and changes to stakeholders' needs and expectations. Evaluation should include reviewing all outputs from the surveillance system to ensure they are appropriate for those who need them and sufficient to inform any public health actions that may be required. A plan for regular evaluation of the surveillance system should be considered when designing any new system.

New opportunities for surveillance

Surveillance systems have been able to take advantage of recent developments in information technology, the ability of communities to access the Internet, and new molecular technologies. As further developments occur, public health authorities and owners of surveillance systems need to be aware of new opportunities to improve the information available to inform public health action.

Genomics

The past 20 years have seen a huge technological shift from phenotypic culture-based microbiological diagnoses towards molecular methods that provide genotypic information. Techniques within the field of genomics—such as multilocus sequence typing (MLST), multilocus variable-number tandem repeat analysis (MLVA), and WGS—increase the amount of information that can be elicited about individual pathogens (see ➲ Chapter 10).

Molecular typing techniques provide information to discriminate between different strains of a particular bacteria or virus to a much higher degree than older phenotypic methods. This provides an opportunity for earlier identification of outbreaks, detection of strains with higher virulence or pathogenicity, identification of linked cases or likely routes of transmission, and monitoring of the spread of genes for multidrug resistance or virulence. Currently, no one technique is used across all microbiological species, with certain techniques preferred for different organisms.

WGS will provide maximal discrimination of strains and can be linked to clinical and epidemiological phenotypic information. Currently, WGS is time-consuming, labour-intensive, and costly, which limits its use in many countries. However, the emergence of benchtop sequencing technology and the ability to process rapidly the amount of data developing in the future mean that WGS is likely to play an increasing role in the typing of microorganisms and surveillance systems.[11]

Event-based surveillance

The concept of event-based surveillance (EBS) has developed as an important part of early-warning and -response systems. It is defined as the organized collection, monitoring, assessment, and interpretation of mainly unstructured ad hoc information regarding health events or risks to health that may represent a potential acute risk to human health.

EBS sits alongside the traditional indicator-based surveillance systems, which are defined as the systematic collection, monitoring, analysis, and interpretation of structured data. The two systems are complementary, and both will play a role in a public health system's ability to detect significant issues early.

EBS can collect information from multiple, diverse, official, and unofficial sources, which may include the media, schools, workplaces, non-governmental organizations, and other informal health networks (Box 2.3). Data collection in EBS is usually an active process, which then requires a defined method to triage the information and determine

Box 2.3 Event-based surveillance (EBS) in action at the London 2012 Olympic and Paralympic Games

The Health Protection Agency used EBS as an integral part of its surveillance strategy during London 2012 Olympic and Paralympic Games. Local health protection teams across England were asked to report any events of interest from any source that might have an impact on the games to the regional operational cells. This information, together with information entered into the national electronic public health case management database, was reviewed by the EBS team daily for 73 days between July and September 2012.

The most commonly reported events were related to food-borne pathogens or diseases, followed by events relating to vaccine-preventable diseases.[13] EBS was found to be an effective way of identifying timely information on potentially significant events.[14]

what is, and is not, relevant. A verification process follows; an assessment of risk to human health is carried out, and the information is fed back to stakeholders.[12] The investigation and verification stage is significantly more important for EBS than traditional indicator-based surveillance, because of EBS's sensitive nature and potential to identify false rumours or hoaxes.

EBS is particularly useful for detecting rare or new events that would not be picked up by traditional indicator-based surveillance, as well as in communities that do not have access to formal healthcare organizations.

Big data

Big data is the name given to large amounts of information that might overload traditional database systems because of their volume, variety, and rate of change.[15] These data are often identified from search queries on the Internet or through social networks, such as Facebook or Twitter, but they are not easily analysed without the use of complex computer algorithms. The utility of big data for epidemiology and surveillance of infectious disease is beginning to be realized, and, as technology continues to develop novel ways to store, manage, and analyse large complex data sets, it is likely to provide greater opportunities to use different types of data for public health surveillance.

Google Flu Trends, which produces weekly graphs of influenza activity in 25 countries worldwide by aggregating specific search queries relating to influenza is one example of big data being used for surveillance of infectious disease.[16] However, this type of data is subject to many different influencing factors and may not always project future trends accurately. Understanding how best to leverage this voluminous (but variable-quality) data for public health benefit remains a challenge. Other uses of big data have included crowdsourcing techniques to carry out surveillance of influenza in the European Union (EU).[17] Supermarket loyalty cards contain large amounts of data that have potential uses for infectious disease surveillance and outbreak investigation. These data have been used to identify food items linked to an outbreak of hepatitis A in British Columbia[18] and to look at changes in purchasing behaviour for non-prescription medications during the influenza pandemic in 2009.[19]

Big data could provide many additional sources of information for surveillance. The challenges in using this type of data include addressing potential issues and concerns about data confidentiality and privacy, and the development of hardware, software, and statistical methods to, for example:

- extract relevant information from the vast amount of data available
- undertake appropriate statistical analyses to address the unique problems related to big data
- understand the reliability of the data and the different influences on Internet use and social media.

Data protection and governance issues

Data collected should be relevant and sufficient to meet the requirements of the surveillance system and should not include any information that is not essential. Data should be anonymized, wherever possible, but, if patient identifiable information is collected, it should be stored securely, with access granted only to those who require it.

Many instances of data on individuals being lost by organizations or used inappropriately have been reported. These episodes have resulted in most countries across the world bringing in strict data protection laws and guidance on issues around information governance (Box 2.4). These frameworks apply to all forms of surveillance systems, and owners of surveillance systems need to be aware of the legal framework relevant to the processing of data for such purposes. The UK's Data Protection Act (1998)[20] gives individuals the right to know how information about them will be used, the right to object to the use of information about them, and the right to access any information held about them. In 2012, the European Commission proposed the European General Data Protection Regulation,[21] which will establish a single set of data protection rules in all EU member states for all organizations that process personal data belonging to residents of the EU.

Box 2.4 Six key data-management principles based on the Caldicott principles used in the United Kingdom

Justify the purpose for using patient data:

- Do not use patient-identifiable information, unless absolutely necessary.
- Use the minimum necessary patient-identifiable information.
- Access to patient-identifiable information should be on a strict need-to-know basis.
- Everyone involved in use of the data should be aware of their responsibilities to maintain confidentiality.
- Understand and comply with the data protection laws in your country and any region of the world to which the data might be transferred.

Source: data from Health and Social Care Information Centre, *Quick reference guide to Caldicott and the Data Protection Act 1998 principles*, available from http://systems.hscic.gov.uk/infogov/igfaqs/quickreferencef.doc.

References

1. World Health Assembly (2005). *Revision of the International Health Regulations, WHA58.3. 2005*. Available at: http://apps.who.int/gb/ebwha/pdf_files/WHA58-REC1/english/Resolutions.pdf (accessed 19 January 2015).
2. Centers for Disease Control and Prevention Morbidity and Mortality Weekly Report (2001). *Updated guidelines for evaluating public health surveillance systems: recommendations from the Guidelines Working Group*. Available at: http://www.cdc.gov/mmwr/preview/mmwrhtml/rr5013a1.htm (accessed 19 January 2015).
3. Royal College of General Practitioners. *Research and Surveillance Centre*. Available at: http://www.rcgp.org.uk/clinical-and-research/our-programmes/research-and-surveillance-centre.aspx (accessed 19 January 2015).
4. Royal College of Paediatrics and Child Health. British Paediatric Surveillance Unit. Available at: http://www.rcpch.ac.uk/bpsu (accessed 19 January 2015).
5. World Health Organization (2005). *International Health Regulations (IHR)*. Available at: http://www.who.int/topics/international_health_regulations/en/ (accessed 19 January 2015).
6. PulseNet International. Available at: http://www.pulsenetinternational.org/ (accessed 19 January 2015).
7. European Centre for Disease Prevention and Control. *European Legionnaires' Disease Surveillance Network (ELDSNet)*. Available at: http://ecdc.europa.eu/en/activities/surveillance/ELDSNet/Pages/index.aspx (accessed 19 January 2015).
8. ProMED mail. Available at: http://www.promedmail.org/ (accessed 19 January 2015).
9. Farrington CP, Andrews NJ, Beale AJ, Catchpole MA (1996). A statistical algorithm for the early detection of outbreaks of infectious disease. *J R Stat Soc Ser A*, **159**, 49–82.
10. Noufaily A, Enki DG, Farrington P, Garthwaite P, Andrews N, Charlett A (2013). An improved algorithm for outbreak detection in multiple surveillance systems. *Stat Med*, **32**, 1206–22.
11. Sabat AJ, Budimir A, Nashev D, *et al.*; ESCMID Study Group of Epidemiological Markers (ESGEM) (2013). Overview of molecular typing methods for outbreak detection and epidemiological surveillance. *Euro Surveill*, **18**, 20380.
12. World Health Organization Western Pacific Region (2008). *A guide to establishing event-based surveillance*. Available at: http://www.wpro.who.int/emerging_diseases/documents/docs/eventbasedsurv.pdf (accessed 19 January 2015).
13. Health Protection Agency (2013). *Significant events reported by the Event Based Surveillance London 2012 Olympic and Paralympic Games*. Available at: https://www.gov.uk/government/uploads/system/uploads/attachment_data/file/398940/2.1_Event_Based_Surveillance_London_2012_report.pdf (accessed on 20 March 2014).
14. Health Protection Agency (2013). *London 2012 Olympic and Paralympic Games: summary report of the Health Protection Agency's Games times activities*. Available at: http://www.hpa.org.uk/webw/HPAweb&HPAwebStandard/HPAweb_C/1317137693820 (accessed 19 January 2015).
15. Hay SI, George DB, Moyes CL, Brownstein JS (2014). Big data opportunities for global infectious disease surveillance. *PLoS Med*, **10**, e1001413.
16. Google.org Flu Trends. *Explore flu trends around the world*. Available at: http://www.google.org/flutrends/intl/en_us/ (accessed on 19 January 2015).
17. Influenzanet. *Influenzanet*. Available at: http://www.influenzanet.eu (accessed on 19 January 2015).
18. Swinkels HM, Kuo M, Embree G, *et al.* (2014). Hepatitis A outbreak in British Columbia, Canada: the roles of established surveillance, consumer loyalty cards and collaboration, February to May 2012. *Euro Surveill*, **19**, 20792.
19. Todd S, Diggle PJ, White PJ, Fearne A, Read JM (2014). The spatiotemporal association of non-prescription retail sales with cases during the 2009 influenza pandemic in Great Britain. *BMJ Open*, **4**, e004869.
20. The Stationery Office. *Data Protection Act 1998*. Available at: http://www.legislation.gov.uk/ukpga/1998/29/contents (accessed 19 January 2015).
21. European Commission (2012). *Proposal for a regulation of the European Parliament and of the Council on the protection of individuals with regard to the processing of personal data and on the free movement of such data (General Data Protection Regulation)*. Available at: http://ec.europa.eu/justice/data-protection/document/review2012/com_2012_11_en.pdf (accessed 19 January 2015).

References

Chapter 3

Outbreak investigations

Clarence Tam and Walter Haas

Outbreak investigations

The investigation of outbreaks requires specific expertise and is a major task of infectious disease epidemiology. To ensure the best public health outcome during acute outbreak situations, a systematic approach to their timely detection, assessment, investigation, and control is required, together with rapid collation and rigorous interpretation of multiple sources of often imperfect evidence.

This chapter describes the basic principles of outbreak investigations. The epidemiological features of different types of outbreaks are described, together with the use of surveillance for outbreak detection and case ascertainment, the role of the outbreak control team, the major features of epidemiological and environmental investigations, issues in the interpretation of evidence, and considerations in the implementation and evaluation of control measures.

What is an outbreak?

An outbreak is often defined as an increase in incidence of a disease above expected levels in a particular location or population in a given time period. Another common definition is the occurrence of a disease in two or more epidemiologically linked individuals, such as those with a confirmed common source of infection.

Types of outbreaks and epidemic curves

Outbreaks can be common-source, propagated, or both. In common-source outbreaks, a population is exposed to a common source of contamination. Exposure may be restricted to a particular event or point in time (a point-source outbreak), intermittent over an extended period, or continuous. In propagated outbreaks, the infection is transmitted from person to person directly (e.g. influenza) or indirectly (e.g. mosquito-borne transmission of dengue virus (DENV)). Propagated outbreaks can include several waves of transmission resulting from secondary and tertiary spread. A mixed outbreak occurs when a common-source outbreak involves secondary person-to-person spread; this is common for pathogens transmissible through food and the faeco–oral route such as norovirus, hepatitis A virus, and *Shigella*.

The epidemic curve—a plot of the number of new outbreak cases by the time/day of illness onset—is a crucial feature of any outbreak investigation and can provide valuable information on the type of outbreak, mode of transmission, incubation period, exposure period, and transmission potential of the infection (Figure 3.1). The steps required to investigate an outbreak are summarized in Box 3.1.

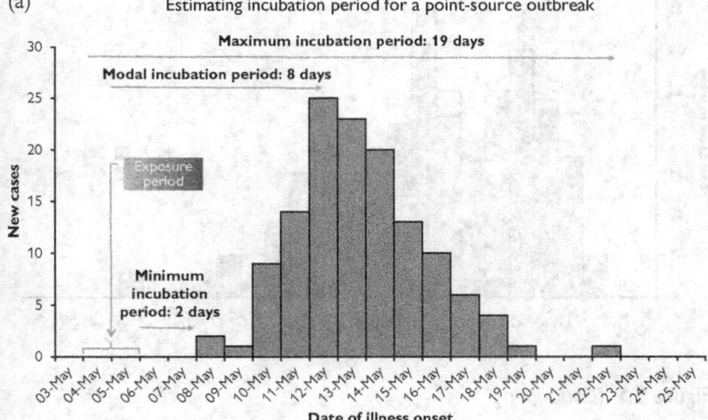

Figure 3.1 Types of outbreaks. Point-source outbreaks: if the exposure period is known, the epidemic curve enables the calculation of the modal incubation period and range, which can be useful for narrowing down the list of likely causal pathogens (a); if the incubation period is known, the exposure period can be inferred (b); extended common-source outbreak (c); mixed outbreak with initial point-source and subsequent propagation through person-to-person transmission (d).

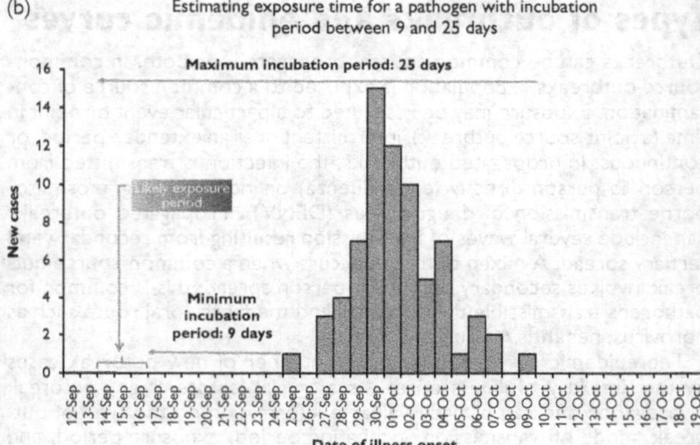

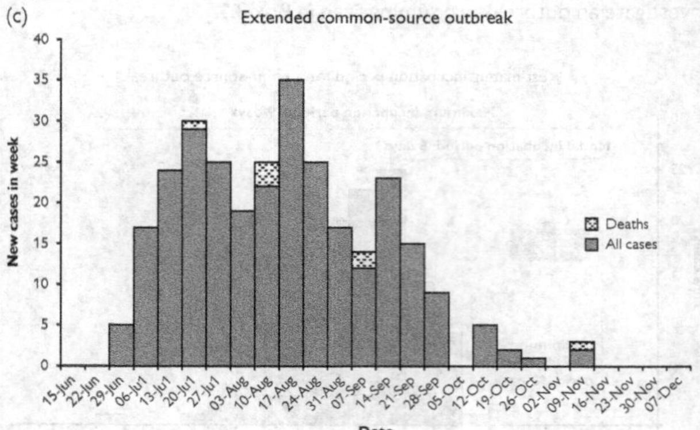

Figure 3.1 (*Continued*)

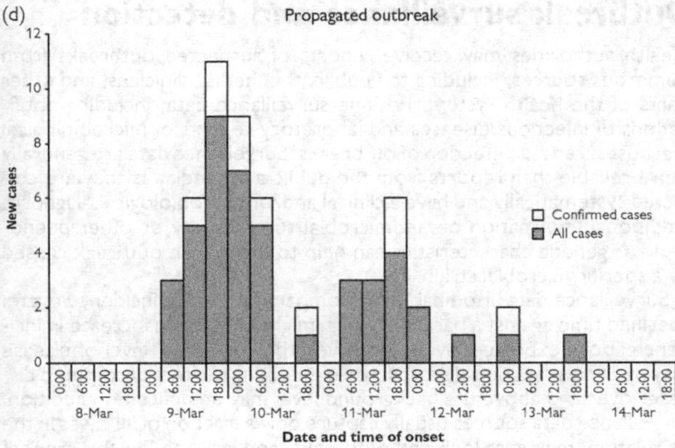

Figure 3.1 (*Continued*)

Box 3.1 Steps of an outbreak investigation

- Conduct outbreak surveillance and detection.
- Confirm the diagnosis, and assess the public health impact.
- Convene an outbreak control team, and establish communication.
- Establish a case definition and mechanisms for case ascertainment.
- Conduct thorough descriptive epidemiological and preliminary investigations.
- Where relevant, conduct contact tracing and environmental investigations.
- If necessary, undertake an analytical study to identify the cause of the outbreak.
- Communicate the findings.
- Implement and evaluate control strategies.

Outbreak surveillance and detection

Health authorities may receive reports of suspected outbreaks from numerous sources, including the public, the media, clinicians, and other parts of the health system. Routine surveillance data, including notifications of infectious diseases and laboratory reports of microbiological diagnoses, can aid detection of outbreaks. Surveillance data are generally more reliable than reports from the public and media, as they are collected systematically and have a clinical and/or microbiological diagnosis. Additional information on antimicrobial susceptibility or other phenotypic or genetic characteristics can help to identify an outbreak caused by a specific microbial strain.

Surveillance data also enable the comparison of case incidence over a specified time against a baseline, which might indicate an increase in incidence above expected levels. However, the 'expected' level of disease may be unclear for rare diseases, while detecting clusters of common diseases over and above the background level may be difficult. In addition, surveillance data sources usually capture only a fraction of all cases in the population, may miss localized outbreaks, and lack the 'on-the-ground' context and detail that clinicians treating patients in hospitals or primary care can provide.

Investigating every potential outbreak report is unfeasible, so systematic collation and review of reports are important to prioritize those that require further investigation.

Assessing the public health impact

Assessing the public health threat is crucial to prioritize responses to specific outbreaks and assign adequate urgency and resources. Important considerations include disease severity (e.g. high risk of mortality), setting (e.g. vulnerable hospitalized populations), outbreak size, transmission potential, and feasibility of containment. Annex 2 of the IHR[1] provides a decision tree to judge the risk of international spread that would require immediate (<24 hours) communication to the WHO and collaboration with international counterparts for a Public Health Event of International Concern (PHEIC).

Special urgency is warranted if the risk of infection is ongoing and the outbreak source has not been identified or where specific interventions could curb exposure, such as ring vaccination in a measles outbreak or decommissioning and disinfection of water systems to prevent spread of *Legionella*. Political interest and implications can also play a role.

Prioritizing infectious diseases helps to allocate surveillance resources and support assessment of the potential impact of an outbreak based on known disease properties.[2] Emerging pathogens, such as influenza A H7N9 and MERS-CoV, pose a special challenge, because knowledge of their epidemic potential is limited at present, so even a single case of imported disease usually warrants thorough investigation to exclude its involvement in an outbreak[3]. ➲ Chapter 6 outlines the investigation of emerging infection outbreaks.

Convening an outbreak control team

Investigation of outbreaks usually requires a multidisciplinary approach, and its coordination is the responsibility of an outbreak control team (OCT). The public health authority in the locality where the outbreak is first detected is generally responsible for evaluating the situation, convening the OCT, and leading the investigation.

The team's composition should be adapted to the specific outbreak, but it usually comprises a public health specialist or an epidemiologist with field experience, a clinician, a microbiologist, a communications officer, and, where relevant, a representative of the affected institution(s). Additional expertise might be required, e.g. if an environmental source is suspected. Not all of these individuals will be part of the core team, but frequent communication (initially once or twice daily) ensures that no information is lost. Decisions and actions taken by the OCT should be documented to facilitate the exchange of information. The OCT should assess early on whether regional- and national-level epidemiologists should be alerted, e.g. if widespread transmission is likely, and whether to bring in specialist expertise not available locally, such as a reference microbiologist.[4] For suspected food-borne outbreaks, the food safety administration should be involved to initiate tracing of food products back through the supply chain.

Mechanisms for active, regular, and transparent communication with relevant authorities, the media, and the public should be established early on. The current status of the outbreak and investigation, affected groups, potential risks, and unknowns should be clearly communicated.

Case definitions

The OCT is responsible for developing clear and appropriate case definitions throughout the investigation. This ensures that cases are systematically identified and reported, and avoids expending resources investigating cases unrelated to the outbreak. Case definitions reflect a balance between sensitivity and specificity. An initial working case definition generally favours sensitivity over specificity, as the public health consequences of missing outbreak-related cases usually outweigh the resource implications of investigating cases not related to the outbreak. As the investigation develops and more information becomes available regarding the clinical and microbiological profile of the disease, the case definition will be tightened, with increasing focus on specificity. The case definition should be easy to interpret and implement, and should include key features of the disease, people affected, and epidemiological circumstances (time period, place, and potential exposure event).

Often information on each individual will be insufficient to classify them definitively as a case; microbiological confirmation may be lacking, and clinical signs and symptoms alone might lack specificity. A hierarchical set of definitions for confirmed, probable, and possible cases can be useful to classify cases based on the strength of evidence (Box 3.2). Where the disease has several clinical manifestations, definitions for a range of outcomes will be required.

Increasingly, microbiological typing and genetic profiling is used to detect unusual strain clusters and improve specificity of case definitions based on genetic relatedness, antimicrobial resistance profiles, and other microbial phenotypes. WGS is a rapidly evolving technique for molecular typing and characterization of outbreak strains in the future. ➲ Chapters 9 and 10 provide further detail on these techniques.

Box 3.2 Case definitions for influenza

- Influenza-like illness (ILI): sudden onset of symptoms with at least one of the following systemic symptoms—fever, malaise, headache, and myalgia—and one of the following respiratory symptoms—cough, sore throat, and shortness of breath.
- Acute respiratory illness (ARI): sudden onset of symptoms judged by a clinician to be due to an infection, with at least one of the following respiratory symptoms: cough, sore throat, shortness of breath, and coryza.
- Possible case of influenza: any person meeting the clinical definition of ILI or ARI.
- Probable case of influenza: any person meeting the clinical definition of ILI or ARI who has an epidemiological link to a confirmed case, which indicates human-to-human transmission.
- Confirmed case of influenza: any person meeting the clinical definition of ILI or ARI and with laboratory confirmation of influenza infection, defined by any of the following:
  - isolation of influenza virus from a clinical specimen
  - detection of influenza virus nucleic acid in a clinical specimen
  - identification of influenza virus antigen by direct fluorescence antibody test in a clinical specimen
  - presence of an influenza-specific antibody response.

Source: data from European Centre for Disease Prevention and control, *Influenza case definitions*, Copyright © European Centre for Disease Prevention and Control (ECDC) 2005–2015. Available from: ℘ http://ecdc.europa.eu/en/activities/surveillance/eisn/surveillance/pages/influenza_case_definitions.aspx.

Surveillance during an outbreak

Surveillance may need to be intensified to ascertain outbreak-related cases, particularly if the outbreak is widely disseminated, illness is severe, or the risk of onward transmission is high (see ➲ Chapter 2). The OCT should alert relevant public health authorities and clinicians and communicate case definitions and reporting procedures. Active surveillance may be required when timely and comprehensive case ascertainment is necessary (e.g. to initiate prompt treatment, containment, or contact tracing). The OCT will contact key personnel at predefined intervals to enquire about new cases of disease. Active surveillance is more feasible when cases are ascertained at a limited number of sites such as tertiary care centres or clinics within a defined location. A minimum set of information should be collected on each case using standardized forms, including contact details, age, sex, residential location, occupation, date of illness onset, laboratory confirmation, hospitalization, outcome, and common risk factors for the suspected pathogen.

Descriptive epidemiology

The epidemic curve should be updated daily to understand the course of the epidemic and to determine its magnitude, whether transmission is increasing or decreasing, and whether secondary or continuous transmission is occurring. The key clinical and epidemiological features of cases should be described, using the principles of person, place and time. The timing, location, and population affected can yield valuable clues regarding outbreak aetiology and control implications. Clustering of cases in time might point to a specific event at which transmission was initiated, such as a function or public gathering. Spatial clustering might indicate a common environmental exposure, while common characteristics of cases can indicate shared risk factors such as consuming food from the same venue, attending the same school, or belonging to a high-risk group.

Preliminary investigations

In-depth interviews with initial cases (or proxy respondents) can provide timely information to develop hypotheses regarding outbreak aetiology. Trawling questionnaires are often used to collect information on a comprehensive list of possible exposures before the onset of illness. Shared behaviours or exposures among initial respondents can lead to specific hypotheses and inform the development of standardized questionnaires for further investigations using analytical study designs. Careful consideration of the intended analysis is needed when designing the questionnaire to ensure that it captures sufficient breadth and detail on exposures, exposure information is specific to avoid misclassification biases, and adequate information is collected on likely confounders and other relevant features such as dose response, vaccination status, or use of personal protective equipment.

Contact tracing

Contact tracing serves to follow up exposed and potentially infected contacts to prevent further spread and to identify the source of infection. Exposure definitions should be standardized, and different risk categories are often assigned, based on relationships to the index case (e.g. household vs community contact) and the intensity and duration of contact. For TB, recommendations are fairly standardized internationally, and contact tracing is prioritized using a combination of diagnostic information (smear or culture positivity) and cumulative exposure time. The risk of contacts progressing to active disease is also considered.[5]

Environmental investigations

Environmental investigations are especially important for pathogens with non-human reservoirs of infection. For example, contamination of cooling systems with *Legionella* and aerosolized spread has caused large outbreaks, sometimes infecting people living several kilometres away from the source.[6,7] Environmental investigations are also important for investigating nosocomial spread via fomites or contaminated medical devices—as in outbreaks among patients in neonatal intensive care. For food-borne outbreaks, inspection of food premises, supply chain integrity, and compliance with established food hygiene standards are integral to the investigation. Detailed knowledge of infection vehicles, pathogen habitats, and transmission routes is necessary to direct environmental investigations. In certain contexts, other information, such as meteorological data on temperature, humidity, and wind direction and velocity, can be useful. Consideration should also be given to the frequency, timing, and location of environmental sampling and the sensitivity of pathogen detection from these samples.

Analytical studies in outbreak investigations

In most instances, descriptive analysis of the data will suffice to inform outbreak control strategies and protect groups at highest risk. Where evidence from initial epidemiological and environmental investigations is insufficient to implement adequate control measures, the OCT may decide to conduct an analytical study. Such studies require considerable resources, so the purpose and aims of the study should be clearly defined and agreed by members of the OCT and other partners involved in the investigation. Analytical studies might be particularly justified when:

- there is a public health imperative to identify the source of infection and prevent further cases
- the investigation could yield novel information regarding the epidemiology or natural history of the disease such as a previously unrecognized risk factor, the effectiveness of an intervention, or the infection serial interval.

Analytical studies involve the use of a comparison group to establish associations between suspected exposures and illness. Cohort studies and case control studies are most commonly used. The choice of study design depends on the specific circumstances. ➲ Chapter 4 provides further details on these study designs, including their limitations.

Cohort studies

Cohort studies are particularly useful for investigating point-source outbreaks in well-defined, relatively small populations such as a food poisoning outbreak among guests at a catered event. Investigators would interview all attendees to collect information on foods consumed at the event and subsequent illness. Associations between exposures and illness are analysed using exposure-specific attack rates and ratios (Table 3.1).

Case control studies

Case control studies are more suitable when cases are disseminated in space and/or time and the population at risk is difficult to define. In other situations, the population at risk may be well defined but too large to investigate using a cohort approach, so a case control study may be conducted by recruiting all, or a random subset of, cases and an adequate control group. Risk factors are identified by assessing exposure-specific odds ratios (ORs).

Appropriate choice of controls is important to minimize bias and depends on the specific outbreak. Because outbreaks often affect specific population subgroups, restriction and matching are commonly used for selection of controls to ensure that they reflect the population from which cases arise. Examples include outbreaks of varicella-zoster infection among patients with cancer, TB in schools, and syphilis detected at a clinic for STIs. For community-wide outbreaks, potential sources of controls include individuals registered at the same medical clinics as cases but who do not have the disease or civil registers such as the electoral roll or population registries. Random-digit dialling is a popular method

Table 3.1 Food-specific attack rates (ARs) and attack rate ratios (ARRs) in an outbreak of *Clostridium perfringens* food poisoning among guests at a hotel dinner party

Food item	Ate food item			Did not eat food item			ARR
	Cases	Total	AR (%)	Cases	Total	AR (%)	
Beef stew	42	47	89	1	14	7	12.51
Rice	41	49	84	2	12	17	5.02
Green salad	28	40	70	15	21	71	0.98
Bread	30	46	65	13	15	87	0.75
Cured meat sausage	3	6	50	40	55	73	0.69

The food-specific attack rate (AR) is the risk of disease among individuals eating a particular food item (the percentage of individuals eating a particular food item who subsequently fell ill). This is compared with the risk of disease among those who did not eat that particular food by means of a food-specific attack rate ratio (ARR; actually a ratio of risks). In the example, in this table, the AR is 42/47 = 89% among those eating beef stew and 1/14 = 7% among those not eating beef stew. Comparing the two gives an ARR of 89/7 = 12.51. People eating the beef stew were therefore 12.51 times more likely to become ill than those who did not eat the stew. A food item with a high food-specific AR and large ARR is a likely candidate for a contaminated food vehicle, as this implies that the food is strongly associated with illness and that it was consumed by a large proportion of cases.

Adapted with permission from Wahl E, Rømma S, Granum PE. A Clostridium perfringens outbreak traced to temperature-abused beef stew, Norway, 2012. *Euro Surveill.* 2013;18(9):pii=20408. Available online: http://www.eurosurveillance.org/ViewArticle.aspx?ArticleId=20408.

for selecting controls when a sampling frame is unavailable but is increasingly challenging (and potentially biased), given recent increases in the use of mobile phones. For reasons of expediency, some investigators ask cases to nominate peers as controls. Case-nominated controls are easier to identify, and acquaintance with the case can be an incentive to participate. However, acquaintances are likely to be similar to cases in terms of area of residence and certain behaviours that might be related to infection risk, so overmatching is a potential problem and could limit the ability to detect the exposure of interest.

Inference in analytical studies

Statistical evidence of the strength of association between exposures and illness can be assessed using *p* values and 95% confidence intervals for effect measures (ARRs or ORs), which are available in most statistical software (see Chapter 13). Mantel–Haenszel stratified analysis or multivariable regression models can be used to adjust for confounding factors. Matched study designs require specific analysis methods such as McNemar's test for matched pair designs or conditional logistic regression.

Outbreak size is usually a limiting factor in the analysis. Study power in an outbreak investigation is limited by the number of cases affected and the resources available for recruitment of controls. With modest case numbers, statistical support may be weak, yielding borderline *p* values and wide confidence intervals. However, analytical studies of outbreaks aim to provide evidence for timely public health action, not estimation of parameters. Statistical evidence and the strength of the association should be interpreted alongside other evidence, including results of microbiological and environmental investigations and the known biology of the suspected pathogen. For outbreaks of food-borne diseases, evidence from an analytical study implicating a specific food vehicle, identifying the same pathogenic strain in cases and implicated foods, and corroborating evidence of contamination from environmental investigations are considered the gold standard for establishing causation. Potential sources of bias, summarized in Table 3.2, should be considered when interpreting evidence from analytical studies.

Table 3.2 Common sources of bias in analyses of outbreaks

Type of bias	Description
Poor recall	Respondents' recall of exposures may be inaccurate, particularly for organisms with a long incubation period, such as *Giardia* or hepatitis A virus, or if there is a delay between onset of illness and the interview.
Recall bias	Exposure recall may be more accurate among cases than healthy respondents, because their illness has prompted them to think more carefully about possible exposures.
Selection bias	In case control studies, selection bias can occur when the control group does not adequately reflect the population from which cases arise. An example would be an investigation in which cases are recruited from a genitourinary medicine clinic, but controls are selected from the community, as it is not possible to know whether community controls would have attended the clinic had they developed the disease in question.
Participation bias	The incentive to participate in an outbreak investigation may be less for those who have not been ill, so respondents could be a selected, non-representative sample of healthy individuals.
Social desirability bias	Respondents may not be willing to provide information on risk factors that may be sensitive or stigmatizing, such as sexual activity, drug use, or potentially illicit behaviours, or they may provide responses that they feel are more socially acceptable.

Implementation and evaluation of control strategies

The OCT should decide and coordinate the implementation and evaluation of adequate control strategies. For any given strategy, consideration should be given to existing evidence for its effectiveness, resources and infrastructure available for implementation, and methods used for its evaluation. For example, a community-wide outbreak of TB would require consideration of resources and priorities for contact tracing, region-specific evidence for adherence to and effectiveness of chemotherapy in different risk groups and mechanisms for its delivery, the use of laboratory resources for molecular typing to identify chains of transmission, and mechanisms for prompt case finding and detection.

The OCT is responsible for declaring the end of an outbreak. The team should consider whether control strategies implemented are adequate to prevent new cases or whether there is a continuing threat to the population. The OCT should also discuss implications for:

- changes to existing control policy
- changes to guidelines for private enterprises, public bodies, and the general public
- procedural issues to facilitate future investigations
- legal issues arising from the outbreak
- future mitigation of risk
- further research into specific areas.

The OCT should arrange to complete a written report of the outbreak investigation, including implications and recommendations.

Conclusions

Outbreak investigations require a balance between epidemiological rigour and pragmatism, as circumstances often dictate the quality of available information and the scope and sophistication of the investigation. Geoffrey Rose's view that epidemiologists work with dirty hands, but a clean mind, and make concessions to rigour, always aware of the implications of each concession,[8] is no truer than when applied to outbreak situations. The acute nature of outbreaks, their capacity to cause great social disruption, and the need to identify the causes and implement adequate control measures rapidly means that investigators must often work with, and make decisions based on, descriptive analysis of imperfect data. Development of clear questions and systematic assessment of all the strands of evidence, with its associated limitations, should be guiding principles for making sound inferences. Fortunately, circumstances often work in our favour; for many outbreaks, the exposure effect is strong and can be detected in analytical studies with a modest sample size, and results should be robust against various forms of bias, particularly when considered in the context of other evidence. However, because outbreaks often affect specific population subgroups and result from unusual circumstances, results are not easily generalizable to other settings.

References

1. World Health Assembly (2005). *Revision of the International Health Regulations, WHA58.3. 2005*. Available at: http://apps.who.int/gb/ebwha/pdf_files/WHA58-REC1/english/Resolutions.pdf (accessed 19 January 2015).
2. Balabanova Y, Gilsdorf A, Buda S (2011). Communicable diseases prioritized for surveillance and epidemiological research: results of a standardized prioritization procedure in Germany, 2011. *PLoS One*, **6**, e25691.
3. Reuss A, Litterst A, Drosten C (2014). Contact investigation for imported case of Middle East respiratory syndrome, Germany. *Emerg Infect Dis*, **20**, 620–5.
4. Gregg M (2008). *Field epidemiology*, 3rd edn. Oxford University Press, New York.
5. European Centre for Disease Prevention and Control (ECDC). *Risk assessment guidelines for infectious diseases transmitted on aircraft (RAGIDA)—tuberculosis*. ECDC, Stockholm.
6. Nguyen TMN, Ilef D, Jarraud S (2006). A community-wide outbreak of Legionnaires' disease linked to industrial cooling towers—how far can contaminated aerosols spread? *J Infect Dis*, **193**, 102–11.
7. White PS, Graham FF, Harte DJG, *et al.* (2013). Epidemiological investigation of a Legionnaires' disease outbreak in Christchurch, New Zealand: the value of spatial methods for practical public health. *Epidemiol Infect*, **141**, 789–99.
8. Coggon D, Rose G, Barker D (2003). Measurement error and bias. In: Coggon D, Rose G, Barker D (eds). *Epidemiology for the uninitiated*. BMJ Publishing Group, Chennai, pp. 21–8.

Chapter 4

Study design

Punam Mangtani

Introduction to study design

Epidemiological studies provide evidence that helps us understand the natural history, clinical prognosis, transmission, and control of infectious disease. The controlled trial is the most rigorous design and commonest type of intervention study. Allocation is usually randomized or quasi-randomized. Trials can provide strong evidence on which to act and are invaluable to monitor and evaluate interventions, uptake, screening programmes, to assess the risk of infections and to control outbreaks.

Often, however, observational designs are the only possible studies for ethical and logistical reasons. The choice of study design will be affected by the characteristics of the diseases, what is already known, and the urgency of the response required.

Identifying a question and a clear set of objectives is a key first step in designing both trials and observational studies (Box 4.1). The questions to be answered in relation to infectious diseases using epidemiological studies include:

- Who is at risk of acquiring an infection or developing an infectious disease?
- How is infection acquired?
- Why does infection progress to disease, sequelae, or death?
- Which of the possible interventions is the most effective?

Box 4.1 Formulating the question and objectives: a key first step

- Construct a clear question (aim) or hypothesis to test:
  - Discuss with colleagues, nationally responsible bodies, and/or funders to ensure the question is relevant and fits identified priorities.
  - The aims include the general question, the risk factor, the outcome, and the population to be examined; develop separate questions if there is more than one risk factor or outcome.
- Develop a clear set of objectives:
  - The objectives list the individual tasks to answer the question.
- Be specific:
  - Specify the target population (the population to which the findings can be generalized) and source population (from which the study subjects are recruited), and define inclusion and exclusion criteria for the study population.
  - Define the outcomes and risk factors and how they will be measured.
- Measure outcomes and risk factors with as much accuracy as possible.
- Confirm that objectives can be fulfilled by the design selected.

Outcomes can be colonization, carriage, infection, disease, positive serology or strain, sequelae, or death. Infection can thus be the risk factor causing disease in one study, and the outcome after being 'exposed' to a source of infection in another.

Epidemiological studies answer three main types of questions:

- What is the distribution of the disease or condition, i.e. what are the patterns by person, place, and time?
    - Patterns can suggest the possible infectious cause, target groups affected, and priority recipients for interventions, as well as assess the burden of the infection. The latter informs decisions about resource allocation and the benefits of intervention, compared to its risks. These are descriptive studies.
- What are the determinants of an infectious disease, and what are the factors that may affect these?
    - These may be the host, the agent, or environmental factors at the population or individual level. The level of importance and interplay between them will vary substantially by disease and intervention. For example, host and viral factors strongly influence the zoonotic potential of avian influenza viruses, while social factors influence the ability to quarantine patients with possible severe acute respiratory syndrome (SARS) to reduce onward transmission. These are analytical studies.
- What are the effect and impact of an intervention?
    - An evaluation has four main stages—stage 1 is formative research that assesses the feasibility of the materials used or activities planned; stage 2 examines process measures such as uptake of the intervention; stage 3 measures the impact on knowledge, attitudes, and practices; and stage 4 assesses the effect or impact on outcomes. Epidemiological study design contributes mostly to the last three stages. These are evaluation studies.

Some questions are best answered by other important public health-related sciences. For instance, social science or anthropological methods are often needed to understand why an intervention is taken up or whether it is acceptable. Economic analyses help assess the most efficient use of resources (see ➔ Chapter 17).

The main study designs

Epidemiological studies are divided into two main types: observational (non-experimental) and interventional (experimental) studies (Figure 4.1). In the latter study type, the researcher allocates the intervention. In both study types, the data can come from groups or individuals. Observational studies can be descriptive, e.g. descriptive studies of TB may use routine surveillance data to assess burden and trends by time, place, or person. They may also be analytical (aetiological), in which information on risk factors is examined in relation to the outcome, e.g. rates of TB in a sample of areas may be examined in relation to the average level of deprivation or overcrowding.

A key criterion for all study designs is the ability to control for confounding (Box 4.2).

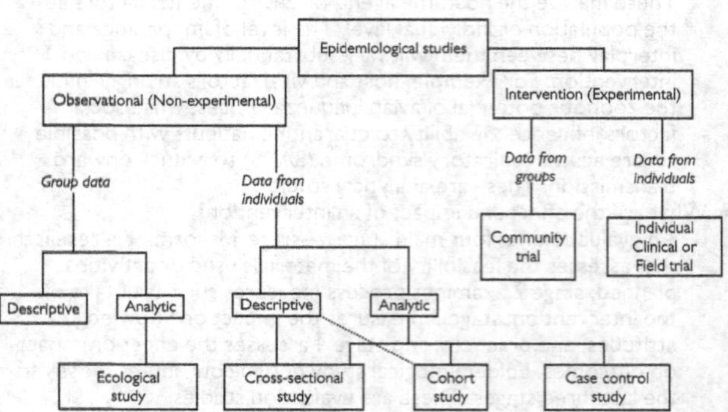

Figure 4.1 Typology of studies.

Box 4.2 Confounding

- A key source of error in epidemiological research is confounding, i.e. an alternative explanation in the population under study, for all or part of the association between a potential risk factor and disease. Alternative explanations are factors that are closely associated with both the risk factor and outcome of interest and are not in the causal chain (either between the exposure and the outcome or a consequence of the outcome). For instance, circumcision reduces the risk of HIV infection but, in some populations, is closely linked with later age of sexual debut, which also reduces risk.
- The main ways to control for confounding are:
  - via study design (e.g. restriction of the individuals who can be included, randomization in trials, matching in observational studies)
  - during the analysis (e.g. collecting information on potential confounders in observational studies and controlling for them using stratification or multivariable analysis; see ➲ Chapter 13).

Trials

When ethical and practical, well-designed and well-conducted trials provide clear evidence of a cause-and-effect relationship. They are often seen as a separate endeavour, with their own logic, conduct, tools, and vocabulary. ➲ Chapter 5 covers trials in greater detail.

Cohort studies

Main features

The starting point for a cohort study is to identify a group of people free of the outcome of interest and define their risk factor status. They are then followed over time to see who develops the outcome, disease, or condition. Importantly, this design provides evidence of the temporality of an association—a key criterion for assessing causality.

The design of cohort studies is prospective, with incidence measured over the follow-up period. An historical cohort study for which risk factors and outcomes have already been measured and the cohort can be assembled from records is still prospective, because the incidence of disease is ascertained over time.

Inclusion in the cohort must be independent of future outcome status, in order to avoid selection bias. Information on the main risk factors and confounders can be collected at the commencement of prospective cohort studies, but follow-up can be costly. For acute infections, in which follow-up periods are not prolonged, this is of less concern. Historical cohort studies have the opposite considerations; data already collected may be less precise, and data on important confounders may be missing, but they tend to be cheaper to conduct.

The cohort design can provide descriptive information on the burden of disease and the patterns of occurrence in the population. If the investigator is interested in identifying the determinants of disease, a comparison group is required. These individuals should be as similar as possible to the exposed group, except for their exposure status. The outcome must be ascertained in the same way in both groups. Ascertainment can be:

- active: through repeated contact to collect outcomes or measure seroconversion from susceptible to infected
- passive: using data already being collected by others.

Active ascertainment of outcome can provide more precise data; however, the passive approach is less costly.

Incidence in cohorts with the risk factor can also be compared with incidence in the general population. Again, outcome ascertainment needs to be the same for both the cohort and the general population, e.g. by using death certificate data.

General population-based cohort studies collect data on a number of risk factors and then divide the cohort at the analysis stage, with incidence assessed in those with the risk factor and those without. A particular advantage of this approach is being able to examine a number of different outcomes simultaneously. For example, the Karonga Prevention Study in Malawi was set up to look at leprosy as an outcome but has since included TB, HIV, and other disease outcomes. The accuracy of outcome ascertainment depends strongly on the methods to measure them; linkage to electronic routine data may be possible in high-income and some middle-income countries, but, in poorer countries, routine data may be non-existent or incomplete.

One advantage of cohort studies is their greater power to examine the effect of rare risk factors, which is difficult in case control studies. The population impact of the risk factor on the burden of disease may be small, e.g. the risk of pneumococcal pneumonia in welders, but such studies can give an insight into biological mechanisms of disease.

Notes on presenting results

Risk and rates can be calculated, depending on the denominator data available. If baseline data on the population at risk are available, the risk of the outcome is calculated. If person–time data are available, rates can be calculated. The latter is useful for repeated events. Risk or rate ratios are calculated to summarize how much more likely the outcome is in one risk factor group compared to another. The absolute number of extra events that occur can be summarized using risk or rate differences. ➲ Chapter 13 provides further detail on statistical methods.

Case control studies

Main features

The starting point with a case control study is to define a group of people with the particular disease or condition of interest ('cases'), so that their past history can be compared with a group of people without the disease or condition ('controls'). Information on suspected risk factors must be collected in the same way from both groups. Whether risk factors are collected after the outcome is defined or from records before the outcome was defined has implications for vulnerability to bias.

A case control study can be based on cases already diagnosed at the start of the study (prevalent cases) or be concurrent recruiting incident cases, i.e. cases are recruited into the study as they are diagnosed. Recruitment of incident cases is preferred if the study is looking for causes. Usually it is not possible to get a measure of disease incidence, but the researcher can investigate the distribution of the disease by age or other subgroup compared to baseline. This design is not simple, and three key considerations are given in Box 4.3.

Box 4.3 Key considerations when designing case control studies

- Clearly define the source population (i.e. know the underlying cohort) with a known period of time.
- When selecting subjects, ensure the exposure varies freely (i.e. do not select cases and controls on the basis of the risk factor of interest).
- Reduce selection bias by making sure that controls are selected from the underlying or source population/cohort in such a way that, if a control had developed the disease, they would have been selected as a case.

Types of controls

The choice of the control group is an important potential source of selection bias, and the decision should be taken after rigorous consideration. Population-based controls are recruited at random from the source population; a sampling frame is required, which may not always be available. Neighbourhood controls are sometimes used due to the ease of local enumeration. If the risk factor under study is clustered, this may reduce the study power. For example, water sources may be similar in the local area, which will reduce the study's ability to detect an effect on gastrointestinal infections. Controls from the same catchment area of a primary healthcare provider as the case may also be more similar to the case than a randomly selected control.

Controls based in hospitals or other health facilities may be easier to recruit but should be considered only if the cases come from such facilities, as factors affecting help-seeking behaviour may bias the type of cases seen in such institutions to more severe cases or those living close to a facility. Depending on the setting, the latter may be richer or poorer than those living further away. When selecting controls from patients with other conditions, it is important to avoid conditions similar to the main outcome, e.g. to assess vaccine effectiveness, controls with other vaccine-preventable diseases should not be selected, as not having the vaccine of interest is likely to be related to not having other vaccines.

Test-negative studies

Test-negative studies often take advantage of surveillance data already collected on people tested but found not to have the infection, e.g. patients with ILI attending primary care services. Risk factors in those with polymerase chain reaction (PCR)-positive nasal swabs are compared with controls who are PCR-negative. However, selection bias may be a problem—it is a strong assumption that those attending with symptoms due to other infections are similar to those patients attending with the infection of interest—and can affect the validity of such a design.

Controlling for confounders

Instead of collecting data on confounders and controlling for them in the analysis of case control studies, known confounders are sometimes matched. There are two types of matching:

- Frequency matching: frequency matching involves recruiting controls in roughly equal numbers to cases in a category of a confounder. Analysis of the association of the risk factor with the outcome within the categories (or strata) of the confounder controls for that confounder. Frequency matching is usually only by broad age ranges or sex. As a rule of thumb, if there are >10 subjects in each category, the matched factor can be examined using methods such as Mantel–Haenszel across the strata or logistic regression models. When well executed, these methods help maximize the use of all subjects by reducing the number of strata with only cases or only controls.
- Individually matched controls: individual pair-wise matching produces confounder, risk factor, and outcome associations that do not

exist in reality. The analysis is more stringent, as each case control pair is a stratum. Only pairs discordant for the risk factor provide information and are analysed. Conditional logistic regression or Mantel–Haenszel for pair matched data, which preserves the strata produced by individual matching, is also required to control for other unmatched confounders. The matching factor in this situation cannot be examined for its association with disease.

The need to collect information on factors to match is time-consuming and may waste subjects for whom matches are not available.

Information bias

Another key source of bias in case control studies is information bias, as information on risk factors is usually obtained after the event has occurred. Past records (e.g. vaccine records) or biomarkers (e.g. serological evidence of past infection) are ideal. If not otherwise available, information should be collected using standardized and, if possible, validated questionnaire instruments. Such data are still subject to recall bias. Recall may be non-differential, with memory fading over time, or differential, e.g. when cases are more interested in, and able to recall, the past more readily than a control or have developed their own theory as to why they have the outcome.

Notes on presenting results

The odds of having the risk factor is compared between cases and controls. This is mathematically equivalent to the odds of the disease, given the risk factor (Box 4.4). ➔ Chapter 13 provides detail on calculating ORs.

When interpreting the results, the main question is 'Is this a causal association?'. In case control studies, where exposure information is collected after the disease has occurred, there is the potential for reverse causality, i.e. the disease may have resulted in the presence of the risk factor.

Box 4.4 Calculating the odds ratio

Number of people	Cases	Controls
Exposed to factor	*a*	*b*
Not exposed to factor	*c*	*D*
Total	*a* + *c*	*b* + *d*

$$OR = (a/c)/(b/d) = ad/bc$$

If the outcome is rare, the odds ratio (OR) is numerically very similar to the risk ratio. If the disease is not rare, the OR is usually further away from 1 than a risk or rate ratio. When controls are sampled concurrently, i.e. controls are sampled at the same time as cases occur, the OR approximates the rate ratio, whether or not the disease is rare.

Hybrid designs

These study designs are sometimes classified as case control studies, and sometimes as cohort studies. The last two are case series exploring risk and no-risk periods in the cases and do not require a control group.

Nested case control studies

These are case control studies nested within cohorts and take advantage of the cohort design, as the cohort becomes a well-documented 'population that gave rise to the cases', avoiding selection bias, and in which the temporal relationship between risk factor and outcome is preserved. Cases are identified within the cohort, and controls are a sample of non-diseased individuals from the same cohort. Researchers can carry out more detailed assessments of risk factors in both types of subjects, using samples of data too expensive to analyse for the whole cohort. Information on confounders will also be collected at the time of exposure, rather than after exposure or after disease has occurred. This is analysed as a case control study. A nested case control study is different from a case cohort in that the analysis is similar to a case control study and ignores the person-years at risk of cases and controls.

Case cohort studies

A more recent design, this is a study in which subjects are selected on the basis of their diseases status (so as cases and controls), but in which the analysis compares person-years experience of cases and controls (treating controls as a random sample of the 'population presumed to have given rise to the cases'). This approach combines the design of a case control study with that of a cohort analysis. It is cheaper than a full cohort study (because, similarly to case control studies, only a sample of the population that produced the cases is studied). This is different from a nested case control study in that the person-years experience of cases and the sample of non-cases are analysed. A key issue is the risk of exposure changing over time, if it is not measured at baseline, on all participants. Analysis is more complex, based on Cox proportional hazards modelling.

Self-controlled case series and case cross-over studies

These are two very similar designs, the first commonly used to evaluate interventions and the second more commonly used to study the effect of a risk factor. Both designs use information on cases only, and different periods of the case experience are used as controls. A comparison group is not needed, as long as the postulated minimum and maximum time between an exposure and the outcome are clearly defined (so the risk and no-risk periods are defined, based on time before outcome).

Self-controlled cases series

The case series determines, for each case, a risk period and non-risk periods and calculates the incidence of disease in the risk and non-risk periods. An example of a case series study: an attenuated mumps vaccine can only lead to aseptic meningitis between 15 and 35 days after vaccine; this is the 'risk period'. A series of cases of aseptic meningitis is collected. Person–time information before and after each case developed the disease is collected. The time of follow-up is divided into the number of days in 'risk periods' (15–35 days after vaccination) and the number of days not in 'risk periods'—the remaining days of follow-up—and the incidence rate in risk and non-risk periods, and incidence rate ratios calculated. The main advantages are that this can be done in cases only, without the need for controls, even when all cases are exposed and an individual's experience is compared across time, so non-time-varying confounders are automatically controlled for and the sample size is smaller. Vaccine safety studies and some surveillance-based studies take advantage of this approach to improve efficiency by avoiding the need to recruit more individuals. A key issue is the definition of the risk period (see ➲ Chapter 12).

Case cross-over studies

Case cross-over studies are a version of the self-controlled case series where the information on a transient risk factor is used only for a short follow-up, so that each case has similar risk and non-risk periods. The odds of exposure in the risk period can be compared with the odds in the non-risk period.

The screening method

The screening method is frequently used to assess vaccine effectiveness. This involves comparing vaccine coverage data in cases to routinely available vaccine coverage data in the population from which cases arose (see ➲ Chapter 12).

Cross-sectional studies

Main features

Cross-sectional studies collect information on disease prevalence, risk factors, or both, at one point or a period of time from a sample of individuals. The study is descriptive if, for example, immunity or past or current burden of disease patterns is examined. The study becomes analytical when infection or disease prevalence is compared between those with and without a risk factor. As both risk factors and disease are measured at the same time, it is not possible to determine whether exposure preceded disease. Using a random sample of the population allows inferences to be made about prevalence in the general population for a smaller cost. Sampling from the general population can be made easier by using cluster sampling methods. Measuring prevalence then needs to take the clustering into account.

Cross-sectional surveys can be a one-off event or can be repeated. This may be necessary, for example, in serological studies monitoring changes in prevalence of immunity, as changes in susceptibility in cohorts not old enough to be vaccinated and not gaining natural immunity may occur due to vaccination of older age groups.

Quality control measures and standard thresholds of assays for defining infection play an integral part in the design of serological surveys; otherwise comparability across studies is compromised (see ➲ Chapter 11 for more detail on serological surveys).

Notes on presenting results

Assessment of risk factors, say for prevalence of an infection, can be carried out using a case control logic, e.g. calculating the OR and using logistic regression to control for confounders, but the design is still cross-sectional. Prevalence ratios are also calculated directly.

Ecological studies

Main features

Ecological studies use a group as the unit of analysis. Risk factors and outcomes are examined at the group level, usually using descriptive data. Frequency of outcomes in the groups is compared using scatter plots and correlation methods to average levels of the risk factor in the same populations. The risk factor can be time (which may be analysed using time-series methods) or place (which may be analysed using spatial analyses), as well as more classical risk factors. The design is useful for factors that cannot be assessed at the individual level such as the weather or season.

Notes on presenting results

Patterns can often generate interesting hypotheses to test further. Justification for investigation can be particularly strong when differences in the level of risk factors between areas are larger than those between individuals in one area.

A key concern with this design is attributing an association that does not actually exist at the group level or is the opposite of that at the individual level. This application is called an ecological fallacy. Ecological bias occurs when outcome rates between groups are affected by another factor that has not been taken into account or when the association at the group level is modified by the presence of another factor.

Descriptive studies

Main features

These studies are often carried out, for example, to assess the burden of disease or to determine the presence and characteristics of an outbreak. They often use routinely collected data, including infectious disease surveillance data, and systematic collections for administrative purposes such as vital statistics. Types of routine numerator data may include mortality records, hospital admissions, disease registers, statutory notifications of infectious diseases, laboratory reports, electronic healthcare records, health insurance data, absenteeism records, and data from routine surveys such as the Health Survey for England and National Health and Nutrition surveys in the USA. Denominator data may be derived from births, deaths, and, in some countries, census data, population registers, and sentinel surveys.

Notes on presenting results

Temporal and/or geographical clustering can provide the first clues about the nature of an outbreak (see ➔ Chapter 14). Patterns by time include epidemic curves, which are key in outbreak investigations. Time trends are used to assess indirect effects, e.g. the protective effect of vaccines in unvaccinated age groups and hence the impact of vaccine programmes. Time-series graphs controlling for age or other confounders, based on direct standardization, are often useful. Graphical presentation by age, calendar period, and cohort is also increasingly possible with newer software. Care is required with secular trends and artefacts e.g. due to changes in classification or diagnostic fashions.

Systematic reviews

The challenge of risk factors with small, rather than large, effects drives not only the need for trials with large sample sizes, but also the science of meta-epidemiology. Evidence from several trials can be summarized in a clear and standardized way by systematic reviews and, if data are sufficient and appropriate, meta-analyses. Such summaries can be of raw individual subject data pooled across trials or effects pooled at the study level. They are useful when numbers in a single study are insufficient to exclude the role of chance. The availability of such a review is often key before a trial or a new study is considered for funding (see ➔ Further reading, p. 69). Data from observational studies can also be reviewed systematically but should be presented separately from data from trials.

Which study design?

A good study design balances rigour, appropriateness, and feasibility. Internal validity is the first aim and is achieved by reducing the play of chance, minimizing the scope and extent of bias (Box 4.5) and controlling for confounding (Box 4.2).

A sample size estimate can help the researcher decide whether undertaking a new study is a sensible decision. The size required will depend on the likely magnitude of an association and will aim to minimize type I (e.g. a 5% probability of rejecting the null hypothesis when it is true) and type II errors (e.g. a 10% probability of accepting the null hypothesis when, in fact, there is a true effect) (see ➲ Chapter 4 for more detail).

External validity or generalizability to other populations is a secondary important aim and should be kept in mind when considering the main advantages and disadvantages of the key study designs (Table 4.1).

Reporting the results

The designs described above provide quantitative data that, depending on the design (Table 4.2), can provide measures of the frequency of outcomes and measures of the effect of a risk factor.

Statistics are used to summarize the size of the effect using the point estimate, as well as the study size or precision with which the effect has been assessed. The latter is displayed by the confidence interval.

Statistical tests cannot ascertain the impact of confounding. As it may not be possible to completely control for confounding factors and eliminate bias, their likely direction and strength should be discussed explicitly to determine whether they could account for the observed findings. A judgement on their importance is required and will depend on the study design and conduct.

Results and their interpretation should also be presented in a way that answers the aims and objectives of the study. Reporting of study findings is increasingly standardized, and journals expect researchers to be aware of the reporting guidelines for presenting the findings of a study such as the Consolidated Standards of Reporting Trials (CONSORT), Strengthening the Reporting of Observational Studies in Epidemiology (STROBE), and Meta-analysis of Observational Studies in Epidemiology (MOOSE) guidelines. These provide a clear structure for accurately presenting the findings to justify the conclusions.

Box 4.5 Bias

Two main types of bias:

- selection bias—who is recruited into the study, losses to follow-up of subjects with certain characteristics, and differences in how outcome is ascertained in the comparison groups
- information or measurement error—recall bias, observation bias, and inaccurate test measurements.

Bias is produced by the researcher through poor design or conduct of a study, unlike confounding, which is a real effect in the population that must be taken into account separately.

Table 4.1 Advantages and disadvantages of each type of observational analytical study

Study	Advantages	Disadvantages
Cohort	• Can establish the temporal sequence, which is important for causal inference • Can examine multiple outcomes • Best design for examining rare exposures • Measure of exposure less biased (not subject to recall bias) • Can be used to obtain population risk or rates	• Expensive • Long duration (depending on type of outcome) • Losses to follow-up are common and can cause selection bias if differential between those with and without the risk factor • Not good for examining rare outcomes • Biases (selection or information) and confounding are still issues
Case control	• Can look at several exposures • Quick, so especially useful for diseases of long latency • Information collected for only a sample of population (controls) • Helps test current hypotheses	• Greater potential for selection bias, especially from control selection at design stage or during conduct of study • Information bias is important problem • Risk of reverse causality • Difficult to examine rare risk factors • Usually no estimate of disease frequency
Cross-sectional	• Relatively cheap, so often used for descriptive information on trends in infection risk for planning purposes	• Presence of risk factor may have followed the outcome (e.g. low weight for age due to TB, rather than vice versa) • Power is limited by the number of cases, so sample sizes may be larger than the corresponding case control study
Ecological studies	• Good for hypothesis generation • Uses secondary data, which makes it quick and cheap	• As with descriptive studies, main problem is data quality: completeness of reporting, over- or underenumeration, differential survival, and classification systematically differing between groups • Ecological fallacy cannot be excluded • Ecological bias is often present

Table 4.2 Measures of outcome occurrence and risk factor effect in analytic study designs

Study	Outcome occurrence	Measure of effect
Trials	• Rate • Risk • Odds • Mean • Median	• Rate ratio • Risk ratio • Odds ratio • Rate difference • Risk difference • Vaccine efficacy • Difference between means or medians
Cohort	• Rate • Risk • Odds • Mean • Median	• Rate ratio • Risk ratio • Odds ratio • Rate difference • Risk difference • Vaccine effectiveness • Difference between means or medians
Case control	• None (unless sampling fractions known)	• Odds ratio (depending on design, equivalent to risk or rate ratio) • Vaccine effectiveness
Cross-sectional	• Prevalence	• Prevalence ratio • Prevalence difference • Odds ratio
Ecological	• Rate • Risk • Prevalence	• Correlation or regression coefficient

Conclusions

Apart from the main question to be answered, controlling for confounding and the rarity of the risk factor or disease is key in the choice of study design. A trial is best for giving clear evidence for or against a causal relationship if ethical and feasible, well designed, and well conducted. If it is not possible to perform a trial, an analytic observational study needs to be chosen. The rule of thumb in Box 4.6 is often helpful.

After a study is completed, the first crucial next stage is to assess validity and then to assess whether any association is causal. For microbiological causes of diseases, decisions can sometimes be based on Koch's postulates. Formulated in 1892, these require that the agent consistently be demonstrated in diseased individuals, that the agent can be isolated from the diseased person and grown in pure culture, and that inoculation must induce the disease experimentally. However, these postulates do not help when there is no scope or technical methods for identifying or growing the organism.

Other criteria proposed by Sir Austin Bradford Hill in 1965 are still applicable today, e.g. demonstrated temporal sequence (i.e. the proposed cause has been shown to come before the effect), reversibility (i.e. the risk of the outcome is reduced if it is possible to remove the risk factor agent), consistency of any association in different studies, and strength of associations. For example, many such criteria had to be fulfilled before *Helicobacter pylori* was accepted as the cause of stomach cancer. Given the associations already discovered, nowadays there are more challenges from risk factors with small effects than large-order associations. This makes application of the Bradford Hill criteria to assess the evidence for causation even more important.

Box 4.6 Which analytic observational study is best?

- A case control study is best if examining a rare outcome.
- A cohort study is best if examining a rare exposure.
- A cohort study is best if examining >1 outcome.
- A case control study is best if examining >1 risk factor.
- Cohort logic is essential if the time relationship between a possible determinant and an outcome needs to be shown.

Further reading

Eggar M, Davey Smith G, Altman DG (2001). *Systematic reviews in health care*. BMJ Publishing Group, London.

Maclure M (1991). The case-crossover design: a method for studying transient effects on the risk of acute events. *Am J Epidemiol*, **133**, 144–53. Available at: http://aje.oxfordjournals.org/content/133/2/144.long (accessed 23 January 2015).

Prentice RL (1986). A case–cohort design for epidemiologic cohort studies and disease prevention trials. *Biometrika*, **73**, 1–11.

Samet JM, Muñoz A (1998). Evolution of the cohort study. *Epidemiol Rev*, **20**, 1–14. Available at: http://epirev.oxfordjournals.org/content/20/1/1.long (accessed 23 January 2015).

US Department of Health and Human Services, Centers for Disease Control and Prevention, Office of the Director, Office of Strategy and Innovation (2011). *Introduction to program evaluation for public health programs: a self-study guide*. Centers for Disease Control and Prevention, Atlanta. Available at: http://www.cdc.gov/eval/guide/index.htm (accessed 23 January 2015).

Wacholder S, Silverman DT, McLaughlin JK, Mandel JS (1992). Selection of controls in case-control studies. II. Types of controls. *Am J Epidemiol*, **135**, 1029–34. Available at: http://aje.oxfordjournals.org/content/135/9/1029.long (accessed 23 January 2015).

Whitaker HJ, Farrington CP, Spiessens B, Musonda P (2006). Tutorial in biostatistics: the self-controlled case series method. *Statistics Med*, **25**, 1768–97. Available at: http://statistics.open.ac.uk/sccs (accessed 23 January 2015).

Chapter 5

Clinical trials

Patrick P.J. Phillips and Andrew J. Nunn

History of clinical trials

Evaluation of medical treatments and therapeutic procedures dates back thousands of years,[1] but the clinical trial, as we know it today, was first developed in the middle of the 20th century. Earlier trials, such as those evaluating treatments for scurvy by James Lind,[2] were flawed in one vital respect: they failed to include a robust system of randomization. An evaluation of streptomycin in pulmonary TB conducted by the British Medical Research Council (MRC) is widely acknowledged as the first properly conducted randomized trial.[3] This trial was different from previous trials, because allocation was concealed before randomization, thus preventing knowledge of the randomization schedule before enrolment, leading to bias which would have seriously compromised the trial and invalidated its results[4] (see ➲ Methods to avoid bias, p. 80).

Although only 107 patients were randomized in the streptomycin trial, this was sufficient to demonstrate a significant benefit in mortality and radiological improvement at 6 months. In addition to concealment of the allocation, other features of this trial are worthy of note. The chest radiographs were assessed by a radiologist who was blind to the allocated treatment, as were the laboratory technicians performing the bacteriological assessments. Of particular importance was the 5-year follow-up, which showed that the early beneficial effects were not sustained because of the emergence of streptomycin resistance in the treated arm (Table 5.1).[3]

Reflecting on the streptomycin trial many years later, Sir John Crofton commented that: 'For many of those of us who had been involved in the MRC streptomycin trial, randomised trials became a way of life, and provided much of the evidence upon which rational treatment policies came to be based'.[6] The streptomycin trial became the model on which the assessment of subsequent new drugs and regimens for TB were evaluated—a model that spread to many other areas of medicine and has become the gold standard by which new treatments are expected to be assessed. However, the presence of randomization is not sufficient in

Table 5.1 Mortality at 6 months and 5 years in the first properly conducted randomized trial evaluating streptomycin in patients with pulmonary tuberculosis

	6-month results[3]				5-year results[5]			
	Streptomycin (*n* = 55)		Bed rest (*n* = 52)		Streptomycin (*n* = 55)		Bed rest (*n* = 52)	
	n	%	*n*	%	N	%	N	%
Mortality	4	7	14	27	32	58	35	67

Source: data from Medical Research Council, Streptomycin treatment of pulmonary TB: a Medical Research Council investigation, *British Medical Journal*, Volume 2, Issue 4582, p. 769, Copyright © 1948; and Fox W. *et al.*, A five-year assessment of patients in a controlled trial of streptomycin in pulmonary tuberculosis: Report to the Tuberculosis Chemotherapy Trials Committee of the Medical Research Council, *Quarterly Journal of Medicine*, Volume 23, Issue 91, p. 347, Copyright © 1954.

itself if the design or conduct of the study is flawed[7] (Table 5.2). Because of the historical importance of TB in clinical trials, and the many challenges posed by its natural history and the prolonged treatment required to cure it, examples from trials in TB are used to illustrate the concepts described in this chapter.

Table 5.2 Possible limitations in randomized trials and observational studies

Randomized trials	Observational studies
• Lack of allocation concealment • Lack of blinding • Incomplete accounting of patients and outcomes • Selective outcome reporting bias • Others, including early stopping and unvalidated outcomes	• Failure to apply appropriate eligibility criteria • Flawed measurement of exposure and outcome • Failure to adequately control confounding • Incomplete follow-up

Adapted from *Journal of Clinical Epidemiology*, Volume 64, Issue 4, Guyatt G. H. *et al.*, GRADE guidelines: 4. Rating the quality of evidence—study limitations (risk of bias), pp. 407–15, , with permission from Elsevier, http://www.sciencedirect.com/science/journal/08954356.

The importance of randomized controlled trials

The limitations of observational studies

A well-conducted trial is the most rigorous study design. However, it is not ethical or feasible to conduct trials in some situations (e.g. when there is no clinical equipoise, or when estimating the risk associated with certain lifestyle behaviours or occupations). Observational studies are discussed in detail in ➲ Chapter 4. In some situations where both study designs can be undertaken, observational studies might seem an attractive alternative to randomized trials, as they may be more representative of the patient population and much simpler, require fewer resources, and usually can be completed in a shorter period of time. However, observational studies do have limitations and need to be interpreted with caution because of potential biases.[8] As a case study, consider a randomized trial and an observational study that compared the same two antiretroviral regimens using death as the endpoint, where unexpected results in the observational study were probably caused by patients with a poorer prognosis being given one regimen in preference to the other.[9]

A frequent criticism of randomized trials is that they do not reflect real life.[10] An advantage of observational data, as long as they are systematically collected, is the potential completeness of coverage, as patients who do not satisfy the eligibility requirements or those who are unwilling to participate in a randomized trial are not excluded. Valuable information on outcomes of different interventions may be obtained from medical records of high quality, as long as the limitations inherent to observational studies are considered when interpreting the results.

Pragmatic and explanatory trials

A trial is described as pragmatic if the objective is to evaluate the intervention under conditions that are close to usual care and as explanatory if the objective is to evaluate the intervention under optimal conditions, merely to test the principle of whether an intervention actually works. This distinction is more a continuum than a dichotomy, with trials having features that could be considered more or less pragmatic or explanatory.[11] Very loose eligibility criteria for entry into a study, e.g. including all patients who would require treatment irrespective of other comorbidities, would make a trial more pragmatic, whereas regular follow-up visits outside of usual care would make a trial more explanatory. Both types of trials are of value—explanatory trials provide proof of concept that an intervention is efficacious and can be delivered safely, while pragmatic trials show what is likely to happen when it is introduced in practice.

Initial trials of short-course chemotherapy for TB conducted by the British MRC in East Africa were more explanatory than pragmatic, as they were conducted under strictly controlled conditions and patients were hospitalized throughout treatment and followed intensively throughout treatment and for a further 24 months.[12] A subsequent trial conducted in Algeria under routine national TB programme conditions, with patients seen mostly as outpatients with limited supervision of their treatment, gave results consistent with the findings of previously published studies,[13] thus strengthening the evidence base for the regimen.

Results of another controlled trial and the survey of the national TB programme, both conducted in Kenya, were contrasting, which highlights the limitations of highly explanatory trials. Although the survey confirmed the poor results obtained in the trial with a regimen of thiacetazone and isoniazid alone, the results of a regimen with an initial supplement of streptomycin were substantially better in the trial—96% of patients were culture-negative at 1 year, compared to only 78% in the programme. The difference in outcomes was attributed to poorer adherence to treatment in the continuation phase of treatment under routine conditions in the TB programme.[14]

Types, phases, and designs of trials

Traditionally, clinical trials are divided into four separate phases, although the fourth phase is often observational in nature (Table 5.3).

In the development of a drug to treat TB, a short (14-day) early bactericidal activity (EBA) study to evaluate safety and compare doses in 12–15 patients per arm would be a Phase IIA trial. A study that evaluated the decline in TB-causing bacilli over 8–12 weeks in 60–100 patients per arm would be a Phase IIB trial. A Phase III trial would evaluate treatment failure and relapse over 18–24 months of follow-up as the primary endpoint, with hundreds of patients per arm and usual standard of care as the comparator.

Classifying trials into phases can be overly restrictive. The development pathway may not always be the same, as an intervention with promising results could move from a small early-phase trial directly into a large confirmatory trial.

Superiority and non-inferiority

The commonest type of late-phase (II–III) trial has a superiority design, in which the aim is to evaluate whether the intervention has superior efficacy to a standard treatment control. However, non-inferiority designs, which evaluate whether an intervention has efficacy that is as good as that of the control, are increasingly used. To demonstrate non-inferiority, it is necessary to show that the intervention is not inferior by more than a prespecified amount, which is called the margin of non-inferiority. A non-inferiority trial is appropriate only when the intervention has additional benefits over the control such as less toxicity, lower costs, or shorter treatment duration. The use of non-inferiority trials for

Table 5.3 Phases of clinical trials

Phase	Description
I	• First time a drug is given to humans • Participants are healthy volunteers • Aims to assess safety and achieve some indication of the maximum tolerated dose of the drug
II	• Participants are patients with disease being studied • Aims to achieve a preliminary evaluation of efficacy and further explore safety over a longer period of time in a larger group of patients • Often split into Phase IIA, which focuses more on dose selection and safety, and Phase IIB, which focuses more on efficacy, often using an intermediate endpoint
III	• Pivotal Phase III trials involve treatment with a new drug for its intended duration and with enough patients to demonstrate efficacy unequivocally on definitive patient-relevant outcomes
IV	• Aims to collect longer-term safety data in much larger numbers of patients than enrolled in previous trials • Often embedded into routine practice post-licensing

interventions with no additional benefit has led to some over-reactive criticism, with some authors describing any non-inferiority trial as unethical.[15–20] The current treatment of MDR-TB is an area for which non-inferiority trials are appropriate. Current treatment of MDR-TB involves daily combinations of toxic drugs for 20–24 months, which severely limits a patient's ability to return to work and resume other daily activities. Trials are evaluating less toxic regimens with substantially shorter treatment durations, which would result in major patient benefit, even if the efficacy is only at least as good as that of the current treatment.[21]

Phase III trials for new treatments for drug-sensitive TB commonly have a non-inferiority design, because the excellent efficacy of the standard 6-month regimen in clinical trials does not always translate well into clinical practice due to the long duration of treatment. A shorter 4-month regimen that had efficacy as good as the standard of care would likely translate into much improved outcomes in practice due to improved adherence.

The rest of this chapter now focuses on superiority trials.

Adaptive trial designs

In a traditional fixed-sample trial, data are analysed only at the end of the trial, once all patients have completed follow-up and all data have accrued. An alternative to this approach is an adaptive design, in which one or more interim analyses during the course of the study are used to adapt the study design. Possible adaptations include changing the sample size, stopping a trial early because of overwhelming efficacy or lack of benefit, and dropping arms in a multi-arm study. Importantly, such adaptation should never be used to attempt to salvage a failing trial, and procedures for adaptation must be prespecified in the study protocol before the study begins (see ➔ Trial monitoring, p. 82). Consideration must be given to the impact of any interim analyses on overall type I and type II errors (see ➔ Power and sample size, p. 78).

When there are several promising new interventions, but limited resources, a particularly attractive design is the multi-arm multi-stage (MAMS) design, in which multiple arms are simultaneously compared with a single control. The MAMS design allows for multiple interim analyses to facilitate the early termination of poorly performing arms, so that resources can be focused on the more promising arms. This method was developed for cancer trials[22,23] but is being adapted for use in trials of new drugs to treat TB.[24,25]

Other trial designs

In most randomized controlled trials (RCTs), individual participants are allocated randomly to treatment arms. The cluster randomized trial is an alternative design, in which 'clusters' of patients—at the community or health system level—are randomized to receive one of the interventions, rather than individual participants.[26] Improved methods for TB case-finding would be an intervention better suited to a cluster randomized trial than an individually randomized trial.

Other trial designs not covered here include step-wedge cluster randomized trials, factorial trials, and sequential multiple assignment randomized trials (SMARTs).

Power and sample size

The sample size of a clinical trial is the minimum number of participants required to be enrolled to achieve the trial's objective. It is unethical to enrol either insufficient patients to achieve the trial objective or many more patients than are necessary.

Sample size calculations are driven by minimizing the probability of type I and II errors. In a superiority trial, a type I error is the probability of demonstrating a difference when no difference exists, while a type II error is the probability of failing to show a difference when there is a real difference between interventions (Figure 5.1). It is common to maintain a low type I error rate of 5%, but a type II error rate of 10–20% usually is acceptable. The power of a trial is the probability that an effective intervention will be shown to be effective and is calculated by subtracting the type II error rate from 100%, so a power of 90% corresponds to a type II error rate of 10%.

When a trial includes multiple interventions or multiple primary endpoints, or when multiple analyses have been conducted (such as in an adaptive design), the chance of falsely finding a statistically significant difference is increased if a conventional significance level of 5% is used for each comparison. In this context, it is appropriate either to adjust the individual significance levels to maintain an acceptable overall type I error rate or to take multiple testing into account when interpreting the results.[27,28]

Having decided on values for the type I error rate and power, the targeted effect size or difference between treatments is another key driver for the sample size. A trial designed with adequate power to detect a small effect size will be larger than one designed to detect a large effect size. It is good practice to link the targeted effect size to the minimum clinically important difference (MCID), so that the trial is designed to detect effect sizes at least as large as the MCID and only miss effects not considered to be clinically important. This highlights the distinction between statistical significance, when there is evidence that a difference, however small, does exist, and clinical significance when the difference is considered large enough for the intervention to change practice.

The expected outcome in the control arm is an important factor that influences the sample size. If this turns out to be very different to what

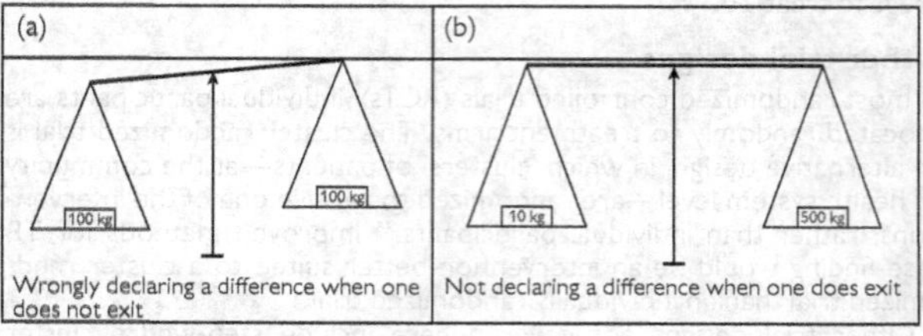

Figure 5.1 Type I (a) and type II (b) errors.

was assumed when the trial was designed, the trial may turn out to be underpowered. It therefore is recommended to use a realistic estimate from previous trials, if available.

It is usually necessary to enrol more patients than is required for the analysis to account for loss to follow-up. It is important to be realistic about the expected rate of loss to follow-up when designing a trial, as it needs to be kept as low as possible during the trial because the true outcome of such patients remains unknown. Differential losses to follow-up may indicate that one treatment regimen is less acceptable or more toxic than another and results in bias in interpretation of the data. Other sources of bias are described in the following section.

Methods to avoid bias

The estimated effect of an intervention from a clinical trial is said to be biased if a systematic error means that it does not reflect the true intended effect of the intervention. Bias can result from a number of sources, with corresponding measures available to avoid it.

Randomization is the most important way to prevent bias in an RCT, because, if properly implemented, it ensures that any known and unknown confounders that might affect outcomes are balanced between arms, with any imbalance occurring by chance. Proper implementation of randomization requires adequate concealment of the allocation to ensure that neither the patient nor the investigator is aware of which arm a patient will be allocated to before consent to enrol in the trial has been obtained. This avoids selection bias where patients are selected for particular arms, e.g. an investigator concerned about the efficacy of a novel treatment may allocate sicker participants to the control arm.

Blinding (sometimes called masking) is a well-established method to avoid bias in clinical trials by keeping the treatment a patient is taking secret. In the strongest form of blinding, known as double-blind, none of the patients, clinicians, investigators, or any other individuals carrying out assessments (such as laboratory technicians) know to what arm the patient has been allocated until the trial is complete. The purpose of blinding is to ensure that every aspect of patient management and data collection is unaffected by knowing to which arm a patient has been allocated. Blinding is particularly important when the primary endpoint has a subjective element, such as a quality-of-life measure, and less important when the primary endpoint is objective such as all-cause mortality.

Blinding in a treatment trial is achieved by giving patients in the control arm identical inactive tablets (placebo) identical in appearance to the trial drug at the same frequency as those in the intervention arm. A double-blind trial can be very difficult to achieve in some settings; for example, it is challenging to produce an inactive perfectly matched placebo for the anti-TB drug rifampicin, which turns a patient's urine and bodily fluids an orange colour. Blinding also substantially increases the complexity and cost of a clinical trial due to the need to manufacture matching placebo and to have central drug packing facilities separate from the trial sites.

Even when it is not feasible or desirable to blind patients and clinicians (in which case the trial is sometimes designated as open-label), it is still important to limit endpoint assessors' knowledge of patient allocation wherever possible and also to ensure that only members of the Independent Data Monitoring Committee (IDMC) (see ➲ Trial monitoring, p. 82) are aware of aggregated data by treatment arm. If the primary endpoint involves some clinical judgement, e.g. identifying an AIDS-defining illness, an endpoint review committee of experts blinded to treatment allocation and independent of the trial could be convened to review the data and classify outcomes.

To ensure that no trial procedures change during the course of a trial as a response to accruing data (particularly important in an open-label study), key aspects of the trial, such as trial objectives, primary endpoint, and primary methods of analysis, should be clearly prespecified in the protocol and remain unchanged once the first patient has been enrolled. The statistical analysis plan, which provides details of the analysis of the primary and secondary endpoints, should also be finalized and signed off early in the trial and before any analysis is done.

Publication bias occurs when trial outcomes are selectively reported to favour the intervention or when whole trials with unfavourable results are not reported. For this reason, most clinical trial funders now expect a trial to be registered—namely, key details logged with publicly available registries (such as ClinicalTrials.gov or International Standard Randomised Controlled Trial Number Register, ISRCTN)—before the study starts. In this way, individuals conducting systematic reviews or those wanting to find out about a particular disease or intervention can search registries to find a more comprehensive picture of which trials are being or have been conducted.

Trial monitoring

Unless the quality of the data obtained in a clinical RCT can be relied on, the results of the trial will be of no value. If a trial is being conducted according to the principles of the International Conference on Harmonisation of Technical Requirements for Registration of Pharmaceuticals for Human Use (ICH)'s *Guideline for good clinical practice* (GCP),[29] regular monitoring is essential. This can be performed in a number of ways and to varying degrees. The GCP guideline requires monitors to be appropriately trained and to have the scientific and/or clinical knowledge needed to monitor a trial adequately.[29] In the past, monitoring often only involved monitors visiting study sites and reviewing data and documentation, with little regard to a strategy of prioritization within the process. More recently, alternative approaches have been advocated,[30] which include central statistical monitoring[31,32] and a risk assessment at the start of a trial to identify the most appropriate monitoring strategies for the trial overall and its individual sites.[30] A risk assessment should be reviewed on an annual periodic basis throughout a clinical trial, and the monitoring techniques employed should be considered and updated accordingly. Monitoring—whether on site, centrally, or both—may highlight the need for additional training of site staff or changes in trial procedures.

Safety monitoring and expedited reporting

In addition to determining efficacy, an essential assessment in clinical trials is the safety of the interventions being studied. It is recommended that patients should be asked at each trial visit about any disability, incapacity, or adverse events that have occurred, as well as hospitalizations and consultations with other medical practitioners. The ICH's GCP guideline sets out the investigators' responsibilities for notifying adverse events to sponsors.[29] These include reporting any defined serious adverse events (SAEs) within an agreed time frame, with particularly expedited requirements for sponsors to report suspected unexpected serious adverse reactions (SUSARs) to regulatory authorities.

Independent Data Monitoring Committee and Trial Steering Committee

All trials of medicinal products are expected to have an IDMC, the purpose of which is to protect the safety of the trial participants, the credibility of the study, and the validity of the study results.[33] The membership, which is often no more than three to five people, should be totally independent of the trial and include clinical trial, statistical, and relevant clinical expertise. The IDMC is expected to meet regularly—commonly every 6 months during the trial—to review study progress and unblinded data on safety and efficacy. At the end of each meeting, the IDMC will make recommendations to an executive decision-making body, such as the Trial Steering Committee (TSC), as to whether the trial should continue as designed or whether modifications should be made. Modifications could include early termination of one or more study arms on account of safety concerns or proof beyond reasonable doubt of differences in efficacy between one of the study arms and its comparator.

The TSC provides expert oversight of the trial, monitoring progress on a regular basis, and receiving the recommendations of the IDMC. Most members of the TSC, including the chair, should be independent of the trial, although additional observers may be present at meetings of the TSC. In addition to deciding on the appropriate response following receipt of the IDMC recommendations, the TSC may be required to attend to issues of concern regarding trial conduct. These include poor recruitment or poor data quality, approval of proposed protocol amendments or new trial substudies, approval of requests for early release of data or external applications for the use of stored samples, and approval of study reports or presentations.

Ethical approval and informed consent

Before starting a trial, approval needs to be obtained from an independent research ethics committee to protect the rights and interests of the trial's participants. This approval will usually be from more than one committee, typically including a central ethics committee, often based in the same country as the trial sponsor, and ethics committees in each participating country or site. For example, in the UK, only central committee approval is required for all sites. Any amendments to be made to the study protocol need to be approved by the ethics committee(s) before they can be introduced.

Informed consent must be obtained from all people being considered for enrolment to the trial before they undergo any investigations, including investigations to assess their eligibility for admission to the trial. Key information that needs to be conveyed to the patient includes the rationale for the study, potential risks and benefits, trial treatments, randomization process, follow-up schedule, and right of participants to withdraw at any time. Before enrolling in the study, a patient consent form needs to be signed. If the person cannot read patient information documentation, an independent witness should be present during the consent process.

Dissemination and impact

It is important for the results of a clinical trial to be published in peer-reviewed journals (there is a recommended standardized format for reporting trials, CONSORT (http://www.consort-statement.org)) and disseminated in scientific conferences, but this is insufficient, as it will only reach the scientific community. As an ethical obligation, the results of the trial should also be shared with the trial participants and the communities in which the trial was conducted, including the investigators and other site staff. This can sometimes take the form of a community meeting to celebrate completion of the trial.

The impact of a clinical trial is often measured by the profile of the journal in which the paper is published and how many times it is subsequently cited in other scientific publications. This is only one component of impact, which can also be measured by, among other things, the extent to which national and international treatment guidelines are changed as a result of the trial, whether practitioners are actually using the new intervention to treat their patients, or resulting advocacy activities by patient and community groups. Funding agencies, such as the British MRC, now require groups conducting clinical trials to include steps to increase impact beyond publication of the results in a peer-reviewed journal.

To have impact broader than in the scientific community alone, additional methods of dissemination can include press releases, videos posted on YouTube, policy briefing documents for governments and health ministries, and direct contact with organizations that produce treatment guidelines such as the WHO. Publishing the reports in journals with open access, such that the publication is freely available to everyone without subscription, also increases dissemination.

References

1. Bull J (1959). The historical development of clinical therapeutic trials. *J Chronic Dis*, **10**, 218–48.
2. Lind J (1757). *A treatise on the scurvy: in three parts, containing an inquiry into the nature, causes, and cure, of that disease*. A. Millar, London.
3. Medical Research Council (1948). Streptomycin treatment of pulmonary TB: a Medical Research Council investigation. *BMJ*, **2**, 769.
4. Student (1931). The Lanarkshire milk experiment. *Biometrika*, **23**, 398–406.
5. Fox W, Sutherland I, Daniels M (1954). A five-year assessment of patients in a controlled trial of streptomycin in pulmonary tuberculosis: Report to the Tuberculosis Chemotherapy Trials Committee of the Medical Research Council. *QJM*, **23**, 347.
6. Crofton J (2006). The MRC randomized trial of streptomycin and its legacy: a view from the clinical front line. *J R Soc Med*, **99**, 531–4.
7. Guyatt GH, Oxman AD, Vist G, *et al.* (2011). GRADE guidelines: 4. Rating the quality of evidence—study limitations (risk of bias). *J Clin Epidemiol*, **64**, 407–15.
8. Grimes DA, Schulz KF (2002). Bias and causal associations in observational research. *Lancet*, **359**, 248–52.

9. Dunn D, Babiker A, Hooker M, Darbyshire J (2002). The dangers of inferring treatment effects from observational data: a case study in HIV infection. *Control Clin Trials*, **23**, 106–10.
10. Schwartz D, Lellouch J (2009). Explanatory and pragmatic attitudes in therapeutical trials. *J Clin Epidemiol*, **62**, 499–505.
11. Thorpe KE, Zwarenstein M, Oxman AD, *et al.* (2009). A pragmatic-explanatory continuum indicator summary (PRECIS): a tool to help trial designers. *J Clin Epidemiol*, **62**, 464–75.
12. Fox W, Ellard G, Mitchison D (1999). Studies on the treatment of tuberculosis undertaken by the British Medical Research Council tuberculosis units, 1946–1986, with relevant subsequent publications. *Int J Tuberc Lung Dis*, **3**, S231–79.
13. Algerian Working Group/British Medical Research Council (1984). Controlled clinical trial comparing a 6-month and a 12-month regimen in the treatment of pulmonary tuberculosis in the Algerian Sahara. *Am Rev Respir Dis*, **129**, 921–8.
14. Kent P, Fox W, Miller A, Nunn A, Tall R, Mitchison D (1970). The therapy of pulmonary tuberculosis in Kenya: a comparison of the results achieved in controlled clinical trials with those achieved by the routine treatment services. *Tubercle*, **51**, 24–38.
15. Garattini S, Bertele V (2007). Non-inferiority trials are unethical because they disregard patients' interests. *Lancet*, **370**, 1875–7.
16. Soliman EZ (2008). The ethics of non-inferiority trials. *Lancet*, **371**, 895.
17. Nunn AJ, Meredith SK, Spigelman MK, Ginsberg AM, Gillespie SH (2008). The ethics of non-inferiority trials. *Lancet*, **371**, 895.
18. Menten J, Boelaert M (2008). The ethics of non-inferiority trials. *Lancet*, **371**, 896.
19. Gandjour A (2008). The ethics of non-inferiority trials. *Lancet*, **371**, 895.
20. Chuang-Stein C, Beltangady M, Dunne M, Morrison B (2008). The ethics of non-inferiority trials. *Lancet*, **371**, 895–6.
21. Nunn AJ, Rusen I, Van Deun A, *et al.* (2014). Evaluation of a standardized treatment regimen of anti-tuberculosis drugs for patients with multi-drug-resistant tuberculosis (STREAM): study protocol for a randomized controlled trial. *Trials*, **15**, 353.
22. Royston P, Barthel F, Parmar M, Choodari-Oskooei B, Isham V (2011). Designs for clinical trials with time-to-event outcomes based on stopping guidelines for lack of benefit. *Trials*, **12**, 81.
23. Sydes MR, Parmar MK, James ND, *et al.* (2009). Issues in applying multi-arm multi-stage methodology to a clinical trial in prostate cancer: the MRC STAMPEDE trial. *Trials*, **10**, 39.
24. Phillips PP, Gillespie SH, Boeree M (2012). Innovative trial designs are practical solutions for improving the treatment of tuberculosis. *J Infect Dis*, **205**(Suppl 2), S250–7.
25. Bratton DJ, Phillips PP, Parmar MK (2013). A multi-arm multi-stage clinical trial design for binary outcomes with application to tuberculosis. *BMC Med Res Methodol*, **13**, 139.
26. Hayes RJ, Moulton LH (2009). *Cluster randomized trials*. Chapman & Hall/CRC, Boca Raton/London.
27. Freidlin B, Korn EL, Gray R, Martin A (2008). Multi-arm clinical trials of new agents: some design considerations. *Clin Cancer Res*, **14**, 4368–71.
28. Wason JM, Stecher L, Mander AP (2014). Correcting for multiple-testing in multi-arm trials: is it necessary and is it done? *Trials*, **15**, 364.
29. International Conference on Harmonisation of Technical Requirements for Registration of Pharmaceuticals for Human Use (ICH) (1996). *Guideline for good clinical practice*. Available at: http://www.ich.org/fileadmin/Public_Web_Site/ICH_Products/Guidelines/Efficacy/E6/E6_R1_Guideline.pdf (accessed 25 January 2015).
30. Baigent C, Harrell FE, Buyse M, Emberson JR, Altman DG (2008). Ensuring trial validity by data quality assurance and diversification of monitoring methods. *Clin Trials*, **5**, 49–55.
31. Venet D, Doffagne E, Burzykowski T, *et al.* (2012). A statistical approach to central monitoring of data quality in clinical trials. *Clin Trials*, **9**, 705–13.
32. Bakobaki JM, Rauchenberger M, Joffe N, McCormack S, Stenning S, Meredith S (2012). The potential for central monitoring techniques to replace on-site monitoring: findings from an international multi-centre clinical trial. *Clin Trials*, **9**, 257–64.
33. Ellenberg SS, Fleming TR, DeMets DL (2003). *Data monitoring committees in clinical trials: a practical perspective*. John Wiley & Sons, Chichester.

Chapter 6

Investigating emerging infectious diseases

Ibrahim Abubakar, Molebogeng X. Rangaka, and Marc Lipman

Introduction to investigating emerging infectious diseases

On 13 June 2012, a 60-year-old Saudi man was admitted to a private hospital in Jeddah, Saudi Arabia, with a 7-day history of fever, dyspnoea, and productive cough. The patient's symptoms, signs, and laboratory and radiological investigations were consistent with an infectious cause. He was severely ill, requiring management in intensive care, and died 11 days later. Serological tests and WGS identified the cause of this fatal illness as a previously unrecognized virus, which is now known as Middle East respiratory syndrome coronavirus (MERS-CoV).[1]

Since then, the epidemiology and clinical features of the infection caused by this pathogen have been identified, and a putative zoonotic source determined. The high mortality observed in the MERS-CoV outbreak illustrates the potential for emerging pathogens to cause human illness and challenge public health systems globally.

Newly identified infectious agents, such as MERS-CoV, are constantly being detected. Emerging and re-emerging infectious diseases thus pose an ongoing threat to global health security. It is not a question of if, but when, the next pathogen that will lead to a local outbreak or pandemic will arise. The study of emerging infections and how to detect and contain them is therefore an essential component of public health practice globally.

What are emerging and re-emerging infections?

No consensus definition exists for emerging or re-emerging infectious diseases. Similarly, the timescale within which a particular infection may be considered existing or re-emerging has not been defined. Emerging infectious diseases is thus a broad term coined to describe the occurrence of infections whose incidence is increasing due to new pathogens appearing in a population, or as a result of previously known organisms rapidly increasing in incidence or geographic range.[2] Figure 6.1 shows select examples of recent emerging/re-emerging pathogens.[3] Infectious diseases may emerge or re-emerge due to:

- a new species of pathogen arising, such as HIV or the coronaviruses responsible for SARS and Middle East respiratory syndrome (MERS)
- organisms that were previously unrecognized as human pathogens such as *Helicobacter pylori* (which is now known to be associated with chronic gastric ulcers)
- an altered form of a previously known pathogen, such as new strains of the influenza virus, including avian and swine forms that have acquired the ability to cause severe disease in humans and can be transmitted from person to person. Emergence of drug-resistant pathogens and their widespread distribution, such as drug-resistant *Mycobacterium tuberculosis, Escherichia coli, Neisseria gonorrhoeae, Pneumococcus* spp., *Shigella* spp., *Plasmodium falciparum*, and *Staphylococcus aureus*, which have turned previously manageable microbes into new threats to global health. A recent review commissioned by the government in the UK estimated that drug-resistant pathogens could cost the global economy trillions of dollars by 2050 if action is not taken.

Re-emerging diseases are known diseases that have reappeared after a significant decline in incidence. Such infections are not caused by new pathogens but result from the re-emergence of microbes or diseases that had previously been controlled successfully. Moreover, many important infectious diseases have never been controlled adequately on either the national or international level, so infectious diseases that have posed ongoing health problems in developing countries may re-emerge in more developed countries (e.g. TB, poliomyelitis, food- and waterborne infections, Ebola virus, West Nile virus infection).

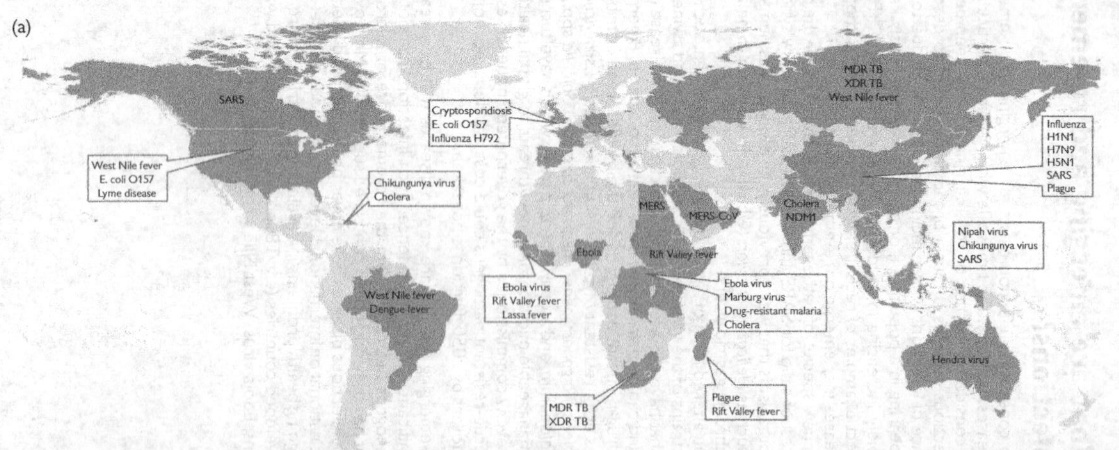
(a)
SARS
West Nile fever
E. coli O157
Lyme disease
Chikungunya virus
Cholera
West Nile fever
Dengue fever
Cryptosporidiosis
E. coli O157
Influenza H792
Ebola virus
Rift Valley fever
Lassa fever
Ebola
MDR TB
XDR TB
MERS
MERS-CoV
Rift Valley fever
Ebola virus
Marburg virus
Drug-resistant malaria
Cholera
Plague
Rift Valley fever
Cholera
NDM1
MDR TB
XDR TB
West Nile fever
Influenza
H1N1
H7N9
H5N1
SARS
Plague
Nipah virus
Chikungunya virus
SARS
Hendra virus

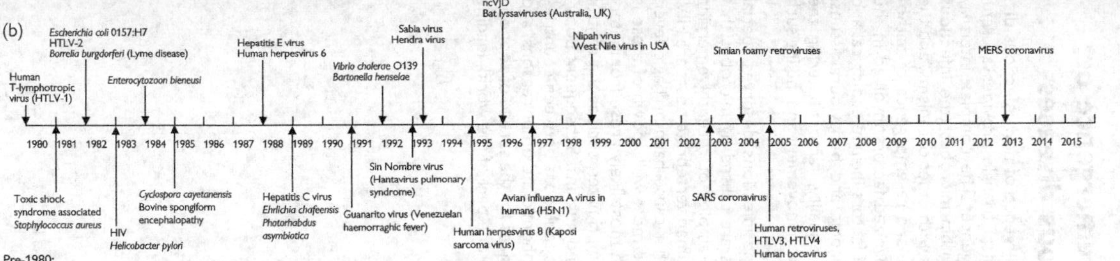

Figure 6.1 (a) Emerging and re-emerging infectious diseases, 2005–15. The map shows countries (shaded) with at least one case of a newly recorded emerging or re-emerging infectious disease in the Global Outbreak Alert and Response Network (GOARN) database between 2005 and 2015 (data accessed in February 2015); (b) Timeline for emergence of new pathogens.

(a) Made with Natural Earth. Free vector and raster map data @ naturalearthdata.com. Source: data from *Global Outbreak Alert and Response Network (GOARN)*, World Health Organization, Geneva, Switzerland, Copyright © WHO 2015, available from http://www.who.int/ihr/alert_and_response/outbreak-network/en/.

Factors involved in the emergence or re-emergence of infectious diseases

Many factors contribute to the (re-)emergence of new infectious diseases. The concept of the epidemiological triangle provides a useful model for understanding disease emergence. The complex interplay of factors in the human **host**, factors within **microbes** (the **infectious agent**), the genomes of both, interactions with other organisms, and the **environment** determines the emergence and re-emergence of pathogens. Table 6.1 summarizes widely recognized factors involved in the emergence of infectious diseases.[4] These factors include ecological and environmental changes, human demographic and behavioural issues, technological advances, poverty and inequality, factors altering the immunity of the human host, and population movement and mixing such as at mass gatherings.

The zoonotic origin of many emerging infections deserves special consideration. Some emerging infections are caused by microbes that originate in non-human vertebrates. Examples of recently emerging viruses that probably originated in non-human vertebrate hosts are HIV, SARS, MERS-CoV, and several viruses that cause haemorrhagic fever, including Ebola virus and Lassa virus. The most well-known of these is HIV—the virus that causes AIDS—which most likely arose from interspecies transmission between non-human primates, such as the central chimpanzee *Pan troglodytes troglodytes*, and humans. Subsequent population movement—such as migration of populations between countries and different world regions, travel for economic and other reasons, and mass gatherings (Box 6.1)—provides avenues for the spread of zoonotic or other pathogens that have emerged in one part of the world, leading to the potential for a pandemic.

Table 6.1 Factors involved in the emergence of infectious diseases

Factor	Description (with examples)
Environment	

Ecological changes (voluntary or involuntary; includes land use)	• Environmental factors such as climate change
	  • Global warming caused by human activities may influence emergence of viral and bacterial vector-borne diseases
	• Farming practices that change the habitat of vectors
	  • Factors affecting animal density, antibiotic use in animals, and changes in animal diet
	  • Dams
	  • Irrigation
	  • De/reforestation
	  • Flood/drought

Human demographics (include economic development)	• Economic and cultural drivers
	  • Increased population growth
	  • Overcrowding
	  • Changing levels of poverty
	  • Poor housing
	  • Poor sanitation
	  • Increased mobility
	  • Intercontinental transport of cargo

(Continued)

Table 6.1 (*Contd.*)

Factor	Description (with examples)
Human behaviour (includes intent to harm)	• Human behaviour plays an important role in re-emergence • Overuse of pesticides and antibiotics, as well as poor stewardship of commonly prescribed antibiotics, may result in emergence of drug-resistant pathogens, allowing many diseases that were formerly treatable with drugs to make a comeback (e.g. tuberculosis, malaria, and nosocomial and food-borne infections) • Recently, decreased compliance with vaccination policy has led to re-emergence of previously controlled diseases such as measles and pertussis • Increased risk of exposure to zoonotic agents through animal or human displacement (voluntary or involuntary) • Changes in activity period of wild animals (under pressure of hunting) • Increased contact between human and livestock/wild animals or other reservoirs (may be associated with outdoor activities such as hunting or may expose humans to bacteria excreted by healthy animal carriers) • Bioterrorism, in which previously controlled microbes are considered for deliberate release into general population; use of deadly pathogens, such as smallpox and anthrax, as agents of bioterrorism is an increasingly acknowledged threat
International travel, commerce, and mass gatherings	• Population movement and mixing is a key determinant of subsequent spread of infections (Table 6.2) • Air travel has revolutionized the rate at which human populations move between regions of the world and so also the potential for spread of infections • Mass gatherings provide unique contexts within which infections can be spread and novel strains transferred to new populations
Technology and industry	• Although technological development and industry has mostly contributed to better living conditions and reduced global burden of infections, some aspects of technology and industry have played a role in emergence and re-emergence of infections • Medical technologies such as transfusion and hypodermic needles • Rapid mechanization of farming leading to deforestation and spread of vector-borne and other infections such as Lassa fever • Dams and waterborne diseases • Globalization of food supply • Iatrogenic immunosuppression

Breakdown in public health measures (includes lack of will, war, and famine)	• Poor public health infrastructure, which may result from poor governance and conflicts • Lack of coordination or harmonization of control systems between neighbouring countries
Poverty and social inequality	• Many infections are spread more effectively within context of poverty through overcrowding in urban slums and malnutrition, which increases susceptibility
Human host	
Increased susceptibility	• Healthy immune systems are required to protect against infection or disease, and changes in human immunity may arise from infectious diseases such as HIV, iatrogenic reasons such as treatment for cancers, and as a consequence of age and even poor nutrition
Microbe (infectious agent)	
Microbial adaptation and change	• Evolution of pathogens through acquisition of new genes by mutations or exchange between organisms (e.g. New Delhi metallo-β-lactamase gene), which could result in response to selection in an environment • Natural genetic variations, recombinations, and adaptations could allow emergence of new strains of known pathogens to which the human immune system has not been previously exposed and that it is therefore not primed to recognize (e.g. influenza)

HIV, human immunodeficiency virus.

Source: data from Morse SS and Schluederberg A., From the National Institute of Allergy and Infectious Diseases, the Fogarty International Center of the National Institutes of Health, and the Rockefeller University. Emerging viruses: the evolution of viruses and viral diseases, *Journal of Infectious Diseases*, Volume 162, Issue 1, pp. 1–7,

Box 6.1 Mass gatherings and emerging infections

Mass gatherings may be defined as 'events attended by a sufficient number of people to strain the planning and response resources of a community, state or nation'.[5] They include religious festivals, sporting events, music concerts, and trade meetings.

Crowding and lack of sanitation at mass gatherings can lead to the emergence of infectious diseases. Food- or waterborne outbreaks have the potential to spread infections efficiently and rapidly on a large scale. Factors that determine the spread of these infections include the types of infection endemic to the host country, those that are endemic to the home countries of the visitors, and mixing of infectious and susceptible populations.[6]

Rapid population movement also means that infections can spread quickly across the world. Air travel can lead to the rapid dissemination of infectious diseases faster than the incubation period of almost all infections.

The context of the gathering is also an important determinant in the spread of infections. Mass gatherings provide an opportunity to engage in public health action that will benefit host communities and the countries from which participants originate.

Surveillance and control of emerging infections

The detection of, and subsequent response to, an emerging or re-emerging infection depends on the pathogen concerned, the disease syndrome caused, how and when it was detected, existing infrastructure for surveillance and public health action available at the site of detection, and the local, national, and global context within which it has emerged. Infections with high morbidity/mortality and potential for spread that emerge over a relatively short period of time require an appropriate initial response, including risk assessments, and measures designed to tackle acute public health emergencies, which will differ depending on the suspected aetiology of the disease. The US CDC's response to the SARS coronavirus (SARS-CoV) outbreak is provided as an exemplary case study in Table 6.2.[7]

Control measures for less acute conditions are just as challenging, and successful implementation may take several years or decades. This is illustrated by several ongoing epidemics in poor settings, including those caused by HIV and TB, where global action has been essential to the control of these infections.

For all infections, irrespective of how fast or slow the epidemic evolves, the following are essential:

- local, national, and global surveillance systems to detect new infections and monitor control efforts (see ➔ Chapter 2)
- disease control systems
- a programme of applied research, including field epidemiology and applied microbiology
- an infrastructure that allows a rapid response to emergencies and is robust enough to sustain the control of longer-lasting epidemics.

Initial clinical response and assessment of risk

Health personnel are often the first to respond to a potential threat of a new pathogen. This places them at direct risk, sometimes leading to significant illness and possibly death. Health personnel accounted for a substantial proportion of deaths in the 2014 Ebola outbreak in West Africa.[5] Transmission within the healthcare setting and beyond is also possible if the infectious nature of the new pathogen is not realized quickly and dealt with systematically. Both SARS and MERS spread successfully in healthcare settings.[6,8] An early systematic assessment of risk therefore is essential to trigger the correct epidemic response and deal with public concern.

Initial patient assessment includes, in the first instance, attending to the patient and providing rapid medical attention. Patients should be asked about potential risk factors and details of their contacts and recent travel history. In the case of a newly emerging pathogen, working case definitions may not exist yet. If an infectious nature is suspected, immediate actions should include isolating the patient and introducing infection prevention and control measures, while a detailed risk assessment is carried out. Local standard operating procedures on conducting initial

Table 6.2 Centers for Disease Prevention and Control (CDC)'s response to outbreak of severe acute respiratory syndrome (SARS)

Year	Month	Day	Description
2002	November	16	• First case of atypical pneumonia reported in Guangdong province of southern China
2003	March	12	• WHO issued global alert for severe form of pneumonia of unknown origin in people from China, Vietnam, and Hong Kong
		14	• CDC activated its EOC
		15	• CDC issued first health alert and hosts media telebriefing about atypical pneumonia, which had been named severe acute respiratory syndrome (SARS) • CDC issued interim guidelines for state and local health departments on SARS • CDC issued 'health alert notice' for travellers to USA from Hong Kong, Guangdong Province, China
		20	• CDC issued infection control precautions for aerosol-generating procedures in patients suspected of having SARS
		22	• CDC issued interim laboratory biosafety guidelines for handling and processing specimens associated with SARS
		24	• CDC laboratory analysis suggested new coronavirus may be cause of SARS • 39 suspected cases identified in USA to date, 32 of which had travelled to countries where SARS was reported
		27	• CDC issued interim domestic guidelines for management of exposures to SARS for healthcare and other institutional settings
		28	• SARS outbreak had become more widespread • CDC began utilizing pandemic planning for SARS
		29	• CDC extended travel advisory for SARS to include all of mainland China and Singapore • CDC quarantine staff began meeting planes, cargo ships, and cruise ships coming directly or indirectly to USA from China, Singapore, and Vietnam and began distributing health alert notice to travellers

April	4	• 115 suspected cases of SARS reported from 29 states in USA; no deaths among these suspected cases
	5	• CDC established community outreach team to address stigmatization associated with SARS
	10	• CDC issued specific guidance for students exposed to SARS
	14	• CDC published sequence of virus believed to be responsible for global epidemic of SARS, as identifying genetic sequence of new virus is important to treatment and prevention efforts; results came just 12 days after team of scientists and technicians began working around clock to grow cells taken from throat culture of one patient with SARS
	22	• CDC issued health alert notice for travellers to Toronto, Ontario, Canada
May	6	• In USA, no new probable cases had been reported in past 24 hours, and there had been no evidence of ongoing transmission beyond initial case reports in travellers for more than 20 days; containment in USA had been successful
	20	• CDC lifted travel alert on Toronto because more than 30 days (or three SARS incubation periods) had elapsed since date of onset of symptoms for last reported case
	23	• CDC reinstated travel alert for Toronto, because Canadian health officials reported cluster of five new probable SARS cases on 22 May
June	4	• CDC removed travel alert for Singapore and downgraded traveller notification for Hong Kong from travel advisory to travel alert
July	3	• CDC removed travel alert for mainland China
	5	• WHO announced global SARS outbreak was contained
	10–15	• CDC removed travel alert for Hong Kong, Toronto, and Taiwan
	17	• CDC updated SARS case definition, excluding cases in which blood specimens collected more than 21 days after onset of illness tested negative, which halved number of cases in USA

(Continued)

Table 6.2 (*Contd.*)

Year	Month	Day	Description
	December	31	• WHO had received reports of SARS from 29 countries and regions globally; this comprised 8096 people with probable SARS and 774 deaths • Eight SARS infections in USA were documented by laboratory testing and additional 19 probable SARS infections were reported
2004	January	13	• CDC issues 'Notice of embargo of civets', which banned importation of civets, after SARS-like virus was isolated from civets captured in areas of China where SARS outbreak originated
2012	October	5	• National Select Agent Registry Program declared SARS coronavirus a select agent (defined as a bacterium, virus, or toxin that has potential to pose severe threat to public health and safety)

CDC, Centers for Disease Control and Prevention; EOC, emergency operations centre; SARS, severe acute respiratory syndrome; USA, United States of America; WHO, World Health Organization.

Reproduced from Centres for Disease Control and Prevention (CDC), *CDC SARS response timeline*, CDC, Atlanta, GA, USA, available from http://www.cdc.gov/about/history/sars/timeline.htm.

risk assessment of a potential threat should exist and would be helpful. Examples of such frameworks include the Advisory Committee on Dangerous Pathogens (ACDP)'s risk assessment guidance and algorithm on VHF,[9] which is issued by the government in the UK, and the ECDC's rapid risk assessment tools.[10]

In resource-rich contexts, an early consultation with a local infection specialist may be possible. Local hotlines, such as the UK's 24-hour imported fever service and rare and imported pathogens laboratory, may offer further advice on testing and clinical management. In the case of a suspected zoonosis, it is essential to assess the risk of transmission to humans. A qualitative risk assessment tool that assigns levels of confidence of risk of zoonotic transmission of animal diseases is available in the UK.[11] Once a risk assessment has been completed and a substantial threat is identified, the public will need to be informed.

Informing the public

Concern is fuelled by the public's perception of their own risk of exposure and infection, the availability of treatment for themselves and their dependents, and local efforts to mitigate the new threat. The media has an important role to play in conveying correct, up-to-date information as part of an organized public health response to the emerging infection.

Managing an acute public health emergency

The public health response to a newly emerged pathogen with potential to cause an outbreak or pandemic usually requires the prompt institution of measures to contain its spread, including the following actions:

- Identify the problem: use descriptive epidemiology, 'soft' intelligence gathering, desktop review of available information, sentinel surveillance (if necessary), and outbreak investigation measures, including microbiological investigations, as summarized in Box 6.2 and outlined in ➔ Chapter 3.
- Set up the required structure and organization: this includes an emergency operating centre and relevant command-and-control infrastructure and assigning roles and responsibilities. In an emergency, this may be the critical factor that determines whether there is chaos or successful disease control.
- Conduct rapid hazard and health risk assessment: tools developed by governmental and non-governmental bodies for rapid assessment of the hazards and risk should be utilized, and the information gathered analysed to inform subsequent actions.
- Establish related surveillance and emergency information systems for ongoing monitoring: this may initially include sentinel surveillance and clinical criteria for establishing the diagnosis; it is essential to establish laboratory surveillance as soon as this is feasible.
- Set up communications systems for healthcare workers and the general population: messages communicated in the early phase of an emerging infection may determine population behaviour and may be essential to prevent nosocomial spread among health workers; provided information should include what to expect, how the disease might be prevented, and how to seek care.

Box 6.2 Investigating an outbreak of a zoonotic or emerging infection

- Identify the problem.
- Undertake a rapid health needs assessment.
- Define information needs.
- Instigate information-collecting approaches (interviews with officials and health workers, rapid surveys, routine sources if available, and verbal autopsies).
- Perform preliminary or descriptive analyses.
- Generate hypotheses.
- Collect further data, and institute outbreak control measures.
- Undertake analytical epidemiological studies and ongoing surveillance (identify zoonotic or other sources, and identify mode of transmission).
- Control emerging infections.

See ➲ Chapter 3 for more detail.

- Plan interventions based on findings of rapid review, surveillance, and aetiology of the outbreak: this may include environmental and occupational health; infection control; and behavioural, medical, and other measures.
- Target specific vulnerable populations, core groups, and other drivers of spread: for many outbreaks and epidemics, the focus of spread is a particular core group or vulnerable population, so tackling the disease in such subpopulations may be the key to disease control; until such a reservoir is addressed, efforts to control and possibly eliminate the outbreak as a public health problem may not be possible.
- Plan for recovery and reconstruction while managing the outbreak: it is never too early to set up plans for recovery, and this is particularly critical for outbreaks or epidemics that have been detected after they have caused considerable morbidity and mortality in the population.
- Set up systems to evaluate the response and learn lessons to prevent future public health emergencies.

National or regional surveillance systems

The organization of national or regional systems for emerging infections is based on the analysis and synthesis of information collected by official public health institutions of health such as Public Health England in the UK and the US CDC. Data are often provided to health officials through partnerships and networks involving medical practitioners and veterinary agencies.

Global mechanisms

At the global level, a number of recognized systems aid the detection of emerging infections.

World Health Organization systems

The IHR[12] are an agreed set of policies, and WHO member states that have signed up to these obligations are required to implement them. This includes a range of measures, implementation of which may require new or modified legislation in some countries. Implementation of IHR began in 2007 and has led to a framework within which the WHO has established an international advisory committee. All member states are expected to foster global partnerships; strengthen national disease prevention, surveillance, control, and response systems; improve public health security in travel and transport; support the WHO global alert and response systems; ensure the management of specific risks; sustain rights, obligations, and procedures; conduct studies; and monitor progress towards implementation of the measures. The WHO runs the Global Outbreak Alert and Response Network (GOARN) which effectively provides global intelligence on emerging infections.

Early Warning and Response System

The Early Warning and Response System (EWRS) is a mechanism established by the EU to allow the competent public health authorities of the EU member states to exchange information on public health incidents promptly, allowing public health actions to be taken to contain threats across the EU.

Programme for Monitoring Emerging Diseases

Programme for Monitoring Emerging Diseases (Pro-Med) is an Internet-based system that allows the rapid global dissemination of information on outbreaks of infectious diseases and acute exposures to toxins that affect human health. It is less formal than GOARN and EWRS and operates as a programme of the International Society for Infectious Disease.

GeoSentinel and European Travel Medicine Network

GeoSentinel (http://www.istm.org/geosentinel) is a worldwide communication and data collection network for the surveillance of travel-related morbidity. It was initiated in 1995 by the International Society of Travel Medicine (ISTM) and the US CDC as a network of ISTM member travel/tropical medicine clinics. GeoSentinel is based on the concept that these clinics are ideally situated to detect geographic and temporal trends in morbidity among travellers, immigrants, and refugees.

The ISTM also initiated the European Travel Medicine Network (EuroTravNet; http://www.istm.org/eurotravnet) to create a network of clinical experts in tropical and travel medicine to support the detection, verification, assessment, and communication of infectious diseases that can be associated with travelling, specifically tropical diseases. The goal of EuroTravNet is to build, maintain, and strengthen a multidisciplinary network of highly qualified experts with demonstrated competence in diseases of interest, ideally in the fields of travel advice; tropical medicine; clinical diagnosis of the returned traveller; and detection, identification, and management of imported infections. The founding core sites and members of EuroTravNet belong to the GeoSentinel surveillance network.

Future priorities

The current approach, in which we wait for new pathogens to emerge before responding, needs to be replaced by a more proactive system that includes prevention of such outbreaks, rapid detection and response by a well-resourced system, and resilience to tackle the longer-term consequence of such outbreaks. Heymann *et al.*[13] have described a model that should help achieve this, based on the 'OneHealth' approach, which depends on collaboration between local, national, and international experts to address human, animal, and environmental health issues.

The response to the threat of emerging and re-emerging infectious diseases requires a global plan that builds on current mechanisms, such as GOARN, and that relies on existing agreements, such as the IHR, to create robust systems to support research, training, surveillance, and control. One element of this plan is the need to strengthen developing countries' health systems, especially those that are weak due to previous conflict or underdevelopment. The contrast between Nigeria and other West African states in containing the outbreak of Ebola fever in 2014 illustrates the importance of health infrastructure and manpower in limiting the spread of emerging infectious diseases.

Consistent with the 'OneHealth' approach, wider determinants of emerging infections would also need to be addressed, including antimicrobial resistance, zoonotic origin of new and re-emerging infections, and changing environmental and population-level factors that determine the emergence and spread of pathogens.

Finally, the development of an applied research infrastructure—including generic protocols that are pre-approved by ethics governance committees, funding agreements, and the formation of international consortia such as the International Severe Acute Respiratory and Emerging Infection Consortium—and of an inclusive global clinical trials programme would be essential to prevent or, if that fails, to contain the next pandemic.

References

1. Zaki AM, van Boheemen S, Bestebroer TM, Osterhaus ADME, Fouchier RAM (2012). Isolation of a novel coronavirus from a man with pneumonia in Saudi Arabia. *N Engl J Med*, 2012, **367**, 1814–20.
2. Morse SS, Schluederberg A (1990). From the National Institute of Allergy and Infectious Diseases, the Fogarty International Center of the National Institutes of Health, and the Rockefeller University. Emerging viruses: the evolution of viruses and viral diseases. *J Infect Dis*,**162**, 1–7.
3. Koenig KL, Schultz CH. The 2014 Ebola virus outbreak and other emerging infectious diseases. In: *Koenig and Schultz's disaster medicine: comprehensive principles and practices*, 2nd edn, p. 10. Available at: http://www.acep.org/uploadedFiles/ACEP/practiceResources/issuesByCategory/publichealth/The%202014%20Ebola%20Virus%20Outbreak.pdf, Oct 21, 2014, (accessed 25 June 25 2015).
4. Morse SS (1995). Factors in the emergence of infectious diseases. *Emerg Infect Dis*, **1**, 7–15.
5. WHO Ebola Response Team (2014). Ebola virus disease in West Africa—the first 9 months of the epidemic and forward projections. *N Engl J Med*, **371**, 1481–95.

6. Seto WH, Tsang D, Yung RWH, *et al.* (2003). Effectiveness of precautions against droplets and contact in prevention of nosocomial transmission of severe acute respiratory syndrome (SARS). *Lancet*, **361**, 1519–20.
7. Centers for Disease Control and Prevention (CDC). *CDC SARS response timeline*. CDC, Atlanta. Available at: http://www.cdc.gov/about/history/sars/timeline.htm (accessed 18 February 2015).
8. Assiri A, McGeer A, Perl TM, *et al.* (2013). Hospital outbreak of Middle East respiratory syndrome coronavirus. *N Engl J Med*, **369**, 407–16.
9. Public Health England, Department of Health (2014). *Viral haemorrhagic fever: ACDP algorithm and guidance on management of patients*. Public Health England and Department of Health, London. Available at: https://www.gov.uk/government/publications/viral-haemorrhagic-fever-algorithm-and-guidance-on-management-of-patients (accessed 18 February 2015).
10. European Centre for Disease Prevention and Control (ECDC) (2014). *Rapid risk assessment: outbreak of Ebola virus disease in West Africa*. ECDC, Stockholm. Available at: http://www.ecdc.europa.eu/en/publications/Publications/Ebola-Sierra%20Leone-Liberia-Guinea-Nigeria-23-09-2014-rapid-risk-assessment.pdf (accessed 18 February 2015).
11. Palmer S, Brown D, Morgan D (2005). Early qualitative risk assessment of the emerging zoonotic potential of animal diseases. *BMJ*, **331**, 1256–60.
12. World Health Assembly (2005). *Revision of the International Health Regulations, WHA58.3. 2005*. Available at: http://apps.who.int/gb/ebwha/pdf_files/WHA58-REC1/english/Resolutions.pdf (accessed 19 January 2015).
13. Heymann DL, Dar OA (2014). Prevention is better than cure for emerging infectious diseases. *BMJ*, **348**, g1499.

Chapter 7

Investigating hospital infection outbreaks

Robert Aldridge and Barry Cookson

Introduction to investigating hospital infection outbreaks

Hospital and other HAIs are important patient safety issues. Patients who acquire such infections experience increased morbidity and mortality, and costs associated with HAI constitute a substantial fraction of healthcare spending.[1] HAIs also pose occupational hazards to healthcare workers, as they are exposed to infected/colonized patients and microbial hazards in the healthcare environment.

Estimates of the burden of HAIs vary by study and location, but the ECDC, using national and multicentre point-prevalence surveys, calculated that, on average, 7.1% of patients in acute care hospitals have an HAI on any given day.[2] This chapter provides an introduction to the investigation of outbreaks of HAIs. Other chapters are also relevant to this topic, including ➲ Chapters 3, 9, 10, and 21.

After reading this chapter, you will have a better understanding of:

- approaches to the dynamics of HAIs
- preventing nosocomial transmission
- types of hospital outbreaks
- identifying transmission of hospital infections
- managing hospital outbreaks.

Approach to the dynamics of healthcare-associated infections

Three main types of HAIs are recognized:

- auto-infection—acquired from an endogenous source
- cross-infection—acquired from an exogenous source
- environmental—acquired from the environment.

All three types of HAI can result in temporal clusters of cases, and the sources/routes of transmission can be identified only through further investigation, as discussed later in this chapter (see ➔ Identifying transmission of hospital infections, p. 112).

The concept of the 'cycle of infection' (Figure 7.1) describes the components of a 'chain' or related factors that must be considered when determining whether a possible HAI outbreak has occurred. The scenario starts with an affected patient. The implicated organism or organisms will have various possible origins ('reservoirs'), which will depend on the particular microbe. One or more of these possible reservoirs will eventually be proved to be the origin ('source') of the HAI. It could be, for example, an already infected/colonized patient, an item of contaminated medical equipment or pharmaceutical product, or an infected/colonized healthcare worker or other member of staff carrying the organism, albeit transiently, on their unwashed hands.

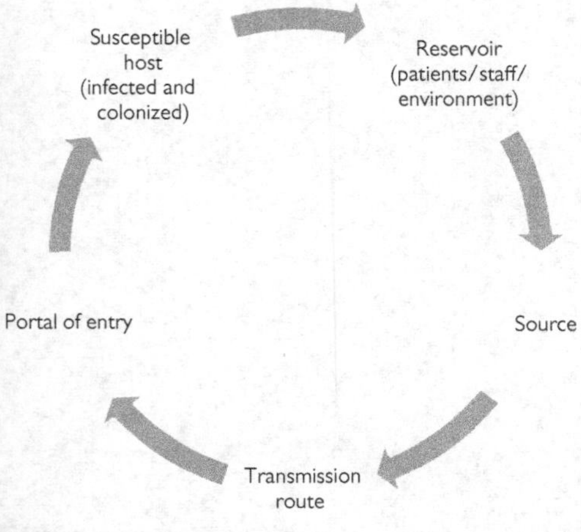

Figure 7.1 Cycle of healthcare-associated infection.

Adapted with permission from Public Health England, *General Information on Healthcare associated infections (HCAI)*, © Crown Copyright 2014, available from http://webarchive.nationalarchives.gov.uk/20140722091854/ http:/www.hpa.org.uk/Topics/InfectiousDiseases/InfectionsAZ/HCAI/GeneralInformationOnHCAI/.

The pathogen requires a 'transmission route' to be able to move from the source to the patient. This is often via direct contact with staff hands, but it might also be via the airborne route, ingestion, or inoculation (e.g. via needles or intravenous/urethral catheters). The 'portal of entry' is the opening via which the microbe enters the host. This can be parenteral (via inserted tubes such as central venous lines or urinary catheters) or through mucous membranes or open wounds. The microbe then has access to the patient, who may be more susceptible to colonization and to infection due to a variety of conditions such as extremes of age and various causes of immunosuppression (e.g. therapeutic, congenital, oncological, or chronic medical conditions).

Importantly, newly affected patients may become part of the reservoir for the microbes associated with the HAI, thus contributing towards their onward transmission. The microbes that typically cause HAI are usually low-virulence pathogens, with <25% of affected patients becoming infected. Most affected patients will only be colonized by the pathogen, but, depending on the case mix and healthcare unit involved, they may also become sources for further transmission to new patients.

Preventing nosocomial transmission

Many strategies have been proved to prevent transmission of HAIs. In general, they can be subdivided into those that reduce person-to-person transmission and those that reduce transmission from the environment.

Types of hospital outbreaks

Hospital infection outbreaks can be simple in their epidemiology e.g. cross-infection of MRSA between patients may result from transient carriage of MRSA on staff hands. Another example is a report of *Pseudomonas aeruginosa* in water outlets causing infections in different hospital neonatal units in several different hospitals.[3]

However, an outbreak can also be far more complex, involving several different sources over time and even different strains and/or microbial species. Such outbreaks can be particularly difficult to detect and are more likely to remain undetected for longer periods of time, as they do not present as an obvious cluster of similar cases. An example of such complexity would be an outbreak due to lack of appropriate antibiotic prophylaxis on a colonic surgery unit; in this situation, a cluster of post-operative infections would occur, with the many different microbes and implicated strains occurring over a potentially long period of time.

Identifying transmission of hospital infections

Identifying hospital-acquired infections requires an effective surveillance programme. Effective surveillance requires attention at different scales of observation, including the clinical unit (typically a hospital ward), hospital, regionally, and nationally.[4] Often an outbreak will be identified by local surveillance, e.g. from analysis of clinical specimens. By collecting and analysing data at these different levels, various types of transmission may be identified, and the connections between data sources complement each other within a coherent surveillance programme. For example, residents of a nursing home may acquire MRSA at a hospital, but the infection may only become apparent after they are discharged into the community. Regional analysis of surveillance data from these community-based patients may cause an initial alert and facilitate identification of the hospital as the source, which may have been missed if data had not been collected and analysed in this way.

The use of standardized definitions for HAIs is crucial to ensure the reliability of the data collected, but also to establish that an infection is hospital-acquired and was not present or incubating at the time of admission. The CDC's National Healthcare Safety Network provides surveillance definitions for specific types of HAIs, which are widely used internationally.[5] In Europe, definitions have also been established by the ECDC.[6] These two sources of definitions were recently compared.[7]

A hospital infection surveillance system comprises several components, including planning, implementation, analysis and feedback, and interventions driven by surveillance (Table 7.1). Data for surveillance systems will be collected from several sources such as patient notes, electronic health records, clinical examinations, and microbiological specimens.

Table 7.1 Hospital infection surveillance system

Surveillance steps	Components
Planning	• Assess available expertise, facilities, and resources • Identify specific objectives, scope, and methods, according to the local situation • Select standardized definitions and preparation of surveillance protocols
Implementation	• Collect clinical data • Conduct other investigations conducted • Complete and finalize data collection forms • Perform ongoing laboratory surveillance of sentinel microorganisms
Analysis and feedback	• Analyse data and interpret results • Adapt local feedback to most appropriate means
Interventions driven by surveillance	• Identify appropriate and feasible interventions and priority areas according to specific results of surveillance • Repeat surveillance activities to assess impact of interventions and adjust them according to results

Reproduced with permission from World Health Organization (WHO), *The burden of health care-associated infection worldwide*. WHO, Geneva, Switzerland, Copyright © 2005, available from http://www.who.int/gpsc/country_work/burden_hcai/en/.

Surveillance systems designed to identify transmission of hospital infections should be monitored continuously.[8]

Surveillance data that indicate an increase in infections and colonizations serve as early warnings that action needs to be taken to prevent additional outbreaks of these and other conditions (see ➲ Chapter 2). 'Alert conditions' (e.g. cellulitis) and 'alert organisms' (e.g. *Streptococcus pyogenes; Staphylococcus aureus*, including MRSA), and antimicrobial-resistant organisms (e.g. gentamicin- or carbapenem-resistant organisms) should be the bedrock of outbreak surveillance activities, with lists of agreed alert conditions (Box 7.1) and alert organisms (Table 7.2) made available to infection control teams (ICTs). The ICTs should visit or call the affected ward each day to discuss the epidemiology (time, place, and person) and clinical status of affected individuals. Changes in commoner infections may, in some settings, serve as useful proxy markers to evaluate how well infection control measures are working in 'real time'.[4]

Box 7.1 Suggested 'alert conditions' that may give rise to hospital outbreaks

- Food poisoning
- Dysentery (amoebic or bacillary)
- Pyrexia of unknown origin
- Severe soft tissue infections
- Tuberculosis
- Legionellosis
- Chickenpox/shingles (herpes zoster)
- Measles
- Mumps
- Rubella
- Whooping cough (pertussis)
- Scarlet fever
- Scabies
- Meningitis
- Meningococcal septicaemia
- Viral hepatitis
- Ophthalmia neonatorum
- Paratyphoid fever
- Typhoid fever
- Diphtheria
- Poliomyelitis
- Viral haemorrhagic fever
- Cholera
- Plague

Adapted from Hospital Infection Working Group, *Hospital infection control*, Department of Health, London, UK, Copyright © 1988, with permission from Public Health England.

Table 7.2 Suggested 'alert organisms' that may give rise to hospital outbreaks

Type of organism	Alert organisms
Bacterial	• MRSA • VISA and VRSA • *Staphylococcus aureus* resistant to other antibiotics, e.g. glycopeptides (GISA and GRSA), gentamicin, and fusidic acid • *Streptococcus pyogenes* • Penicillin-resistant *Streptococcus pneumoniae* • Aminoglycoside- and glycopeptide-resistant enterococci • *Pseudomonas aeruginosa* • *Strenotrophomonas maltophilia* (*Xanthomonas maltophilia*) • Gentamicin-resistant, extended-spectrum β-lactamase-resistant, and quinolone-resistant Gram-negative rods • Other multi-antibiotic-resistant Gram-negative rods • *Clostridium difficile* and/or detection of its toxins • *Legionella* spp. (including serology results) • VTEC (e.g. *Escherichia coli* 0157) • *Salmonella* and *Shigella* spp. • Other bacterial isolates with unusual antibiotic resistance (e.g. *Haemophilus influenzae* resistant to ampicillin and trimethoprim)
Viral	• Rotavirus • Respiratory syncytial virus • Influenza A and B • Herpes zoster • Parvovirus B19
Fungal	• In special units, *Candida* and *Aspergillus* spp.

GISA, glycopeptide-intermediate *Staphylococcus aureus*; GRSA, glycopeptide-resistant *Staphylococcus aureus*; MRSA, methicillin-resistant; VISA, vancomycin-intermediate *Staphylococcus aureus*; VRSA, vancomycin-resistant *Staphylococcus aureus*; VTEC, verotoxin-producing strains of *Escherichia coli*.

Adapted from Hospital Infection Working Group, *Hospital infection control*, Department of Health, London, UK, Copyright © 1988, with permission from Public Health England.

Managing hospital outbreaks

Identifying a hospital outbreak can be a complex process. Once detected, actions should be taken to identify the source and mode of transmission in as timely a manner as possible in order to reduce risk to others. Steps should also be taken to implement control measures to prevent further spread. Reflections and lessons learnt from the outbreak should be disseminated as widely as possible to minimize the likelihood that such outbreaks recur.

The steps involved in managing a hospital outbreak follow the general principles of any outbreak investigation. Specific tasks and issues that should be considered when an outbreak occurs in a hospital setting are described below.

Outbreak control team

An appropriate group of healthcare workers—the outbreak control team (OCT) should be convened. These should include members of the ICT, any infection control ward 'liaison' staff, clinical leads, and other appropriate staff, e.g. pharmacists and senior nurses. This group should agree upon case definitions and discuss the known epidemiology and the hypothesis for ongoing transmission (cycle of infection).

Evaluation of the certainty of an outbreak

Efforts to evaluate data to confirm the outbreak should be conducted immediately. Exclusion of a pseudo-outbreak (i.e. an increase in laboratory cases which cannot be corroborated by other surveillance or clinical data) can avert a costly and time-consuming investigation. Such pseudo-outbreaks may result from poor quality control during the processing of laboratory samples leading to cross-contamination. After excluding a pseudo-outbreak, appropriate initial prevention and control measures should be implemented, particularly if serious infections or infections or colonizations with highly antimicrobial-resistant organisms have been encountered. Control measures might include isolating known cases (e.g. in side rooms or by quarantining similarly infected/colonized patients together, with or without their own nursing staff), increasing hand hygiene, and other infection control audits.

Effective communication between healthcare workers in the hospital and infection control staff is essential throughout this process; this should include regular meetings of the OCT and distribution of summary reports to agreed staff, e.g. those on affected wards and senior management committees. The media department also needs to be alerted, and representatives should attend meetings as necessary.

Case ascertainment

Work should be undertaken to actively identify cases associated with the outbreak. Medical records may be reviewed, and additional individuals at risk and those exhibiting signs or symptoms should be investigated further to determine whether or not they are a case.

Data collection

Additional data should be collected and analysed to compare rates of infection before and during the outbreak, as these will help confirm that an outbreak has occurred. Epidemiological studies should be undertaken; the choice of study design will depend on the type of data available and other considerations such as time constraints and human resources (see ➲ Chapter 4). Descriptive epidemiology, assembly of line lists, and plotting of an epidemic curve are common first steps in any investigation. Reliable time, place, and person data are vital for all types of study. A case control or cohort study may be undertaken, if possible, given the time and resources available. Hospital information technology (IT) systems, or other clinical records, should be used to identify possible readmissions and transfers of patients from other healthcare facilities. Additional investigations may be required to explore alternative hypotheses such as contamination from air, environment, and equipment; staff monitoring may also be informative. Changes in hospital systems (such as people, procedures, equipment, and training) should be investigated to identify potential causes of the outbreak.

Microbiological data

Microbiological data are needed; however, this can be problematic for wards where patients have very short lengths of stay. In this scenario, clinical infections may not have presented on the ward, leading to possible loss of the ability to identify the alert organism/condition. It therefore may be necessary to begin screening systematically, as patients enter the hospital environment and/or after discharge. Post-discharge surveillance systems comprise a variety of strategies, including telephoning patients or general practitioners (GPs) and liaising with other microbiology laboratories to which clinical samples have been sent.

Use of microbiological typing data to identify nosocomial transmission should specifically be discussed. Molecular typing can be used to test hypotheses of causality, particularly when used in combination with good epidemiological data. Further detail can be found in ➲ Chapters 9 and 10.

Ongoing review of prevention/control measures

It is vital that the effectiveness of prevention/control measures is audited prospectively. Over time, an outbreak can seem to be controlled, but new cases may emerge at any point, so continued vigilance is required. Outbreak dynamics may also change, so epidemiological data need to be reviewed as carefully as at the start of an outbreak. Revisiting audits of prevention and control measures, e.g. screening, isolation measures, hand hygiene, 'bundles' for device usage, decontamination of patients with antiseptics, decontamination of equipment, and additional ward cleaning, need to be continually considered. Guidelines are available on the application of evidence-based tools in situations where both evidence and time are limited.[9] Recurrence of infection/colonization might occur due to readmissions of previous patients who were 'affected', but undetected, during their initial admission. Hospital information systems that 'tag' known affected or exposed patients can identify readmissions, so that screening can be implemented.

Evaluation and communication

Once an outbreak has been controlled and brought to a close, staff involved in the management of an outbreak should take part in a debrief meeting, during which lessons learnt can be discussed and reported. Any ongoing tasks that need to be implemented to prevent future outbreaks should be finalized, and a report should be written and disseminated appropriately for others to learn from the situation.

References

1. World Health Organization (WHO). *The burden of health care-associated infection worldwide.* WHO, Geneva. Available at: ℛ http://www.who.int/gpsc/country_work/burden_hcai/en/ (accessed 3 February 2015).
2. European Centre for Disease Prevention and Control (2008). *Annual epidemiological report on communicable diseases in Europe 2008. Report on the state of communicable diseases in the EU and EEA/EFTA countries.* European Centre for Disease Prevention and Control, Stockholm. Available at: ℛ http://www.ecdc.europa.eu/en/publications/publications/0812_sur_annual_epidemiological_report_2008.pdf (accessed 3 February 2015).
3. BBC News Northern Ireland (2012). *Pseudomonas found in more hospital taps.* Available at: ℛ http://www.bbc.co.uk/news/uk-northern-ireland-16953163 (accessed 3 February 2015).
4. Health Protection Scotland (2009). *Guidance on local healthcare associated infection (HAI) surveillance programmes and producing a local surveillance programme.* Health Protection Scotland, Glasgow. Available at: ℛ http://www.hps.scot.nhs.uk/haiic/ic/publicationsdetail.aspx?id=42506 (accessed 3 February 2015).
5. Horan TC, Andrus M, Dudeck MA (2008). CDC/NHSN surveillance definition of health care-associated infection and criteria for specific types of infections in the acute care setting. *Am J Infect Control*, **36**, 309–32.
6. Suetens C, Savey A, Labeeuw J, Morales I, HELICS-ICU (2002). The ICU-HELICS programme: towards European surveillance of hospital-acquired infections in intensive care units. *Euro Surveill*, **7**, 127–8.
7. Hansen S, Sohr D, Geffers C, *et al.* (2012). Concordance between European and US case definitions of healthcare-associated infections. *Antimicrob Resist Infect Control*, **1**, 28.
8. Public Health England (2014). *Healthcare associated infections (HCAI): guidance, data and analysis.* Public Health England, London. Available at: ℛ https://www.gov.uk/government/collections/healthcare-associated-infections-hcai-guidance-data-and-analysis (accessed 3 February 2015).
9. Palmer S, Jansen A, Leitmeyer K, Murdoch H, Forland F (2013). Evidence-based medicine applied to the control of communicable disease incidents when evidence is scarce and the time is limited. *Euro Surveill*, **18**, 20507.

Chapter 8

Clinical epidemiology

Noel McCarthy and Adrian Smith

Definition of clinical epidemiology

Clinical epidemiology involves the application of epidemiological and statistical techniques to study problems encountered in clinical medicine. The scope of clinical epidemiology is defined both by the type of work clinicians undertake (e.g. prevention, diagnosis, and treatment) and the populations that seek clinical advice (e.g. patients and people at risk of disease). As healthcare has evolved to deliver primary and secondary prevention in addition to tertiary prevention, so has the epidemiological evidence used to inform such clinical activities.

This chapter considers the epidemiologic concepts relevant to this range of clinical activity: evaluation of infection risk, diagnosis, prognosis, and treatment.

Evaluating risk of infection

Clinicians may be called on to assess the risks of infection for an individual before any indication of illness, with a view to advising on preventive actions. This may occur:

- **prior** to a potential exposure to an infection, e.g. a traveller seeking advice before travel; in this case, the aim is to assess the risk that an individual will come into contact with a source of infection and to assess the potential benefit of pre-exposure intervention
- **after** a specific potential exposure to an infection, e.g. a healthcare worker seeking advice after a workplace injury; in this case, the aim of assessment is to quantify the infection risk posed by a specific event and assess the potential benefit of post-exposure intervention.

For any transmission of infectious disease to occur, a **susceptible** individual must make **effective contact** (contact sufficient for transmission to occur) with an **infectious source**. The clinical justification for preventive interventions relies on assessment of these factors; consideration of the clinical severity of the infection to the individual; and knowledge of the efficacy, availability, and risks of the intervention.

The **susceptibility** of the individual may be apparent from their medical and vaccination history and, for some diseases, inferred from historic surveillance data. In some cases, particularly when the probability of immunity is high and/or the intervention is scarce or has a significant risk of side effects (e.g. assessment of pregnant women for human normal immunoglobulin therapy after exposure to measles), direct laboratory assessment of immunity may be indicated.

The need for pre-exposure interventions may relate to a specific **infectious source**. For example, pre-exposure antiretroviral prophylaxis may be recommended to a HIV-negative individual whose partner is known to be HIV-positive. Post-exposure intervention may be guided by identification of a suspected source, e.g. the direct observation of a dog after a human bite for signs of rabies. Local human, veterinary, and environmental surveillance data are often used to estimate the likelihood of source infectiousness in the absence of specific information about the infectiousness of a source and when considering the prospective risk of exposure.

The definition of an **effective contact** differs for different communicable diseases, and the probabilities of transmission of types of contact between an infectious source and a susceptible contact are derived from observational studies. For isolated contacts, detailed characteristics may discern features predictive of a risk of transmission. For instance, the depth and extent of a wound after an animal bite are predictive of the risk of transmission of rabies.

Measuring test performance

Diagnosis is the identification of the nature of an illness through clinical assessment. Diagnostic tests include any kind of clinical measurements performed to help establish the diagnosis. Diagnostic tests include all clinical assessments aimed at narrowing the differential diagnosis, including features of the patient's history, physical examination, and laboratory tests.

Sensitivity and specificity

The validity of a diagnostic test is the extent to which it correctly classifies individuals with and without the disease, compared to the most accurate reference method—the **gold standard**. The concept of a gold standard acknowledges that even the best measure may not be a completely accurate classification of the presence or absence of disease. The validity of a diagnostic test has two components: its sensitivity and specificity (Box 8.1). The sensitivity of a test is a measure of its ability to identify correctly those who have the disease, while specificity is a measure of its ability to identify correctly those who do not have the disease.

For most tests, the consequence of increasing the sensitivity of a diagnostic strategy is an increase in the false-positive rate (thus decreasing specificity). Similarly, aiming to increase the specificity usually results in an increase in the false-negative rate. Given the trade-off between sensitivity and specificity, the relative importance of each should reflect the anticipated clinical purpose of the test. A strategy may prioritize sensitivity at the expense of specificity if the test is being used to rule out individuals with the disease—for instance, when screening blood products for HCV or excluding malaria as the cause of fever.

Positive and negative predictive value of tests

Although sensitivity and specificity reflect the performance of a test in which the disease status is known, clinical decision-making requires understanding of the extent to which positive or negative test results accurately indicate the presence or absence of disease for individual patients.

The positive predictive value (PPV) of a test is the probability that a person who tests positive actually has the disease, while the negative predictive value (NPV) of a test is the probability that a person who tests negative does not have the disease (Box 8.2). The PPV is influenced by the number of false positives, which is the product of the **specificity** of the test and the number of people tested who are free of disease. Similarly, the NPV depends on the **sensitivity** of the test and the number of people who have the disease in the population tested. Predictive values therefore depend on the frequency of disease in the population (prevalence), as well as the test's sensitivity and specificity.

The effect of disease prevalence on PPV and NPV indicates the need for caution when applying research findings to clinical use where the prevalence of disease may be very different. Systematic diagnostic performance may be particularly challenging for infectious diseases with epidemic or seasonal patterns accompanied by considerable fluctuation in population prevalence (Box 8.3).

Box 8.1 Calculation of sensitivity and specificity

Diagnostic test result	Disease status (gold standard)		
	Disease	No disease	Total
Positive	TP (a)	FP (b)	$a + b$
Negative	FN (c)	TN (d)	$c + d$
Total	$a + c$	$b + d$	

- True positive (TP): patients have the disease and test positive.
- True negative (TN): patients do not have the disease and test negative.
- False positive (FP): patients do not have the disease but test positive.
- False negative (FN): patients have the disease but test negative.
- **Sensitivity**: the proportion of people who have the disease and test positive:

  $a/(a+c)$

- **Specificity**: proportion of people who do not have the disease and test negative:

  $d/(b+d)$

- **False-negative rate**: proportion of people with the disease who test negative:

  $c/(a+c)$ or $(1 - \textit{sensitivity})$

- **False-positive rate**: proportion of people without the disease who test positive:

  $b/(b+d)$ or $(1 - \textit{specificity})$

Worked example

- New rapid diagnostic test (RDT) for malaria, compared to gold standard (microscopy)

RDT result	Microscopy		
	Positive	Negative	Total
Positive	340	40	380
Negative	30	1230	1260
Total	370	1270	1640

- Sensitivity of rapid test = 340/370 = 91.9%
- Specificity of rapid test = 1230/1270 = 96.9%

Likelihood ratios of positive and negative tests

A related clinical decision-making question is, 'What information will this test add?' Likelihood ratios (LRs) quantify the increment in information gained from either a positive or negative test result (Box 8.2). The positive likelihood ratio (LR+) is the ratio of the odds of disease after a positive test result to the pretest odds of disease. Similarly, the negative likelihood ratio (LR−) is the ratio of the odds of disease after a negative test to the pretest odds of disease. Both measures can be calculated knowing only the sensitivity and specificity of the test.

LRs can be interpreted in their own right; a LR of 1 indicates no information gain by testing, while a LR+ much greater than one or a LR− much less than one indicates significant predictive values. Alternatively, the information gain can be expressed as the difference in pretest probability of disease (i.e. the prevalence of disease) to the post-test probability of disease, given a positive or negative test result. Nomograms simplify calculations for use in everyday clinical decision-making.[1]

Box 8.2 Calculation of predictive values and likelihood ratios

Diagnostic test result	Disease status (gold standard)		
	Disease	No disease	Total
Positive	TP (*a*)	FP (*b*)	*a* +*b*
Negative	FN (*c*)	TN (*d*)	*c* + *d*
Total	*a* + *c*	*b* + *d*	

- **Pretest probability of disease**: the disease prevalence:

  $(a+c)/(a+b+c+d)$

- **PPV** (or predictive value of a positive test): the probability of truly having the disease if the test is positive:

  $a/(a+b)$

- **NPV** (or predictive value of a negative test): the probability of truly not having the disease if the test is negative

  $d/(c+d)$

- **Positive likelihood ratio** (LR+): the ratio of the post-test odds of disease (given a positive result) to the pretest odds of disease:

  sensitivity / (1 − *specificity*)

- **Negative likelihood ratio** (LR−): the ratio of the post-test odds of disease (given a negative result) to the pretest odds of disease:

  (1 − *sensitivity*) / *specificity*

Box 8.3 Worked example: effect of prevalence on positive predictive value (PPV) and negative predictive value (NPV) of a rapid malaria test with sensitivity of 91.9% and specificity of 96.9% during season with high (a) and low (b) levels of transmission of malaria

(a)

RDT result	Gold standard		
	Positive	Negative	Total
Positive	340	40	380
Negative	30	1230	1260
Total	370	1270	1640

- Prevalence of disease = 370/1640 = 22.6%
- PPV (positive RDT) = 340/380 = 89.5%
- NPV (negative RDT) = 1230/1260 = 97.6%
- LR+ = 0.919/(1 − 0.969) = 29.6
- LR− = (1 − 0.919)/0.969 = 0.08

(b)

RDT result	Gold standard		
	Positive	Negative	Total
Positive	34	51	85
Negative	3	1552	1555
Total	37	1270	1640

- Prevalence of disease = 37/1640 = 2.3%
- PPV (positive RDT) = 34/85 = 40.0%
- NPV (negative RDT) = 1230/1233 = 99.8%

Optimizing diagnosis

Infection versus disease

The range of biomedical techniques available to diagnose infectious diseases is expanding, particularly with the increasing clinical availability of rapid molecular diagnostics. Many techniques have high sensitivity and specificity to quantify the presence of the infectious agent, but, in many diagnostic scenarios, the mere presence of infection does not confirm this as the cause of a clinical illness. Colonization and carriage of coincidental infectious agents (e.g. *Staphylococcus aureus* and *Neisseria meningitidis*) and coexisting latent or subclinical infections (e.g. *Mycobacterium tuberculosis* and *Plasmodium falciparum* in semi-immune adults) may result in diagnosis of infection in the investigation of an illness caused by something else.

In such scenarios, the diagnostic validity of the test for infection is an overestimate of the clinical diagnostic validity. For instance, a throat swab and culture might have acceptable utility to identify streptococci in the nasopharynx of children with sore throats but may have poor specificity and PPV as a definitive clinical test for streptococcal tonsillopharyngitis if coincidental colonization is commonplace. Methods to adjust the predictive value of laboratory tests for the prevalence of incidental carriage[2] or that incorporate discriminatory clinical information into predictive algorithms may help optimize such clinical diagnosis strategies.

Selection of test cut-off

Many clinical and laboratory measures are not dichotomous but are distributed across a range of values (e.g. body temperature, leucocyte count, HIV antibody titre). Receiver operating characteristic (ROC) curves are one method to help inform the selection of an appropriate dichotomous test cut-off from a range of measures.

The ROC curve plots sensitivity against (1 − specificity) (i.e. the proportion of false positives) across different values of a diagnostic test or increments of a diagnostic algorithm. Figure 8.1 plots the performance of an antibody test at nine cut-off titres (points 1 to 9).

The ROC curve may be used to:

- visualize the trade-off between sensitivity and specificity across the range of values of a diagnostic test or algorithm
- identify the value of a diagnostic test at which sensitivity and specificity are optimized
- compare the diagnostic performance of two or more tests for the same disease
- compare the diagnostic performance of one test in different types of individuals (e.g. different age groups or stages of infection).

The area under a receiver operating characteristic (AUC) curve is a summary measure of the ability of a diagnostic test to classify correctly the presence or absence of disease over its range of values (Figure 8.2). The AUC ranges between 1 (a test that classifies all cases correctly) to 0 (a test that classifies all cases incorrectly), with a value of 0.5 indicating

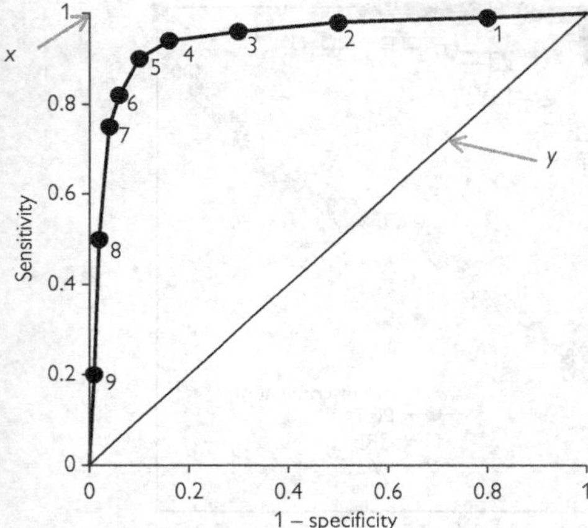

Figure 8.1 Receiver operating characteristic (ROC) curve of laboratory assay.

that the test offers no discrimination. The AUC values of different tests for a disease may be compared in this way, and the test with the AUC closest to 1 would be deemed to be more discriminatory of the presence of disease across its range of values.

Caution must be applied in translating technically optimum cut-off points from ROC curves to clinical practice. The method assumes that sensitivity and specificity are of equal clinical relevance, i.e. the consequences of false-positive and false-negative classifications are equivalent. This is often not the case, and there may be a clear clinical rationale to prioritizing the sensitivity of a diagnostic test over its specificity (for instance, where the disease is severe) or vice versa (for instance, where treatment comes with considerable risk).

Multiple test algorithms

An alternative strategy to optimize diagnostic performance is to combine tests. Where two diagnostic tests of the same condition are used, the effect on net sensitivity and specificity is dependent on the decision rule for discordant results.

- A result is positive if **either** test is positive: a net gain in sensitivity at the expense of increasing the number of false positives (net loss in specificity).
- A result is positive if **both** tests are positive: a net gain in specificity at the expense of increasing the number of false negatives (net loss in sensitivity).

The overall sensitivity, specificity, and cost of complex decision rules can be evaluated in the same way. Diagnostic algorithms may instead be

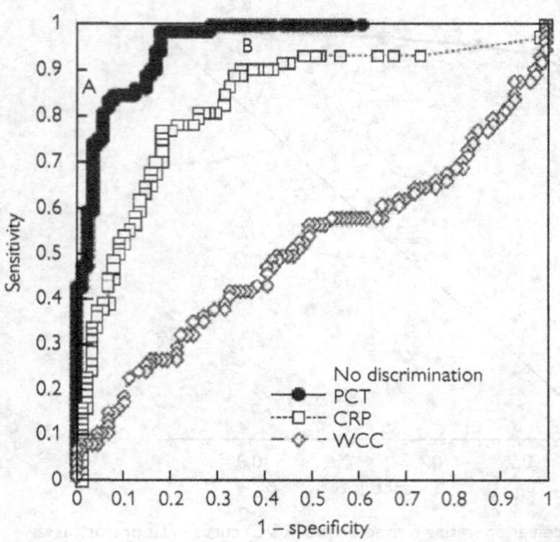

Figure 8.2 Worked example: laboratory predictors of septic shock among paediatric admissions.

A study compared procalcitonin (PCT), C-reactive protein (CRP), and leucocyte counts (WCC) among children on admission to intensive care. The ROC curve displays the validity of the measures in correctly classifying children with and without septic shock (diagnosed by subsequent bacteriology) across the range of reported laboratory values. PCT was more discriminatory of septic shock across its range of values (AUROC 0.96 [95% confidence interval 0.93 to 0.99] than CRP [AUROC 0.83], while WCC was not discriminatory of septic shock. The optimum trade-off between sensitivity and specificity of PCT was a cut-off of 20 ng/mL (sensitivity 83%, specificity 92%, point A). However, the authors concluded that the appropriate clinical application was as a test optimized to rule out septic shock (PCT >2 ng/mL, sensitivity 100%, specificity 62%, point B).

Adapted by permission from BMJ Publishing Group Limited from Hatherill M *et al.*, Diagnostic markers of infection: comparison of procalcitonin with C reactive protein and leucocyte count, *Archives of Disease in Children*, Volume 81, pp. 417–21, Copyright © 1999, BMJ Publishing Group Ltd and the Royal College of Paediatrics and Child Health.

optimized in terms of the information gained from additional tests, which may be more meaningful to clinical decision-makers. In this case, conditional LRs are used to quantify the information gained by sequences of different tests within a diagnostic algorithm, in which the post-test odds of the prior test represent the pretest odds of the following test.

Prognosis and treatment

Prognosis and burden of disease

Disease prognosis for any disease is influenced by patient characteristics as well as treatment. For infections, the outcome in the patient or host is influenced by a range of additional inter-related and dynamic factors (Figure 8.3). Severity and outcome can vary by pathogen subtype and the presence of co-infection with other microbes, which are, in part, features of the population surrounding the host. The interplay between the host's immune system and the pathogen is modified by past interactions between the host and similar organisms or by simulated interactions in the form of vaccination. Infectious diseases are also typically self-limiting, if not fatal during the acute stages, although complications may persist and contribute to a large and increasingly recognized proportion of disease burden for common infections.[3]

A minority of infections can escape adaptive immunity and become chronic or recurrent. Chronicity can be almost universal, as in HIV infection, or relatively rare, such as hepatitis B acquired after the neonatal period. Pathogen, host, and treatment factors that affect prognosis are considered separately below. Their inter-relatedness, the ecological- or population-level effects, and individual effects are illustrated in Figure 8.3.

Pathogen factors affecting prognosis

Some pathogens are monomorphic, and clinical diagnosis identifies a non-diverse organism such as measles, for which there is no variation in clinical outcome due to variation in the infecting organism. In other infections, different clinical patterns associated with variation in stable subspecies are well recognized such as the varying clinical syndromes associated with different serogroups of meningococcal infection and types of influenza.[4] Mobile genetic material can also affect prognosis, including that associated with antibiotic resistance, which can move within, and even between, bacterial species.[5] As rapid WGS of pathogens becomes low cost and big data approaches make it feasible to use routine data to follow prognosis in large groups, the evidence base on pathogen factors that affect prognosis is likely to increase rapidly (see ➲ Chapter 10). Rapid microbial evolution will continue to generate new factors that affect prognosis—including through response to therapy—for many pathogens.

Host factors that affect prognosis

Some host factors that affect infectious disease outcomes are well characterized. Extremes of age and underlying illness are strong predictors of poor outcome for many infections, mainly due to ineffective immune responses to infections. Many more specific host factor–outcome associations have been quantified, such as the approximately fourfold increased risk of severe illness from influenza among pregnant women and the 40-fold increased risk among those with neurological conditions such as cerebral palsy and severe immunosuppression. Table 8.1 maps some varied examples across population groups and pathogens.

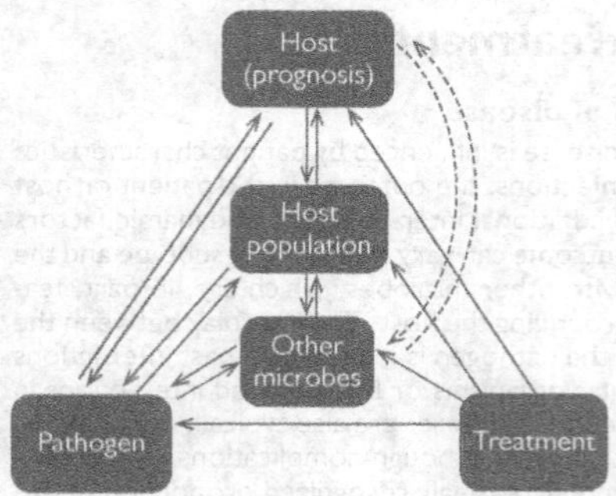

Figure 8.3 Inter-related factors affecting individual patient prognosis.

Table 8.1 Variation in prognosis by patient group and type of infection (poor prognosis represented by a tick)

Patient characteristic	Infection			
	Influenza	Listeria	Varicella	VTEC
Neonate	✓		✓	✓
Child				✓
Pregnant	✓	✓	✓	
Elderly	✓	✓		✓
Immunosuppression	✓	✓	✓	
Cerebral palsy	✓			

VTEC, verocytotoxin-producing *Escherichia coli*.

In addition, some highly specific and well-characterized altered immune responses that affect prognosis include a particular risk of severe TB in patients with immune deficits produced by the anti-tumour necrosis factor (TNF) drugs increasingly used to treat rheumatoid arthritis and the increased risk of meningococcal sepsis in patients with some complement deficiencies. Host factors that affect prognosis do not always correlate with factors that affect incidence of infection, e.g. influenza is commoner, but usually mild, in non-infant children.

Treatment factors

Treatment of infections is dominated by, although not restricted to:

- treatment to remove one of the underlying causes, namely the presence of an infecting organism
- modification of the host's immune response when this can reduce symptoms and complications

- symptomatic and supportive treatments until the host's immune response has controlled the underlying infection.

Features of therapy that are specific to infections are:

- diagnosis of infectious disease can lead to interventions being directed to others, typically close contacts
- the clinical response to treatment can affect the risk of, and prognosis for, potential future cases
- treatment effectiveness can be affected adversely by the treatment histories of others such as when this has promoted resistance to antimicrobial therapies.

These features emphasize the interplay of factors at the individual level with ecological- and population-level factors. This has implications for how interventions should be evaluated. Although licensing of medical interventions is based on benefits and risks at the individual level, indirect benefits can be the main purpose of an intervention against infectious disease. For example, revaccination of children aged 3–4 years against pertussis is undertaken to prevent illness in young infants in contact with these children. In addition, the prevalence of influenza was lower among those remaining unvaccinated in isolated rural communities where some children were vaccinated against this virus, compared with children in communities where vaccination was not used (3.1% versus 7.6%),[6] and this indirect effect (i.e. herd immunity) is a key benefit of vaccination when coverage levels are high enough to achieve this effect.

References

1. Fagan TJ (1975). Nomogram for Bayes theorem. *N Engl J Med*, **293**, 257.
2. Gunnarsson RK, Lanke J (2002). The predictive value of microbiologic tests if asymptomatic carriers are present. *Stat Med*, **21**, 1773–85.
3. Werber D, Hille K, Frank C, *et al.* (2013). Years of potential life lost for six major enteric pathogens, Germany, 2004–2008. *Epidemiol Infect*, **141**, 961–8.
4. Hayward AC, Fragaszy EB, Bermingham A, *et al.* (2014). Comparative community burden and severity of seasonal and pandemic influenza: results of the Flu Watch cohort study. *Lancet Respir Med*, **2**, 445–54.
5. Pontikis K, Karaiskos I, Bastani S, *et al.* (2014). Outcomes of critically ill intensive care unit patients treated with fosfomycin for infections due to pandrug-resistant and extensively drug-resistant carbapenemase-producing Gram-negative bacteria. *Int J Antimicrob Agents*, **43**, 52–9.
6. Loeb M, Russell ML, Moss L, *et al.* (2010). Effect of influenza vaccination of children on infection rates in Hutterite communities: a randomized trial. *JAMA*, **303**, 943–50.

Chapter 9

Public health microbiology

Helen R. Stagg, Nigel M. Field, and Sani H. Aliyu

Introduction to public health microbiology

Public health microbiology contributes toward identifying and controlling the microorganisms responsible for human disease at the population level. Technological evolution over recent decades has led to increasingly sophisticated methods, which may be used to identify different pathogens and discriminate between strains within the same species (typing). This chapter will:

- introduce the key microbiological techniques currently used in public health to control and prevent infectious disease
- describe the key public health applications for these methods, using illustrative examples
- discuss the role of the public health microbiology laboratory in disease prevention.

Techniques

Culture systems

Robert Koch, the inventor of solid culture systems for bacteria, once said 'Pure culture is the foundation for all research on infectious disease' as it is the basis for isolating and amplifying microorganisms. The ability or inability of microorganisms to grow on specific media or under certain environmental conditions may aid their identification, as may their morphology.

Although more sensitive techniques now exist, culturing is still the gold standard for identifying some organisms such as *Bordetella pertussis* and *Neisseria gonorrhoeae*. However, not all organisms grow easily on conventional agar medium, e.g. *Mycoplasma* spp., and competition with normal flora may also affect yield. This has led to the development of selective media containing specific bionutrients. Inhibitors that prevent bacterial overgrowth may be required for some organisms, e.g. *Legionella*. Liquid culture systems include automated blood culture broths in which bacteria (such as *Mycobacterium tuberculosis*) are suspended within a nutrient medium to produce enhanced and more rapid bacterial growth. Traditionally, cell cultures have been used to propagate viruses and screen for the presence of cytopathic effects from the toxins produced by bacteria, e.g. *Clostridium difficile*, but they can be expensive and difficult to maintain, although they are still vital for discovering emerging pathogens, determining novel disease mechanisms, and vaccine development.

Microscopy

Microscopy is used to detect, and subsequently identify, microorganisms on the basis of their morphology or by using organism-specific probes attached to coloured or other tags. Sputum smear microscopy using Ziehl–Neelson stain is still widely used for the diagnosis of *Mycobacterium tuberculosis*, but has poor sensitivity. Fluorescence microscopy with auramine stain is used routinely to detect *Cryptosporidium* oocysts in stool. Technological advances, such as scanning transmission electron microscopy, give a resolution down to a few nanometres to visualize even the smallest viruses.

Serotyping and other immunological tests

Detection of antigens and the response of the host's immune system to such antigens can be useful to identify and type microorganisms and for population-level measures of immunity. The human response to specific surface antigens can be used to classify microorganisms into groups, e.g. serotyping in the investigation of food outbreaks. It requires skilled manpower and is time-consuming and costly, and not all isolates can be typed (see ➔ Chapter 11). The functional response of immunological cells to antigens from the microorganism under investigation can be used as a marker of previous exposure to the organism (e.g. release of interferon gamma (IFN-γ) in response to *Mycobacterium tuberculosis* antigens measured by the IFN-γ release assay).

Biochemical tests

Biochemical tests, such as oxidase, urease, and coagulase tests, are based on specific metabolic characteristics of the organism in question. Colour changes can be scored and converted into a numeric code to aid identification.

Mass spectrometry

Microbial organisms produce a unique signature (or spectral pattern) when subjected to a fixed-pulse laser beam, and this can be fed into a database to allow accurate and rapid speciation of the organism, without the need for prolonged biochemical tests. Mass spectrometry (MS) is increasingly available in well-funded hospital laboratories. The development of new ionization methods for MS, based on examination of whole-cell bacterial chemical composition, such as electrospray (ES) and matrix-assisted laser desorption/time of flight mass spectrometry (MALDI-TOF MS), has revolutionized the field; minimal sample preparation and handling are required, and the technology can be applied to a wide range of organisms, including fastidious and biochemically inert species. However, MALDI-TOF MS has low accuracy for identification of Gram-negative anaerobes, *Shigella* spp., viridans-group streptococci, and *Stenotrophomonas maltophilia*.

Drug sensitivity testing

Drug sensitivity testing, using culture techniques or sequencing of known genetic markers conferring antimicrobial resistance, is vital to identify appropriate treatment regimens for patients.

The role of the public health laboratory

The role of the public health laboratory (PHL) is to support local and national public health programmes through provision of timely and accurate epidemiological surveillance data on food, water, and environmental microbiology. PHLs can identify trends in infectious diseases through surveillance programmes (see ➲ Chapter 2) and analyse the effectiveness of public health interventions, and so are key players in the development and prioritization of national and regional health agendas.

Public health applications

Despite the widespread availability and expansion of molecular diagnostics in microbiology, conventional laboratory tests continue to play a major role in public health and disease prevention, particularly in resource-limited settings.

Sample collection, specimen selection, and choice of tests

Microbiological investigations within a public health setting require good knowledge of sampling and laboratory techniques. It is important that the right type of specimen is collected and processed in a timely manner in order to maximize diagnostic yield. Understanding the pathophysiological process of infectious disease is essential to ensuring that this is done correctly. For instance, *Legionella pneumophila* serogroup 1 is best detected using a urine antigen test, however, expectorated sputum or bronchoalveolar lavage is required for cultures for typing when legionellosis is due to other serotypes. Specimens may need to be taken on more than one occasion before a diagnosis of certain infections can be excluded. The timing of sample collection is also important, as the quality of samples can deteriorate rapidly, e.g. cervical swabs for *Neisseria gonorrhoeae* may require plating directly on to culture media at source before transporting to the laboratory.

Identifying key laboratory tests relevant to investigation

Although it is frequently possible to culture the pathogen responsible for a disease, some agents are difficult to grow (e.g. *Coxiella burnetti*), and diagnosis will depend on the detection of antibodies in the patient. In infections caused by *Clostridium difficile*, the diagnosis is based on detection of toxins, but isolation of the organism by culture is still required for ribotyping (gene fingerprinting using restriction enzymes to digest bacterial ribosomal genes) in outbreak situations. Culture is still considered the gold standard for the diagnosis of most infections, as it is highly specific and enables antibiotic susceptibility to be determined, as well for the performance of key outbreak investigation analyses such as serotyping (e.g. for salmonellosis) and molecular subtyping (e.g. pulse field gel electrophoresis, PFGE).

Surveillance of nosocomial infections and emerging infections

Public health microbiology has a large role in the surveillance of nosocomial and emerging infections (see ➲ Chapters 6 and 7). Reporting of nosocomial infections, such as MRSA bacteraemias, has been mandatory in English hospitals since April 2001. Control of emerging infections, such as MERS-CoV, Ebola virus, and West Nile virus, requires a robust public health microbiology infrastructure with access to the latest molecular diagnostic techniques.

Surveillance of antimicrobial resistance

Antimicrobial resistance is a major cause of morbidity and mortality worldwide. The prevalence of antimicrobial resistance varies for different regions of the world, and monitoring of new resistant strains in a particular area is an important role for public health microbiology. Although antibiotic susceptibility tests have evolved over the years, interpretation of new resistance profiles remains difficult for non-reference laboratories. For example, carbapenemase production cannot be inferred from routine microbiological susceptibility methods based on breakpoints, so the presence of decreased susceptibility to carbapenems among clinical isolates should raise suspicion for carbapenemase-producing *Enterobacteriaceae* (CPE) and prompt confirmatory testing.

Outbreak investigations

Confirmation of an outbreak requires the use of diagnostic microbiological methods and rapid evaluation based on prior laboratory data to detect trends and changes in local epidemiology. Indeed, case definitions in an outbreak setting should always have a microbiological component (see ➲ Chapter 3).

Limitations

Classic microbiological techniques, which are often cheap to implement with relatively little staff training, lack the sophistication of modern microscopic, spectroscopic, and molecular epidemiological techniques and are often much slower (see ➲ Chapter 9). As the costs of the latter fall their improved sensitivity and specificity, and the large amounts of information that can be derived from samples, will likely lead to the rise of in-house molecular testing, with associated challenges at the national level for quality control.

Looking to the future

MALDI-TOF MS is showing great potential as a diagnostic tool for the modern microbiology laboratory. Recent studies have demonstrated its potential applicability in identifying isolates directly from positive blood cultures, thus reducing turnaround time from 24–48 hours to less than an hour. This means that timely and appropriate antibiotic advice can be offered to patients with septicaemia, which could improve patient outcomes.

Polymerase chain reaction-electrospray ionization mass spectrometry (PCR-ESI MS) has been shown to improve the sensitivity of PCR-based direct organism identification from blood culture. The technique uses electronspray (ES) to analyse the nucleotide composition of PCR amplicons. This method can detect important pathogens that would otherwise have been missed by conventional blood culture systems, including aerobic Gram-negative bacteria and *Staphylococcus aureus*. When compared to MALDI-TOF MS, PCR-ESI MS is more complex to use, is considerably more expensive to run, and requires highly skilled manpower in its present form, so it is unlikely to be introduced successfully into the routine laboratory in the near future.

The demands of a modern diagnostic laboratory have resulted in a move away from manual methods of plating organisms, reading plates, and interpreting results towards laboratory automation. As we move from agar plates to microchips, WGS and microarrays may be the new diagnostic tools for the modern microbiology laboratory of the future.

Conclusions

Microbiological techniques are important in public health practice for the identification of pathogens—a process that also aids clinical diagnosis and management. Although routine microbiological methods that rely on lengthy culture and serological techniques will continue to be employed in the routine microbiology laboratory, the scenery is already changing, as more rapid molecular-based techniques become the preferred tools for the diagnosis and prevention of infection.

Further reading

Burnham CD (2013). *Automation and emerging technology in clinical microbiology, an issue of Clinics in Laboratory Medicine*. Elsevier, St Louis.

Christner M, Trusch M, Rohde H, *et al.* (2014). Rapid MALDI-TOF mass spectrometry strain typing during a large outbreak of Shiga-toxigenic *Escherichia coli*. *PLoS One*, **9**, e101924.

Collins CH, Lyne PM, Grange JM, Falkinham JO III (2004). *Collins and Lyne's microbiological methods*, 8th edn. Hodder Arnold, London.

Dingle TC, Butler-Wu SM (2013). MALDI-TOF mass spectrometry for microorganism identification. *Clin Lab Med*, **33**, 589–609.

Frank C, Milde-Busch A, Werber G (2014). Results of surveillance for infections with Shiga toxin-producing *Escherichia coli* (STEC) of serotype O104:H4 after the large outbreak in Germany, July to December 2011. *Euro Surveill*, **19**, 20760.

Johnson AP, Davies J, Guy R, *et al.* (2012). Mandatory surveillance of methicillin-resistant *Staphylococcus aureus* (MRSA) bacteraemia in England: the first 10 years. *J Antimicrob Chemother*, **67**, 802–9.

Murray PR, Baron JE, Jorgensen JH, Pfaller MA, Yolken RH (2003). *Manual of clinical microbiology*, 8th edn. ASM Press, Washington, DC.

Nichols GL, Richardson JF, Sheppard SK, Lane C (2012). *Campylobacter* epidemiology: a descriptive study reviewing 1 million cases in England and Wales between 1989 and 2011. *BMJ*, **2**, e001179.

Chapter 10

Molecular epidemiology

Nigel M. Field, Duncan MacCannell, and Helen R. Stagg

Introduction to molecular epidemiology

Infectious disease molecular epidemiology utilizes molecular typing methods for infectious agents in the study of the distribution, dynamics, and determinants of health and disease in populations.

The following core concepts underpin our understanding of infectious disease molecular epidemiology:

- pathogens with similar molecular typing characteristics are likely to be related
- the degree of similarity between types can be used to make inferences about their relatedness or the number of generations (time) since their most recent common ancestor.

Analysis of molecular typing data, ideally linked with other data sets, provides a powerful means to investigate infectious disease transmission events.

This chapter will:

- summarize the tools and techniques currently available
- introduce the role of molecular epidemiology in public health
- explain specific sources of limitation and bias associated with molecular epidemiological data
- describe legal and ethical and other considerations when using such data.

Techniques

The 'omics' (genomics, transcriptomics, proteomics, and metabolomics)—laboratory techniques that underpin molecular epidemiology—are very rapidly developing fields used to study the structure, function, and dynamic interactions of microorganisms and their genomes:

- **Genomics** is the study of an organism's genome, be that deoxyribonucleic acid (DNA), ribonucleic acid (RNA), or a combination of the two. Genomics is an ever-growing field, particularly since the advent of inexpensive **WGS** using next-generation sequencing (**NGS**) techniques. Approaches can be divided into four major categories:
  - direct comparison of DNA/RNA sequences: WGS of DNA or RNA can be used to identify single-nucleotide polymorphisms (**SNPs**). **16S ribosomal RNA (rRNA) sequencing** (e.g. for the species-specific identification of anaerobic Gram-negative rods) using **multilocus sequence typing** (**MLST**), for example, can distinguish between Shiga toxin-producing strains of *Shigella* and *Escherichia coli*
  - measurement of the accumulation of pathogen-specific genetic targets amplified by PCR using labelled nucleotides
  - gel electrophoresis to examine the size of the products of the digestion of DNA at known cut sites using restriction enzymes, to examine the size of PCR-amplified products (e.g. mycobacterial interspersed repetitive units–variable number tandem repeats (**MIRU-VNTR**), where DNA fragment size relates to the number of repeats for *Mycobacterium tuberculosis*), and to identify restriction fragment length polymorphisms (**RFLPs**) (partially discriminatory for *Shigella* spp.)
  - hybridization, in which single-strand nucleic acid recognition sequences of known composition (probes) attached to a matrix are exposed to single-strand fragments of a microorganism's genome and binding is measured (e.g. DNA microarray or 'gene chip').
- **Transcriptomics** studies the expression of an organism's genes, examining the patterns of individual gene expression and the relative abundance of RNA transcripts, including messenger, ribosomal, and transfer RNAs.
- **Proteomics** involves analysis of the proteins expressed by an organism, which reflect gene transcription, translation, and post-translational modification.
- **Metabolomics** is concerned with a cell's metabolic (i.e. chemical) fingerprint. In multicelled organisms, the transcriptome, proteome, and metabolome may differ substantially between cell types.

A number of important factors have helped to drive innovation in molecular epidemiology and adoption of these 'omics' techniques. Faster acquisition of data, as a result of eliminating the need for slow amplification steps and improved resolution and throughput, has resulted in more relevant and actionable information for patient care and public health. Improving resolution and throughput in a reproducible, epidemiologically concordant, and relatively cost-effective fashion has led not only to greater volumes of high-quality data, but also to easier automation and standardization than conventional techniques.

Tools

Bioinformatics tools are used to curate large data volumes, as well as to analyse molecular epidemiological data. Such tools can be used to identify regions of genetic similarity or variation between pathogen strains or between a strain isolated from a case and a reference strain, as well as to annotate sequences, e.g. *in silico* identification of areas within the genome with particular functionality. Phylogeny (evolutionary relationships) may be depicted using dendrograms (Figure 10.1) to visually represent phylogenetic trees. In addition, other 'omics'-derived data may be analysed to compare patterns of gene expression under different environmental conditions.

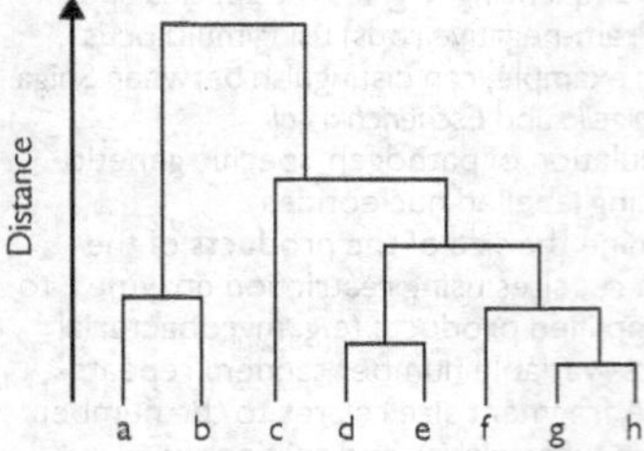

Figure 10.1 Dendrogram. An example dendrogram of eight related yet distinct strains; (a) and (b) are more closely related to each other than (a) and (c).

Analytical challenges

WGS and other high-throughput laboratory technologies are fundamentally changing the practice of public health and clinical microbiology. Although these techniques offer unprecedented resolution, speed, and comprehensiveness, their application and coordinated use present some important new challenges:

- **Data volume**: raw genomic data sets typically comprise millions, or even billions, of short sequence reads, with uncompressed file sizes of several gigabytes or more. This represents a significant increase in data volume over conventional molecular epidemiologic workflows and requires careful consideration of how to best ingest, transmit, analyse, manage, and store vast amounts of sequence data and associated metadata. High-speed networking, peta-scale storage, high-performance computing, virtualization, and cloud computing are all increasingly vital to the analysis and management of microbial genomic data.
- **Bioinformatics capacity**: suitable bioinformatics capacity is critical to the timely analysis and interpretation of complex genomic data sets, and many of these analyses require specialized bioinformatics infrastructure and staff.
- **Limited reference collections**: for many pathogenic microorganisms, only a handful of well-documented and high-quality reference genomes, near neighbours, common commensal organisms, and environmental contaminants exist in public repositories. The relevant features of new sequences may be difficult to recognize without appropriate taxonomic and phylogenomic context. Several activities are currently under way, such as the 100 000 Genomes Project and the US CDC's Advanced Molecular Detection Initiative, which include efforts to sequence important pathogens, including unusual and under-represented species.
- **Data standards and interpretive criteria**: the development of consensus data standards and standardized analytical approaches is critical for information sharing, outbreak detection, investigation, and response. For example, in SNP-based strain typing, interpretation can be significantly impacted by differences in the reference sequence, choice of algorithms and runtime parameters, and the process by which panels of parsimoniously informative loci are identified. Similarly, the interpretation of putative clusters will usually require standardized interpretive criteria, information on baseline diversity and strain-type dynamics of the organism, and a thorough understanding of the epidemiologic context of the isolates (e.g. is a two-SNP difference between isolates significant?).

Other considerations

- **Choice of biological marker**: it is necessary to consider whether the chosen marker has an appropriate molecular clock (Box 10.1), given the public health question at hand. For example, assessment of whether cases arose through local transmission chains over a short time period would typically require a marker that is more discriminatory than a study examining the geographical movement of strains over many years. It is also important to ensure that the methods chosen will not incorrectly disregard highly divergent strains.
- **Differences in the ease of isolation of the organism** may lead to information bias (non-differential misclassification) if one of the strains in question is more difficult to detect or analyse than others under investigation.
- **Multiple infections may be common**, and one strain may overwhelm the received 'signal', leading to under-representation of other strains. Modern WGS techniques, which can detect multiple sequences simultaneously, can take such heterogeneity into account.
- **Legal and ethical** issues may arise, particularly when direct transmission of infection is investigated. In global case law, criminal prosecutions have followed the transmission of STIs, including HIV, hepatitis B virus (HBV), and herpes simplex virus (HSV) type II. Using molecular typing data, it is much easier to disprove, rather than prove, transmission, and such data are of little value without linked epidemiological data.

Box 10.1 Molecular clock

The term 'molecular clock' refers to the basic rate of nucleic acid sequence evolution of a specific molecular marker (rather than a specific pathogen or whole genome). Sequence variation occurs due to mutation and recombination and is highly dependent on the pathogen and the marker under examination.

Public health applications

The public health applications of molecular epidemiology are rapidly expanding. These currently fall into the following categories:

- **Surveillance**: molecular techniques are used to monitor the spread of specific pathogen strains at regional, national, and international levels to inform intervention efforts. For example, the WHO's Global Influenza Surveillance and Response System (GISRS) undertakes continuous surveillance and virus characterization to understand current, and predict future, circulating influenza strains and to inform decisions about the antigenic composition of global influenza vaccines.
- **Tracing the origin of emerging infections**: molecular typing can be used to identify and trace the source of new infections. Sequencing undertaken on respiratory samples from patients with MERS-CoV provided the first evidence that this was a betacoronavirus—similar to bat coronaviruses—and helped public health experts to understand that a patient in London was infected with a virus closely resembling the strain infecting the index case in Saudi Arabia.
- **Outbreak source identification**: valuable public health information may be obtained about the source of outbreaks using molecular analyses that allow strains to be compared and epidemiological hypothesis testing about the most likely source. These include food-borne pathogens (such as Shiga toxin-producing *Escherichia coli*), airborne pathogens (such as *Mycobacterium tuberculosis*), environmental pathogens (such as *Legionella pneumophila*), and bioterrorism threats (such as during the anthrax attack in the US in 2001). The use of WGS to identify an asymptomatic healthcare worker as the source of an outbreak of MRSA in a special-care baby unit in England, which led to the decolonization of this asymptomatic carrier, is an example that defined a paradigm for how genomic data can be used to inform public health decisions. Box 10.2 provides another example of the use of WGS for outbreak investigation.
- **Mapping transmissions in time and place**: genomic methods have been used to map the spread of specific pathogen lineages. In the US, sequencing of *Neisseria gonorrhoeae* isolates has demonstrated the spread of strains with reduced antibiotic susceptibility among sexual networks of men who have sex with men (MSM). Likewise, global transmission of the 'El tor' strain of *Vibrio cholerae* has been mapped to three likely independent waves, including several transcontinental transmission events.
- **Understanding pathogenesis**: molecular techniques are also useful, in a broader scientific sense, to improve our knowledge of the molecular basis for pathogen virulence. Such uses include investigation of the causes of reduced drug susceptibility (only 40–50% of patients with hepatitis C virus (HCV) genotype 1 achieve cure when treated with peginterferon alfa-2b and ribavirin), rapid evolutionary appearance of resistance to new drugs (HIV), vaccine escape mutants (influenza viral drift/shift), and back mutations in live vaccines (live attenuated Sabin polio vaccine).

Box 10.2 WGS for outbreak investigations

Linking traditional 'shoe leather' epidemiological data with biological data, such as from WGS, can provide a very powerful way to understand the transmission of infections within populations.

An example is from Canada where 41 cases of tuberculosis (TB) in 2006–2008 were identified in a British Columbia community through case finding and contact tracing. The outbreak in this small community led to more than a tenfold increase in the annual local incidence of TB.

Using basic epidemiological data, researchers failed to identify an index patient as the source of the outbreak, but a social network approach, using structured interviews with cases, honed in on likely sources for the outbreak. RFLPs and MIRU-VNTR typing was identical for the isolates, which seemed to confirm the clonal nature of the outbreak, but provided insufficient resolution to establish the sequence in time of transmission events. However, WGS (comparing 204 SNPs) unexpectedly identified two separate lineages of *Mycobacterium tuberculosis* consistent with not one, but two, concurrent outbreaks. Moreover, the genomic data suggested that the divergence in strains had occurred before the outbreak, implying that an external factor had precipitated the rapid spread of two strains already present within the population.

Going back to the epidemiological data, the researchers spotted a strong association between infection with *Mycobacterium tuberculosis* and the use of crack cocaine. Using interview data about the timing of symptoms and social interactions, together with the molecular data, which could be used to rule out transmission where people were infected with different strains, 'superspreaders' were identified among the cases.

In this example, data from WGS were used to show that the early assumption that all transmission events in this outbreak were linked was incorrect. The outbreak was caused by two distinct strains—driven by key individuals within the community—and was linked to drug use. Neither the epidemiological data nor the molecular data alone could be used to make these inferences, but together these data provided the evidence for clear public health actions.

Conclusions

The cost of genome sequencing per base pair has fallen by more than 100 million times since the first pathogen genome was published in the 1990s. Richard Resnick, Chief Executive Officer of GenomeQuest, has equated this to filling up your car with petrol in that decade, waiting 20 years, and being able to drive to Jupiter and back...twice! This is a disruptive technology that has enormous potential for exploring interactions between pathogens and their hosts. Although genomics and the other 'omics' have yet to be incorporated fully into everyday public health practice, it seems likely that molecular techniques will increasingly be applied to real-world public health problems and practice.

One of the major difficulties in undertaking genomics and other 'omics' work is in handling the vast quantity of data generated. To this end, multidisciplinary teams of bioinformaticians, statisticians, and epidemiologists will need to work together with microbiologists and basic scientists to make sense of the data. Public health practitioners should be ready to harness these data, while maintaining a critical eye on their interpretation.

Further reading

Attwood T, Parry-Smith DJ (1999). *Introduction to bioinformatics*. Prentice-Hall, Harlow.

Chalmers J (2002). The criminalization of HIV transmission. *Sex Transm Infect*, **78**, 448–51.

Dodds C, Weatherburn P, Hickson F, Keogh P, Nutland W (2005). *Grievous harm? Use of the Offences Against the Person Act 1861 for sexual transmission of HIV*. Sigma Research, London. Available at: http://tiny.cc/bvmlfx (accessed 27 January 2015).

Eurosurveillance (2013). *Special edition: Middle East respiratory syndrome coronavirus (MERS-CoV)*. European Centre for Disease Prevention and Control, Stockholm.

Field N, Cohen T, Struelens MJ, *et al*. (2014). Strengthening the Reporting of Molecular Epidemiology for Infectious Diseases (STROME-ID): an extension of the STROBE statement. *Lancet Infect Dis*, **14**, 341–52.

Gardy JL, Johnston JC, Ho Sui SJ, *et al*. (2011). Whole-genome sequencing and social-network analysis of a tuberculosis outbreak. *N Engl J Med*, **364**, 730–9.

Grad YH, Kirkcaldy RD, Trees D, *et al*. (2014). Genomic epidemiology of *Neisseria gonorrhoeae* with reduced susceptibility to cefixime in the USA: a retrospective observational study. *Lancet Infect Dis*, **14**, 220–6.

Köser CU, Holden MT, Ellington MJ, *et al*. (2012). Rapid whole-genome sequencing for investigation of a neonatal MRSA outbreak. *N Engl J Med*, **366**, 2267–75.

Orengo CA, Thornton JM, Jones DT (2002). *Bioinformatics: genes, proteins and computers*. Bios Scientific Publishers, Oxford.

Roetzer A, Diel R, Kohl TA, *et al*. (2013). Whole genome sequencing versus traditional genotyping for investigation of a *Mycobacterium tuberculosis* outbreak: a longitudinal molecular epidemiological study. *PLoS Med*, **10**, e1001387.

Tsai CS (2002). *Introduction to computational biochemistry*. John Wiley & Sons, New York.

van Belkum A, Tassios PT, Dijkshoorn L, *et al*. (2007). Guidelines for the validation and application of typing methods for use in bacterial epidemiology. *Clin Microbiol Infect*, **13**(Suppl 3):1–46.

Westhead DR, Parish JH, Twyman RM (2002). *Instant notes in bioinformatics*. BIOS Scientific Publishers, Oxford.

World Health Organization (2014). *Recommended composition of influenza virus vaccines for use in the 2014–2015 northern hemisphere influenza season*. World Health Organization, Geneva. Available at: http://www.who.int/influenza/vaccines/virus/recommendations/2014_15_north/en/ (accessed 23 May 2014).

Chapter 11

Immuno-epidemiology

Saranya Sridhar and Ibrahim Abubakar

Introduction to immuno-epidemiology

The host immune system protects against infection and disease after exposure to infectious agents. Studies of the immune status of populations provide critical information about the burden of previous epidemics and risk factors for infection and disease to help predict the risk and nature of future epidemics and pandemics.

Definition of immuno-epidemiology

Immuno-epidemiology is defined as the systematic collection and testing of blood samples and other body fluids from a representative or defined population, using immunological assays to characterize population immune responses following exposure to infections or vaccinations, to assess the distribution and determinants of health outcomes.

Uses of immuno-epidemiology

Immuno-epidemiology contributes to four broad and overlapping areas:

- surveillance to provide data on the incidence and prevalence of disease in the population
- surveillance to provide data on population-level immunity as the basis for deployment and evaluation of immunization programmes
- as an epidemiological tool to investigate risk factors and occurrence of new emerging infectious diseases
- as a surrogate marker or biomarker for treatment/vaccine response.

The underlying principle for the use of immuno-epidemiology is to measure changes in the host immune system as it reacts and adapts to infection and disease. Understanding of the immune system and the laboratory tools used to characterize the immune system thus are essential in the field of immuno-epidemiology.

The immune system

The immune system is broadly divided into innate and adaptive systems. The innate immune system is the first barrier to any pathogen and is rarely assayed for the purposes of sero-epidemiology. The adaptive immune system that responds more specifically to pathogens is broadly divided into the cell-mediated and humoral immune responses.

The cell-mediated arm is formed of T cells, which are broadly of two types: CD8-positive T cells, which are cytotoxic killer cells, and CD4-positive T-helper cells, which provide help to different arms of the immune system. Induction of cell-mediated immune response is particularly important against intracellular parasites, viruses, and bacteria such as *Plasmodium*, HIV, and *Mycobacterium tuberculosis*, respectively, and T cells exert their function by the secretion of different proteins called cytokines such as interleukins (ILs) and IFN. For example, the T cell response to *M. tuberculosis* antigens may be determined by measuring the ability of T cells to secrete the cytokine IFN-γ (IFN-γ release assays). T cells also have an important role to play in B cell-mediated immunity.

The humoral arm of the adaptive immune system is composed of antibodies, which are immunoglobulin (Ig) molecules that are generated and secreted by B cells. The five different types of human immunoglobulins—IgA, IgM, IgG, IgD, and IgE—each have distinct functions. Humoral immunity is particularly important in the response to extracellular bacterial infections such as *Haemophilus* and meningococcal meningitis, and viral infections such as polio and hepatitis B.

An antigen is a protein or part of the pathogen that is recognized by components of the immune system, specifically T or B cell receptors, or antibodies.

Immune response to infection

Immuno-epidemiology relies on measurement of different components of the immune system that define different clinico-pathological stages of infection in order to assess population-level risk of disease. Understanding of the host immune response to infection by different pathogens therefore is necessary for reliable use and interpretation of immuno-epidemiological data.

A key feature of adaptive immunity is 'immunological memory'. This refers to the capacity of T and B cells to respond more rapidly and effectively on re-exposure to a pathogen. Subsequent to infection, an early effector response to clear the pathogen is followed by the development of immune memory. In the acute phase of an infection, effector T cells are induced first, along with short-lived IgM antibodies, and this is followed by delayed induction of long-lived IgG antibodies. As the pathogen is cleared from the body, pathogen-specific, long-lived memory T cells and B cells develop, and these are maintained for an individual's lifetime.

Development and selection of the appropriate test to measure and characterize the immune response is thus important to provide information about the state of infection in individuals. For example, current or recent infection is often diagnosed by measuring IgM antibodies, while levels of IgG antibodies would usually reflect prior infection and cumulative experience of the individual to a pathogen. Clinically mild or asymptomatic subclinical infections can be diagnosed only through the use of immunological tests. Therefore, sero-epidemiology can reveal the total burden of infection (clinical and subclinical) in the population at the time of the test as well as in the past (Table 11.1).

Table 11.1 Sources of human biological material for immuno-epidemiology

Sources	Advantages	Disadvantages
Planned surveys from target populations	• Best approach, as careful selection of representative population possible • Estimate incidence of infection • Estimate immunity to disease to guide vaccine policy or catch-up campaigns • Collection of demographic information allows identification of risk factors	• Expensive • Labour-intensive
Blood donors from blood donation programmes (anonymized blood samples)	• Convenient sampling • Large number of samples available • Useful for screening to look at immunity to specific viruses or presence of outbreak	• Prevalence of infection estimated • Not representative of age and sex structure of population • History of vaccination not available, limiting estimates of burden of infection
Entrance and periodic examination of different groups: military, industry, and healthcare workers	• Repeated surveys of same groups of individuals allow estimation of incidence in the group • Economical • Convenient, as groups require medical checks regularly • Good clinical records available for linkage	• Not representative of entire population • Such groups may have specific exposures that increase risk of infection (e.g. healthcare workers and influenza)
Hospitals and public health laboratories: pathology and microbiology laboratories, and prenatal clinics	• Convenient sampling • Catchment population may be known, allowing estimation of incidence • Can be linked to clinical records	• Target population not known • Not representative of population as potential for hospital bias

Immunological assays

Immunological assays measure either antibodies or T cells that are specific to a pathogen and reflect the experience of the immune system following infection or vaccination. Assays are developed based on testing for the presence of either pathogen-specific antibodies or T cells. Assays to quantify antibodies measure their ability in the biological sample to bind to a specific antigen (e.g. enzyme-linked immunosorbent assay (ELISA)) or the ability to prevent a reaction caused by the pathogen or antigen (e.g. haemagglutination inhibition or microneutralization assays). T cell assays measure the functionality of T cells in secreting cytokines in response to antigen or pathogen (e.g. enzyme-linked immunospot (ELISpot)). Figure 11.1 provides a schematic of ELISA and ELISpot—the two assays most commonly used to measure antibodies and T cells, respectively; Table 11.2 lists some representative examples for the use of these assays.

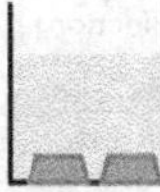

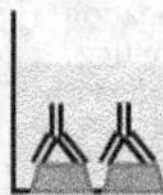

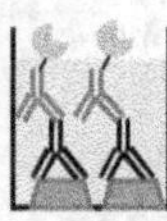

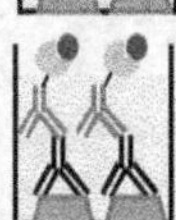

Antigen-coated well

Substrate is added which is converted by enzyme into coloured product. The intensity of colour formation is proportional to the amount of specific antibody

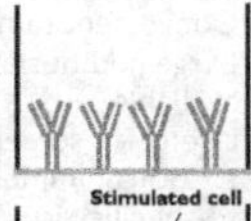

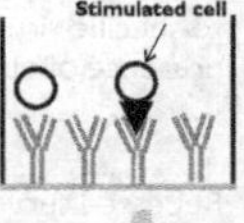

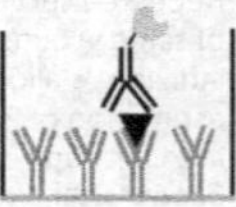

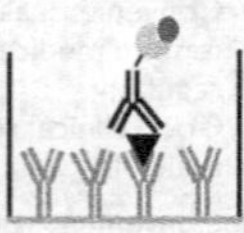

Membrane at bottom of well coated with capture antibody

Stimulated cell
Antigen stimulated cell secretes cytokine which is captured by membrane-bound antibody

Enzyme linked antibody binds to secreted cytokine

Substrate is added which is converted by enzyme into coloured spot. Each spot reflects 1 antigen-specific cell secreting cytokine.

Figure 11.1 Schematic of ELISA and ELISpot.

Table 11.2 Representative examples for the use of different assays

Disease	Pathogen	Assay	Readout	Use
Bacterial infections				
TB	*Mycobacterium tuberculosis*	ELISpot ELISA	IFN-γ release from T cells	Estimate prevalence of latent TB infection in population[1]
Meningitis	*Neisseria meningitides*	Serum bactericidal antibody assay	Complement-mediated lysis by specific antibody	Estimate prevalence of immunity to different strains following introduction of vaccination programme[2]
Pertussis	*Bordetella pertussis*	Indirect EIA	IgG antibodies to pertussis toxin	Estimate prevalence of new and past *B. pertussis* infection[3]
Viral infections				
Influenza	Influenza	Haemagglutination inhibition assay	Antibodies that neutralize viral infection	Estimate incidence of influenza over a season and estimate seasonal and secular trends[4]
Hepatitis	Hepatitis B	ELISA	IgG antibodies to HBsAg	Estimate prevalence of hepatitis B infection in population[5]
Chickenpox/shingles	Varicella-zoster	ELISA	IgG antibodies	Estimate incidence and high-risk age groups for targeting vaccination[6]
German measles	Rubella	Latex agglutination test	IgM or IgG antibodies	Serological diagnosis of rubella infection or immunity[7]
Parasitic and other infections				
Neosporosis	*Neospora*	Inhibition ELISA	IgG antibodies	Investigate zoonotic transmission from canine to humans[8]

EIA, enzyme immunoassay; ELISA, enzyme-linked immunosorbent assay; ELISpot, enzyme-linked immunospot; HBsAg, surface antigen of the hepatitis B virus; IFN-γ, interferon gamma; IgG, immunoglobulin G; IgM, immunoglobulin M; TB, tuberculosis.

Source: data from Zwerling *et al.* 2012[1]; Trotter CL *et al.* 2012[2]; Cherry JD *et al.* 2004[3]; Hardelid P *et al.* 2010[4]; Caley M *et al.* 2012[5]; Vyse AJ *et al.* 2004[6]; Giraudon I *et al.* 2012[7]; and McCann *et al.* 2008[8].

Analysis of immunological data

The readouts from immunological assays are often different to the epidemiological data usually encountered, and they are also presented and analysed differently. The quantity of antibodies in a biological sample is often provided in terms of titres or concentration of antibodies after normalizing it to a reference standard (e.g. titre of 1/32 or 10 mIU/mL). A titre is the lowest dilution of antibody at which no further functional activity of the antibody is observed. The average population-level antibody quantity is expressed as the geometric mean.

In contrast, T cell data using ELISpot are expressed in terms of spot-forming counts/million cells (SFCs/million) and follow a Poisson distribution. More recently, new immunological biomarkers that measure a variety of different immune parameters against the same pathogen are being used. The use of immune biomarkers and their analysis pose different considerations in the analysis of the data.

The analysis of immunological data should take into consideration the following relevant issues.

Structure of immunological data

Most immunological data used in sero-epidemiology are not normally distributed and therefore will not satisfy the data assumptions of common statistical tests. Data thus should be transformed to fulfil assumptions of normal distribution, or parametric methods applicable to the identified distribution or non-parametric methods should be used.

Reproducibility

This refers to the variation in assay results using the same test and sample. Analysis of sero-epidemiological data must take into account the degree of variation and the factors affecting this variation when comparing assay results over time.

Standardization and repeatability

This refers to the variation in assay results between different laboratories or in different studies, and is usually due to differences in protocols and methods of the assay in different laboratories. Standardization across countries and public health centres has become very important to allow comparison of sero-epidemiological data. The European Sero-Epidemiology Network (ESEN2) is an initiative designed to coordinate and harmonize the serological surveillance of immunity to a variety of vaccine-preventable infections across Europe.[9]

Multiple testing

The problem of multiple testing is when investigators undertake multiple statistical testing on different immunological parameters measured in the same data set. This leads to the possibility of statistically significant associations occurring by chance, rather than being reflective of true biological relationships. This issue is gaining increasing importance, as new assays and techniques are developed to measure an increasing number of different immunological parameters.

Differentiating past and current infection

Depending on the type of antibody tested, the durability of the antibody after infection and the maintenance of immune markers after infection allow estimation of current and past burden of infection and disease. For example, in the case of hepatitis B, the prevalence of chronic infection is estimated by measuring serum levels of hepatitis B surface antigen (HBsAg) because of its long persistence and low possibility of chronic cases losing HBsAg, while the burden of past hepatitis infection is often estimated by measuring IgG antibodies to HBsAg and the hepatitis B core (HBc) antigen.

Use of immuno-epidemiology in public health and study design for serological studies

Estimating prevalence of infection

Traditionally, case-based surveillance programmes are used to estimate the burden of disease in a population. Measuring pathogen-specific immune responses, particularly serum antibodies, in a population enables estimation of the prevalence of past or current infection and is termed seroprevalence. In contrast to case-based prevalence, seroprevalence data reflect both clinical and subclinical infection. Seroprevalence studies are particularly useful to identify population groups at risk of infection, rather than those at risk of clinical disease. The commonest study design used to estimate seroprevalence is the cross-sectional study (see ➲ Chapter 4). Cross-sectional study designs do not provide estimates of the incidence of infection.

Examples of public health applications of seroprevalence studies include:

- estimation of the burden of a disease in the population or in particular risk groups (e.g. pregnant women): for example, HIV seroprevalence in the USA was estimated from HIV testing of sera collected as part of demographic and health surveys
- provision of valuable data on the age distribution of immunity and population groups at risk of infection: for example, in settings where Epstein–Barr and dengue virus are prevalent, although Epstein–Barr virus antibodies are acquired very early in life, with 95% of the population positive by age of 5 years, antibodies to DENV tend to develop in most children by the age of 10 years, which is indicative of differences in susceptibility to infection and disease, as well as opportunities for exposure[10,11]
- seroprevalence studies also allow identification of risk groups and modes of transmission: for example, seroprevalence studies on human T-lymphocytic virus 1 (HTLV-1) identified a high prevalence of antibodies in adults, which raised the possibility of sexual transmission, and this was strengthened by high rates in those with a positive test for syphilis[12]
- comparisons across countries: the convenience and ease of cross-sectional seroprevalence studies allow countries to undertake them on a large representative population. For example, comparison of HIV seroprevalence from national surveys in 22 developing countries showed considerable variation between the different countries.[13] However, when comparing across countries, attention must be paid to the standardization of the assays and the representation of the populations in the different countries.

Estimating incidence of infection

Estimating the incidence of infection is particularly important for pathogens that cause high proportions of asymptomatic or subclinical infections, which can drive disease transmission (e.g. influenza, TB), and infections with a long latent period to development of disease (e.g. HIV). Two broad approaches are commonly used to assess recent infection. Seroconversion—usually defined as a fourfold increase in pathogen-specific antibodies before and after infection or over the early course of an infection—enables estimation of the sero-incidence of infection. Measurement of IgM antibodies that are raised recently after infection may also be used to estimate the incidence of some infections.

The most powerful study design to estimate the incidence of infection is the prospective cohort (see ➲ Chapter 4), with samples collected before and after infection in individuals. The advantages of prospective cohort studies for estimating sero-incidence are shown in Box 11.1.

A repeated cross-sectional survey provides an alternative approach to estimating incidence. A change in seroprevalence from cross-sectional surveys repeated over time in a defined population, but not necessarily the same individuals, provides a measure of incidence. These studies are convenient and often used by public health agencies to estimate secular trends in infection or changes in disease burden following the introduction of immunization programmes.

Examples of public health applications of sero-incidence studies include:

- estimation of the incidence of infection and clinical disease separately: for example, large population-based cohort studies, such as the Amsterdam HIV cohort studies, provided key data on the incidence of HIV infection in HIV-negative people and HIV-associated disease[14]
- identification of risk factors for infection: prospective serological studies have been useful in defining the risk of CMV and rubella, which may lead to congenital disease in the newborn, via pregnant women[7,15]
- estimation of subclinical/asymptomatic infection: the serological cohort study design is the only approach that allows the proportion of subclinical/asymptomatic infections to be estimated. For example, a prospective cohort study in the UK found that 50% of all influenza infections were asymptomatic[16]

Box 11.1 Advantages of cohort studies

- Provide level of immunity at the start of the study
- Estimate incidence of infection and clinical disease separately
- Identify reinfections and calculate rate of reinfection
- Calculate proportion of symptomatic and asymptomatic infections
- Define the clinical spectrum of infection and illness in the population
- Identify risk factors and immune correlates of risk of infection and illness
- Understand the host response to infection

- estimating reinfection rates: in individuals followed over time, seroconversion indicates primary infection and repeat seroconversions, offering estimates of the rate of reinfection with the same pathogen[17]
- secular trends: serological cohort studies and repeated cross-sectional serosurveys are able to provide data on secular trends in the incidence of viral infection.

Immunization programmes

Sero-epidemiological data are critically important to determine the need for immunization programmes, as well as to evaluate such programmes. These data may be used to define the burden of infection and to determine risk groups, which is essential to decide cost-effectiveness and target groups for immunization programmes. For example, studies in the UK to estimate the baseline measles–mumps–rubella (MMR) antibody prevalence were undertaken to inform the introduction of the MMR vaccine in 1988.[18] As sero-epidemiological data on measles, mumps, and rubella antibodies in 1991 showed low seroprevalence in children aged 7–14 years, this led to an immunization programme for all children aged 5–16 years in November 1994.[18]

After introduction of vaccines, sero-epidemiology is an important adjunct to other methods of surveillance to monitor the impact of vaccination programmes. This is usually estimated by measuring the reduction in seroprevalence or clinical disease in the population after introduction of the vaccine. Cross-sectional serosurveys can also be used to estimate vaccine coverage in a population. Sero-epidemiological tools can also be used as measures of vaccine efficacy. Immune responses that truly predict the risk of developing infection or disease are termed correlates of protection (see ➲ Chapter 12), although not all immune responses induced by a vaccine are protective or associated with protection. Such correlates of protection in immunization programmes are often used as surrogates of protection against infection and disease.[19] This is particularly useful, as it avoids using clinical endpoints to estimate the efficacy of the vaccine. For example, an antibody titre >1:40 measured by haemagglutination inhibition assay is a correlate of protection against influenza infection. Sero-epidemiological studies to measure the proportion of individuals developing such titres after vaccination are used as a surrogate for vaccine efficacy.

Identification of the source of new aetiological agents

Measurement of immune responses in biological samples collected for routine surveillance is often used to identify the risk of infection, as new pathogens emerge in human populations. For example, seroprevalence of antibodies in sera collected 2 years prior to the outbreak of MERS-CoV demonstrated high prevalence in dromedary camels, but not humans, which suggests potential transmission of this virus from camels to humans.[20]

Future developments

Revolutionary advances in immunology and molecular biology have opened the possibility for intensive analysis of the humoral and cellular immune systems. These techniques include the use of gene expression signatures with transcriptomic techniques, multiplex reverse transcription polymerase chain reaction (RT-PCR) that can measure multiple genes at the same time, and multiplex ELISA. Although these techniques still need to be applied to large-scale applications for routine surveillance, there is a rapid expansion of such techniques and assays to study host–pathogen interactions. Other advances include the use of different biological samples that are less invasive than a blood sample, including saliva and nasal swabs, to assess the immune status. These sampling techniques have their own logistical considerations, including the selection of immune assays to measure the appropriate component of the immune system. The future of immuno-epidemiology would be influenced by the emergence of these new assays. At the same time, as more immune markers are developed and identified, newer approaches will need to be developed to handle the possibility of spurious associations and bias in analysing big data.

References

1. Zwerling A, van den Hof S, Scholten J, Cobelens F, Menzies D, Pai M (2012). Interferon-gamma release assays for tuberculosis screening of healthcare workers: a systematic review. *Thorax*, **67**, 62–70.
2. Trotter CL, Findlow H, Borrow R (2012). Seroprevalence of serum bactericidal antibodies against group W135 and Y meningococci in England in 2009. *Clin Vaccine Immunol*, **19**, 219–22.
3. Cherry JD, Chang SJ, Klein D, *et al.* (2004). Prevalence of antibody to *Bordetella pertussis* antigens in serum specimens obtained from 1793 adolescents and adults. *Clin Infect Dis*, **39**, 1715–18.
4. Hardelid P, Andrews NJ, Hoschler K, *et al.* (2010). Assessment of baseline age-specific antibody prevalence and incidence of infection to novel influenza A/H1N1 2009. *Health Technol Assess*, **14**, 115–92.
5. Caley M, Fowler T, Greatrex S, Wood A (2012). Differences in hepatitis B infection rate between ethnic groups in antenatal women in Birmingham, United Kingdom, May 2004 to December 2008. *Euro Surveill*, **17**, pii: 20228.
6. Vyse AJ, Gay NJ, Hesketh LM, Morgan-Capner P, Miller E (2004). Seroprevalence of antibody to varicella zoster virus in England and Wales in children and young adults. *Epidemiol Infect*, **132**, 1129–34.
7. Giraudon I, Forde J, Maguire H, Arnold J, Permalloo N (2009). Antenatal screening and prevalence of infection: surveillance in London, 2000-2007. *Euro Surveill*, **14**, 8–12.
8. McCann CM, Vyse AJ, Salmon RL, *et al.* (2008). Lack of serologic evidence of *Neospora caninum* in humans, England. *Emerg Infect Dis*, **14**, 978–80.
9. Levy-Bruhl D, Pebody R, Veldhuijzen I, Valenciano M, Osborne K (1998). ESEN: a comparison of vaccination programmes. Part one: diphtheria. *Euro Surveill*, **3**, 93–6.

10. Balmaseda A, Hammond SN, Tellez Y, *et al.* (2006). High seroprevalence of antibodies against dengue virus in a prospective study of schoolchildren in Managua, Nicaragua. *Trop Med Int Health*, **11**, 935–42.
11. Dowd JB, Palermo T, Brite J, McDade TW, Aiello A (2013). Seroprevalence of Epstein-Barr virus infection in U.S. children ages 6–19, 2003–2010. *PLoS One*, **8**, e64921.
12. Riedel DA, Evans AS, Saxinger C, Blattner WA (1989). A historical study of human T lymphotropic virus type I transmission in Barbados. *J Infect Dis*, **159**, 603–9.
13. ICF International (2012). *HIV prevalence estimates from the demographic and health surveys.* ICF International, Calverton, MD.
14. Hendriks JC, Medley GF, Heisterkamp SH, *et al.* (1992). Short-term predictions of HIV prevalence and AIDS incidence. *Epidemiol Infect*, **109**, 149–60.
15. Vyse AJ, Hesketh LM, Pebody RG (2009). The burden of infection with cytomegalovirus in England and Wales: how many women are infected in pregnancy? *Epidemiol Infect*, **137**, 526–33.
16. Hayward AC, Fragaszy EB, Bermingham A, *et al.* (2014). Comparative community burden and severity of seasonal and pandemic influenza: results of the Flu Watch cohort study. *Lancet Respir Med*, **2**, 445–54.
17. Davies JR, Grilli EA, Smith AJ (1984). Influenza A: infection and reinfection. *J Hyg (Lond)*, **92**, 125–7.
18. Vyse AJ, Gay NJ, White JM, *et al.* (2002). Evolution of surveillance of measles, mumps, and rubella in England and Wales: providing the platform for evidence-based vaccination policy. *Epidemiol Rev*, **24**, 125–36.
19. Plotkin SA (2010). Correlates of protection induced by vaccination. *Clin Vaccine Immunol*, **17**, 1055–65.
20. Aburizaiza AS, Mattes FM, Azhar EI, *et al.* (2014). Investigation of anti-middle East respiratory syndrome antibodies in blood donors and slaughterhouse workers in Jeddah and Makkah, Saudi Arabia, fall 2012. *J Infect Dis*, **209**, 243–6.

Chapter 12

Vaccine evaluation: efficacy and adverse events

Laura C. Rodrigues

Introduction to vaccine evaluation

Vaccines are powerful and often cost-effective preventive tools for controlling infectious diseases. Vaccines are most often administered to protect individuals against infection and disease; sometimes they are also effective for reducing infectiousness. In some situations, high population coverage of vaccines can sufficiently reduce transmission, such that even unvaccinated individuals are indirectly protected.

Before a vaccine is licensed for use, it must pass through a complex regulatory process that includes one or more Phase III RCTs to estimate its efficacy (see ➲ Chapter 5). After licensing and implementation in routine use, observational studies (see ➲ Chapter 4) can investigate additional aspects of efficacy, e.g. by time since vaccination, against different serotypes, or in different age groups.

As vaccine-preventable diseases become rarer, public concern may shift towards rare adverse events associated with vaccination. Because trials are designed to be large enough to measure efficacy, only relatively common and immediate adverse events will be detected during the regulatory process; adverse reactions that are rare or take longer to develop tend to be detected only after the vaccine is in routine use. Monitoring systems and observational studies are key to the swift and rigorous evaluation of suspected adverse events and essential to the maintenance of public confidence in vaccines.

This chapter presents the methodological issues concerning the evaluation of vaccine efficacy (VE) and of adverse events. Two notes about terminology:

- No vaccine offers complete protection, so it is useful to distinguish between 'vaccination' (the administration of an antigen) and 'immunization' (the induction of effective protective immunity).
- Trials are designed to measure the maximum protection, and the protection estimated in a trial is often higher than that in routine use; some authors reserve the term 'efficacy' for the protection measured in trials, and 'effectiveness' for that measured in routine programmes; this chapter uses the terms efficacy, effectiveness, and protection interchangeably.

Evaluation of vaccine efficacy

Direct protection

The direct protection of a vaccine is the protection given by the biological effect of a vaccine to a vaccinated individual.

Measurement of overall efficacy

VE is expressed as the percentage reduction in incidence of disease among vaccinated individuals that is attributable to vaccination. It can be estimated in randomized trials, cohort studies (including outbreak investigations and household or contact studies), case control studies, and case population studies (Box 12.1).

- In cohort studies and RCTs, which measure the incidence of the disease the vaccine aims to prevent, VE is estimated by comparing the incidence of disease in the vaccinated and unvaccinated groups.
- In case control studies, VE is estimated based on the relative risk (RR) of the disease in **vaccinated** individuals $_{(v)}$, compared with **unvaccinated** individuals $_{(u)}$: $RR_{v/u}$. In case control studies, RR (or its approximation for rare diseases in the form of the odds ratio, OR) is used, because the incidence of the disease in these studies is not normally known.
- Case population studies compare the proportion vaccinated among cases with the proportion vaccinated among the population (vaccine coverage). The population used must be the same as that from which the cases were drawn, i.e. of the same age and geographical location. Case population studies are also called 'rapid screening' studies, because they are a quick and simplified approach that does not control for confounding. If a case population study finds lower than expected efficacy, a more robust design must be used.

Box 12.1 Estimation of vaccine efficacy (VE) in randomized trials, cohort studies, case control studies, and case population studies

Randomized controlled trials and cohort studies

$$VE = (\text{incidence in unvaccinated} - \text{incidence in vaccinated} \times 100) / \text{incidence in unvaccinated}$$

Case control studies

$$VE = 1 - RR_{(v/u)} \times 100 \quad \text{or} \quad 1 - OR_{(v/u)} \times 100$$

Case population studies

$$VE = (PPV - PCV) / [(PPV(1 - PCV)]$$

OR, odds ratio; *PCV*, proportion of cases vaccinated; *PPV*, proportion of population vaccinated; $RR_{v/u}$, relative risk of vaccinated over unvaccinated.

Efficacy by different aspects of vaccine or against different outcomes

Protection given by a vaccine can vary, depending on the schedule (age at vaccination, number of doses, and interval between doses), time since vaccination, specific outcome (e.g. specific serotypes, severe cases, and site of disease), and situation (e.g. in different continents and with intensity of exposure by the target organism). Some variation will be identified during the licensing process; other variation will be determined in the routine setting using observational studies.

To estimate efficacy according to the number of doses, the interval between doses, and other characteristics, VE is estimated separately for each level of the characteristic of interest by comparing people vaccinated in that level with unvaccinated subjects. For example, a case control study that separately compared children who received two doses and children who received one dose of rotavirus vaccine with unvaccinated children found VE was 76% when children were given two doses of rotavirus vaccine and 65% with only one dose.[1]

To estimate VE against alternative outcomes (e.g. levels of severity, different serotypes, etc.), the usual analysis is performed separately for each outcome. In the same case control study of rotavirus vaccine, VE was 89% against rotavirus genotype G1P[8] and 75% against rotavirus genotype G2P4.[1]

To estimate VE in different settings, separate studies must be conducted in each setting. For example, studies conducted in outbreaks or household contacts will estimate efficacy in settings where exposure to infection is high.

Efficacy against non-specific outcomes

Sometimes it is too costly to use specific endpoints to evaluate VE (e.g. laboratory-confirmed pneumococcal pneumonia, rotavirus diarrhoea, and influenza), but it is possible to evaluate VE against a non-specific endpoint which serves as a sufficiently good surrogate for the outcome of interest (e.g. X-ray-confirmed pneumonia for pneumococcal pneumonia, hospitalized diarrhoea for rotavirus, or influenza-like illness (ILI) for influenza). In this case, the estimated VE is estimated by the observed protection against the non-specific outcome.

For example, in a trial of pneumococcal pneumonia vaccine in Gambia, VE against a first episode of X-ray-confirmed pneumonia was 37%.[2] This measure of VE against the less specific outcome may be of interest in itself from a policy perspective, as it is a measure of the impact of the vaccine on the burden of the non-specific outcome (in this case, indicating that the vaccine would reduce the frequency of the first episode of X-ray-confirmed pneumonia among vaccinated subjects by 37%).

The VE against non-specific outcomes is variable, as it depends on the proportion of the non-specific outcome caused by the specific organism, as well as on the efficacy against the specific outcome. In the example above, 37% protection against X-ray-confirmed pneumonia reflects both efficacy against pneumococcal pneumonia and the proportion of all pneumonias caused by pneumococci in that setting and age group.

It is possible to conduct a study of a non-specific event in a subsample to estimate the proportion caused by the specific organism in order to estimate VE against the specific event.[2]

Immunological correlates/surrogates of protection and bridging studies

As vaccines are agents that provide protection through immunological mechanisms, the specific immune response to vaccination that indicates protection for some vaccines is known. This specific immune response is called a surrogate of protection (when part of the chain of causation between vaccine and protection) and a correlate of protection (when a marker for, but not part of, that chain). Surrogates/correlates of protection are best established in the context of trials.

When an immunological correlate/surrogate of protection is known, the efficacy of a new vaccine can be established in immunological studies, with no need for field trials. For example, assuming that the correlate/surrogate is an antibody and that the antibody level corresponding to protection is known, VE can be estimated as the proportion of initially seronegative subjects who seroconverted after vaccination. In this situation, seroconversion studies can be conducted as bridging trials to compare a new vaccine/formulation/scheme with an older one for which efficacy is established in trials (see ➲ Chapter 11 for more details on sero-epidemiology).

Models of vaccine protection: all or nothing versus partial protection

The same value of VE can result from vaccine protection achieved in different ways. For example, imagine two vaccines—the first offers complete protection to half the vaccine recipients, leaving the other vaccinated individuals with no protection, while the second reduces the incidence of diseases in all vaccine recipients by half. In both cases, the estimated VE will be 50% (Figure 12.1). The first model has been called all-or-nothing protection—50% of vaccine recipients are totally protected, and the other 50% are 'vaccine failures', as susceptible to infection as if they had not been vaccinated. The second model, called partial or 'leaky' vaccination, gives some degree of protection to all vaccine recipients, so the incidence is reduced by 50%.

In the all-or-nothing model, a correlate of protection (if one is known) will identify vaccine recipients that were immunized from those in whom the vaccine failed. In the partial immunity or 'leaky' model, there is no correlate of complete protection, as no one has full protection.

The effect of most vaccines falls between these two extreme cases, with some vaccine recipients being fully protected, some vaccine failures, and some with partial—and possibly varying—degrees of protection. This is discussed in detail in the WHO publication *Correlates of vaccine-induced protection: methods and implications*.[3] These mechanisms of vaccine effect have different implications for the interpretation of estimates of VE with time since vaccination in settings where the disease is very common.[4]

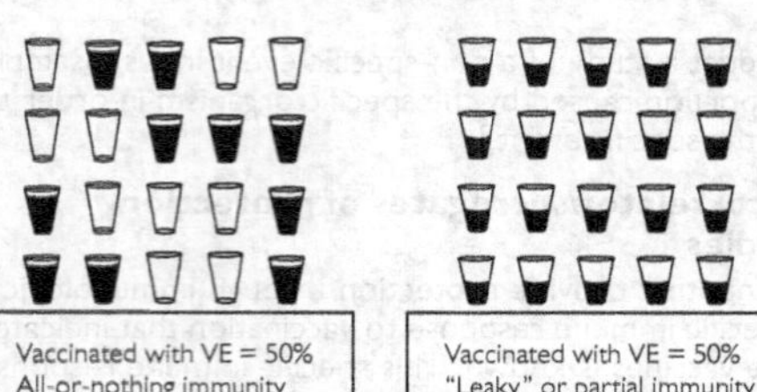

Figure 12.1 Two models of vaccine protection: all-or-nothing and partial (or leaky) immunity. All glasses represent vaccinated individuals; dark glasses represent fully protected individuals; empty glasses represent individuals who are not protected at all, and half-full glasses represent partially protected individuals. VE, vaccine efficacy.

Reproduced courtesy of Laura C. Rodrigues.

Efficacy against infectiousness (VE against disease and VE against infectiousness)

Subjects can be infected and infectious without developing disease, and vaccinated cases can be less or more infectious. The direct effect of a vaccine may not be limited to protecting individuals against infection or disease, as it may also reduce the infectiousness of vaccinated infected individuals. For example, a vaccinated case of pertussis may be less infectious than an unvaccinated case, and a vaccine that renders cases of malaria non-infectious could be developed.

The VE_s (where s stands for susceptibility to disease), which corresponds broadly to the standard measure of efficacy or the reduction in incidence of disease, can be differentiated from VE_i (where *i* stands for infectiousness), which corresponds to the reduction in infectiousness in vaccinated subjects, whether by a reduction in infectiousness per contact (e.g. reduced viral or bacterial load) or a reduction in the duration of the infectious period. The VE_t represents maximum protection in a situation in which a vaccine reduces both the infectiousness of the index case and the susceptibility of the contact. The household contact study is an efficient design for estimating efficacy against infectiousness by comparing the secondary attack rates (SARs) in household contacts of vaccinated and unvaccinated index cases (Box 12.2).

Protection against susceptibility and protection against infectiousness play symmetrical roles in reducing transmission; a vaccine with 90% efficacy against infectiousness and 0% against susceptibility has the same impact on transmission as a vaccine that is 0% effective against infectiousness and 90% against susceptibility. Both are measures of direct protection.

Indirect protection

In evaluating the effects of vaccination programmes, it is useful to differentiate between **direct and indirect protection**. Although direct protection results from the biological effect of the vaccine in individuals

Box 12.2 Estimating efficacy against infectiousness by comparing secondary attack rates (SARs) in household contacts of vaccinated and unvaccinated index cases

$$VE_s = 1 - (SAR_{u-v}) / SAR_{u-u})$$

$$VE_i = 1 - (SAR_{v-u}) / SAR_{u-u})$$

$$VE_t = 1 - (SAR_{v-v}) / SAR_{u-u})$$

$SAR_{u \to u}$, secondary attack rate in unvaccinated contacts of unvaccinated index cases; $SAR_{u \to v}$, secondary attack rate in vaccinated contacts of unvaccinated index cases; $SAR_{v \to u}$, secondary attack rate in unvaccinated contacts of unvaccinated index cases; $SAR_{v \to v}$, secondary attack rate in vaccinated contacts of vaccinated index cases; VE_i, vaccine efficacy against infectiousness; VE_s, vaccine efficacy susceptibility to disease; VE_t, vaccine efficacy of maximum protection.

who received the vaccine, irrespective of any population effects, indirect protection is the protection conferred on vaccinated and unvaccinated individuals by the removal of infectious cases.

An indirect effect is present only when transmission is person-to-person and the target age group for vaccination is responsible for transmission; the magnitude of the effect is variable and depends on the vaccine coverage. Two examples of vaccines that do not cause indirect protection are tetanus, because human tetanus cases do not contribute to transmission, and neonatal bacille Calmette–Guérin (BCG) vaccination, because transmission is mainly by adult cases of TB after neonatal BCG efficacy has waned.

The overall effect of a vaccine on transmission consists of the direct effect and the indirect effect.

Estimation of indirect protection

A trial design based on a combination of individual and group randomization has been proposed to help conceptualize when a trial is measuring direct, indirect, or both effects of vaccination. This is a trial design in which some clusters (e.g. villages or schools) are allocated randomly to one of three options (Figure 12.2):

- cluster in which all subjects are vaccinated
- cluster in which no one is vaccinated
- cluster with individual allocation (each person in the group is allocated to vaccine or no vaccine).

Assuming that members do not mix outside the cluster and that transmission is attributable to the age group vaccinated in the trial:

- direct protection is measured by comparing the incidence of infection in vaccinated and unvaccinated people in the cluster with individual allocation (as both receive indirect protection)

1. Allocation at individual level
compare incidence in vaccinated and unvaccinated subjects

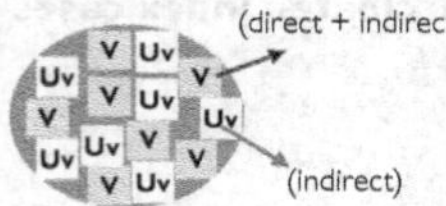

VE: direct effect

2. Allocation at group level
compare incidence in vaccinated and unvaccinated subjects

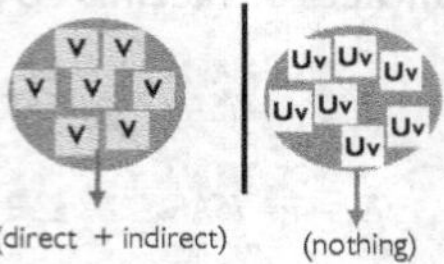

VE: (direct + indirect) effect

Compare incidence in unvaccinated subjects from individual and group level allocation

VE: indirect effect

Figure 12.2 Randomized trials with three allocation groups: (a) cluster in which all subjects are vaccinated, (b) cluster in which no subject is vaccinated, and (c) cluster in which individuals are allocated to vaccination or no vaccination. VE, vaccine efficacy.

Reproduced courtesy of Laura C. Rodrigues.

- indirect protection, which changes according to coverage,[5] is measured by comparing the incidence in unvaccinated individuals in the cluster who received no protection to that in unvaccinated subjects in the cluster with individual allocation (who receive indirect protection only)
- total (indirect plus direct) protection is measured by comparing the incidence in vaccinated and unvaccinated individuals in all the three clusters.

In a simplified application of this approach proposed for cluster randomized trials, the incidence of disease is examined in individuals in the cluster allocated to receive 100% coverage of the vaccination but who were not vaccinated because they refused to participate in the study or did not receive the allocated vaccine (Figure 12.3).[6]

Programme evaluation and demonstration trials

The impact of a vaccination programme is the total long-term effect of the programme on the transmission of infection and the morbidity and mortality attributable to the infection.

The impact of vaccination programmes may become clear only many years after the programme has been introduced for a number of reasons, including changes in the age distribution of susceptible individuals (e.g. pertussis and mumps); an increase in incidence after some time because of a build-up of susceptible individuals (e.g. measles); indirect effects may be stronger than expected, with disease prevented in age groups not directly targeted (e.g. *Haemophilus influenzae* type b (HiB)); protection may wane with time since vaccination (e.g. BCG and pertussis); and

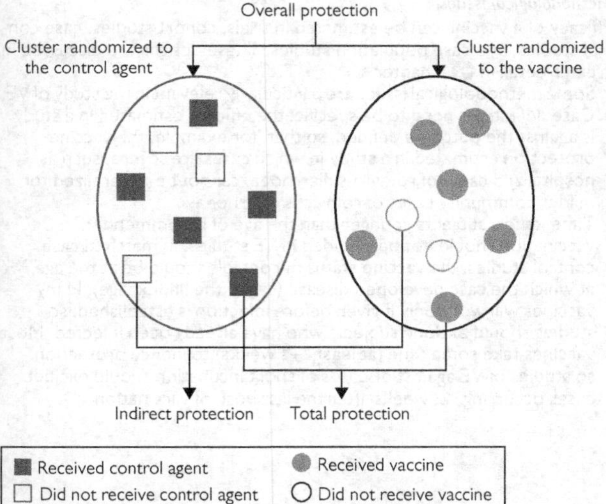

Figure 12.3 Measurement of vaccine-induced herd protective effects in a cluster-randomized vaccine trial. Two hypothetical clusters are shown, and individuals contrasted for measurement of overall, total, and indirect vaccine protection are identified.

complex effects may result from changes in the age distribution of cases (e.g. congenital rubella syndrome (CRS) and varicella-zoster infection). There is no 'formula' for the impact of a vaccine, although vaccine coverage and the direct and indirect effects of the vaccine are important components.

Demonstration trials

In settings where vaccines have been licensed, but not introduced, in routine practice, trials can be conducted not to estimate protection, but to demonstrate to policy-makers the short-term impact that introduction of the vaccine would have on the burden of disease. Demonstration trials often include a component of cost-effectiveness (see ➔ Chapter 17). Because the efficacy is well known, there is no equipoise as to the effect ('clinical equipoise'), so proposers of demonstration trials created the concept of 'public health equipoise'.

Methodological issues

Efficacy of a vaccine can be estimated in trials, cohort studies, case control studies, and case population studies. These designs are discussed in greater detail in ➲ Chapter 4.

Some methodological issues are particularly relevant in the study of VE:

- Case definitions need to be specific: the efficacy estimated in a study is against the outcome defined, so that, for example, the vaccine protection estimated in a study in which cases are severe, such as hospitalized cases of rotavirus diarrhoea, cannot be generalized to milder community cases of rotavirus diarrhoea.
- Time issues: subjects younger than the age of recommended vaccination should not be included in VE studies. In matched case control studies, the vaccine status of controls should be at the age at which the case developed disease (called the 'index' age). Many vaccines will work only if given before infection is established, so studies should exclude subjects who have already been infected. Most vaccines take some time (at least 1–2 weeks) to induce protection, so studies of VE against diseases of short incubation should exclude cases occurring <2 weeks after the last dose of vaccination.

Evaluation of vaccine safety

When high population coverage is achieved with a protective vaccine, the disease that the vaccine aims to prevent may become rare, and public concern shifts from the diseases to events caused, or feared to be caused, by the vaccine itself.

Adverse effects of vaccines that are relatively common and develop shortly after vaccination are usually detected during the licensing process. However, adverse effects may be missed for many reasons, including rarity, time lags between vaccination and the adverse event, and higher incidence in a subgroup not included in the trial.

Many vaccines are given to very young children at an age when developmental abnormalities are first noted. Non-causal temporal coincidence of vaccination and recognition of abnormalities can cause alarm and have dramatic effects on vaccination coverage. An example is the decline in measles vaccination caused by media coverage of a (now retracted and widely discredited) paper describing the association between the MMR vaccine and autism in the UK; coverage increased only when a study disproved the association.[7]

Maintaining public confidence in vaccines requires fast responses to suspected adverse events and appropriate epidemiological studies to investigate whether or not unexpected adverse effects of vaccination are occurring and with what frequency.

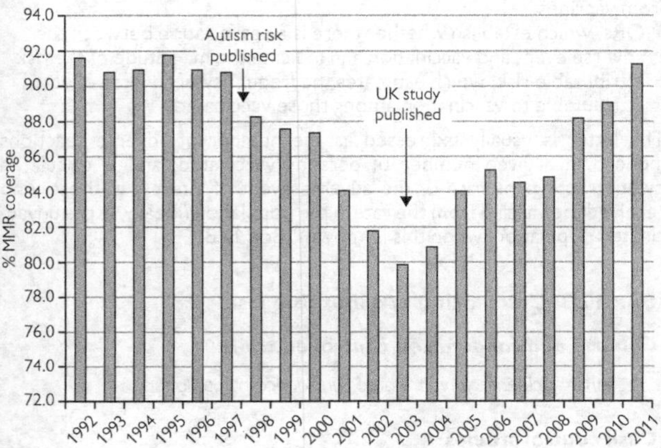

Figure 12.4 Measles, mumps, and rubella (MMR) vaccine coverage in United Kingdom (UK) by the time of the second birthday.

Reproduced from *NHS Immunisation Statistics England 2013–14*, Health and Social Care Information Centre, part of the Government Statistical Service, Copyright © 2014, Health and Social Care Information Centre with permission from Public Health England, available from http://www.hscic.gov.uk/catalogue/PUB14949/nhs-immu-stat-eng-2013-14-rep.pdf.

Monitoring and formulating hypothesis

Reporting systems of adverse events

To monitor the safety of vaccines and other medicines, notification systems are set up for health professionals, patients, and the public to report a suspicion that a vaccine or medicine caused a side effect. This includes the Yellow Card Scheme run by the Medicines and Healthcare products Regulatory Agency (MHRA) in the UK and the Vaccine Adverse Event Reporting System (VAERS) run by the CDC in the USA.

Data scanning

The availability of large amounts of electronic data, with linked individual records of vaccination and morbidity data (e.g. the Vaccine Safety Datalink Project in the USA), has both increased opportunities to identify rare adverse events and raised concerns that undisciplined scanning of the data may uncover spurious associations that may undermine public confidence.[8]

Investigation of suspected adverse events

Studies to establish whether a putative adverse event is linked to a vaccine estimate two measures (OR and attributable risk) and can be conducted using three types of observational studies (case control studies, cohort studies, and case series analyses), in addition to the trials used in the regulatory process.

Measurements

Two measurements are of interest in the investigation of adverse events from vaccines:

- ORs, which establish whether there is an association between the adverse event and vaccination and indicate the magnitude of the risk
- attributable risk, which estimates the frequency of adverse effects attributable to vaccination among those vaccinated.

The latter is usually expressed as the number of adverse reactions induced in a given number of persons vaccinated, and is calculated by subtracting the rate of the adverse event of interest in those who received the vaccine from the rate in the population (ideally, in the unvaccinated population, when this is known) (Box 12.3).

Box 12.3 Calculating attributable risk

Cohorts and randomized controlled trials

$$AR = \text{incidence in vaccinated} - \text{incidence in population}$$

Case control studies

$$AR = r(RR - 1) / (RR - p + 1)$$

AR, attributable risk; *p*, proportion of population vaccinated; *r*, rate of putative adverse event in total population; *RR*, relative risk of adverse event in vaccinated individuals, compared with unvaccinated individuals.

Study designs and methodological issues

Cohort studies, case control studies, and case series are used to investigate suspected adverse events. Cohort studies, case control studies, and self-controlled case series[9] are discussed in ➲ Chapter 4. Of particular relevance for adverse events are large electronic data sets that contain information on both vaccination and the putative adverse event, and all three study designs can be conducted using such data sets.

A particular aspect of the study of adverse events is that some are postulated to occur only during a limited time after vaccination (the 'risk' period). This has two implications.

- Firstly, adverse events in this situation can be evaluated, even in populations in which vaccine coverage approaches 100%, because, although most subjects are vaccinated, only a few would have the adverse event within the risk period after vaccination. A self-controlled case series (see ➲ Chapter 4) can be investigated if this number is higher than expected, establishing whether the putative event is an adverse event of that vaccine.
- Secondly, any observational study must explore the frequency of adverse events only over the risk period, otherwise the frequency of adverse events will be underestimated.

References

1. Ichihara MY, Rodrigues LC, Teles Santos CA, *et al.* (2014). Effectiveness of rotavirus vaccine against hospitalized rotavirus diarrhea: a case–control study. *Vaccine*, **32**, 2740–7.
2. Cutts FT, Zaman SM, Enwere G, *et al.* (1984). Efficacy of nine-valent pneumococcal conjugate vaccine against pneumonia and invasive pneumococcal disease in The Gambia: randomised, double-blind, placebo-controlled trial. *Lancet*, **365**, 1139–46.
3. World Health Organization (WHO) (2013). *Correlates of vaccine-induced protection: methods and implications*. WHO, Geneva. Available at: http://www.who.int/immunization/documents/WHO_IVB_13.01/en/ (accessed 28 January 2015).
4. Smith PG, Rodrigues LC, Fine PEM (1984). Assessment of the protective efficacy of vaccines against common diseases using case-control and cohort studies. *Int J Epidemiol*, **13**, 87–93.
5. Halloran ME, Longini IM Jr, Struchiner CJ (1999). Design and interpretation of vaccine field studies. *Epidemiol Rev*, **21**, 73–88.
6. Clemens J, Shin S, Ali M (2011). New approaches to the assessment of vaccine herd protection in clinical trials. *Lancet Infect Dis*, **11**, 482–7.
7. Smeeth L, Cook C, Fombonne E, *et al.* (2004). MMR vaccination and pervasive developmental disorders: a case-control study. *Lancet*, **364**, 963–9.
8. Chen RT, DeStefano F, Davis RL, *et al.* (2000). The Vaccine Safety Datalink: immunization research in the health maintenance organizations in the USA. *Bull World Health Organ*, **78**, 186–94.
9. Farrington P, Pugh S, Colville A (1995). A new method for active surveillance of adverse events from DPT and MMR vaccines. *Lancet*, **345**, 567–9.

Further reading

Farrington CP (2004). Control without separate controls: evaluation of vaccine safety using case-only methods. *Vaccine*, **22**(15–16), 2064–70.

Halloran ME, Longini IM Jr, Struchiner CJ (2009). *Design and analysis of vaccine studies*. Springer Verlag, New York.

Rodrigues LC, Smith PG (1999). Use of the case-control approach in vaccine evaluation: efficacy and adverse effects. *Epidemiological Rev*, **21**, 56–72.

Basic statistical methods

Laura F. White

Introduction to basic statistical methods

Statistics provide a set of tools to draw conclusions from information (data) such as is collected from epidemiological studies (see ➲ Chapter 4) and surveillance systems (see ➲ Chapter 2). Statistical methods quantify the uncertainty that is inherent in data due to sampling and randomness. This chapter discusses statistical approaches to describing disease transmission and severity.

Transmission

Understanding infectious diseases requires an understanding of transmission, including risk factors for, and intensity of, transmission. This chapter discusses methods to determine characteristics that are associated with transmission and tools to describe how fast a disease is being transmitted.

Associations with transmission events

Epidemiological studies, such as case control, cohort, and household contact studies, and data collected from other surveillance sources can be used to determine factors that are associated with the acquisition of illness. Typically, the outcome variable for these studies is a dichotomous variable that indicates illness or case control status, and characteristics of the environment, infectious individual(s), potential exposures, and/or susceptible individuals that might be associated with the outcome are considered. These simple comparisons can use basic statistical tests, as shown in Table 13.1 (for more detailed information, see ➔ Further reading, p. 190).

Logistic regression methods

In addition, the impact of multiple factors on the outcome of infection can be considered simultaneously. For example, initial analyses may show that age is associated with a food-borne illness at a particular event, but younger and older individuals tend to eat different types of foods, so it is possible that age is independently associated with illness and the main exposure. This phenomenon of alternative explanations, called confounding, can be controlled for in regression models, which all have the same basic form:

$$response = \beta_0 + \beta_1 X_1 + \beta_2 X_2 + \ldots + error$$

In this format, the linear relationship between potential correlates, X_i, and response is assessed while allowing for unexplained error due to sampling or unmeasured covariates. The β_i describes the nature of the assumed linear relationship between X_i and the response. In these models, the outcome is typically a dichotomous indicator of infection status,

Table 13.1 Basic statistical tests when the outcome is a dichotomous indicator of infection or case/control status

Risk factor	Example	Statistical test
Categorical, including dichotomous	• Vaccination status • Gender • Household size • Race/ethnicity	• Chi square
Continuous	• Age • CD4 count	• *t*-test • Wilcoxon test

so the response in the equation above needs to be modified to be linear. This involves logistic regression, which transforms the dichotomous outcome variable to a continuous response by using the log of the odds (called the logit):

$$\text{logit}(p) = \log(p/1-p) = \beta_0 + \beta_1 X_1 + \beta_2 X_2 + \ldots + \text{error}$$

where log(p) indicates the natural log.

The exponential of β_i can be interpreted as the OR. For example, with a single 0/1 covariate, the model is given by:

$$\text{logit}(p) = \log(p/1-p) = \beta_0 + \beta_1 X_1$$

Another way to write this is:

$$\text{logit}(p) = \log(p/1-p) = \beta_0 + \beta_1 \text{ if } X_1 = 1, \text{or } \beta_0 \text{ if } X_1 = 0$$

The OR is calculated as:

$$OR = (\text{odds when } X_1 = 1)/(\text{odds when } X_1 = 0)$$
$$= \exp\{\beta_0 + \beta_1\}/\exp\{\beta_0\} = \exp\{\beta_1\}$$

Correlated data

It is not uncommon for studies on transmission to use information from individuals who are related to, or who are correlated with, one another, which violates the basic assumption of independence of data used in regression modelling. Household contact studies, which gather data from members of the same household who are all exposed to an infectious household member (the index case) are a common example. They enable transmission to be examined by assuming that the household members who are eventually infected with the illness obtained it from the index case. Members of the same household have much in common, such as genetic information, behavioural habits, exposure to the same index case, etc. So in a household of five members, it would be inaccurate to assume that they are contributing five unique pieces of information; instead some overlap in the information they contribute to understanding transmission is likely. The impact of this is that the effective sample size, or the amount of information, is reduced. A household contact study with only 100 individuals might only be equivalent to 90 independent individuals. If the data are assumed to be independent, the standard error estimates will be too small, which will lead to potentially inaccurate inferences.

Two techniques are commonly used to account for correlated data: generalized estimating equations (GEEs) and random (or mixed) effects models. Random effects models estimate the individual or conditional effect, whereas GEE models estimate the population average effect. Other subtle differences exist between the two approaches, but both are widely used for correlated data. Vittinghoff *et al.* provide an excellent introduction and overview,[1] and Fitzmaurice *et al.* provide a comprehensive description of these models.[2] Numerous resources are available to fit these models in standard statistical software packages.

Estimation of the reproductive number

The basic reproductive number is the number of cases a particular infectious individual will lead to in the next link in the chain of transmission when the infection is introduced into a fully susceptible population (see ➔ Chapter 1). Several statistical approaches to estimate the (basic) reproductive number have been developed. Three of these approaches, discussed below, require information only on the epidemic curve, i.e. the number of new cases of disease each day (or over some other appropriate time period such as weeks). These methods make assumptions typical of mathematical models, including homogeneous mixing of individuals, no movement in or out of the population being studied, and complete observation of all of the cases. It should be noted that proposed modifications to the estimation methods discussed below relax each of these assumptions.

A very basic approach to estimating the basic reproductive number comes from work on branching process theory, which was originally developed to determine the probability of a family line going extinct. This approach requires data from the epidemic curve during the period of exponential growth to be grouped into 'generations'. In other words, the initial case(s) is the first observation (or generation), and the second generation is the number of cases infected by the initial case(s). The third generation is the number infected by those in the second generation. If M_i is the number of individuals in the ith generation and the generations used are only those during the period of exponential growth, the estimate of the basic reproductive number is:

$$R_0 = \sum M_i / \left(\sum M_{i-1}\right)$$

The data can be clumped crudely into generations using an estimate of the mean of the serial interval (the amount of time between the onset of symptoms in an infector and infectee pair). Outbreaks with a significantly long serial interval and little variation in its length, which allow the generations to be clearly observed, lend themselves well to this approach during the initial phase of the outbreak.

Wallinga and Teunis[3] provided an approach that requires an estimate of the serial interval. With this information and the complete epidemic curve, denoted as $N_t = \{N_1, N_2, \ldots, N_T\}$, where N_i is the number of new cases on day i out of T total days in the epidemic, they estimate the effective reproductive number on each day of the outbreak as:

$$R_t = \Sigma_i \, p_{ij}$$

Here, p_{ij} is the relative probability that case i has been infected by case j, which can be calculated using the estimate of the distribution of the serial interval. The average of the effective reproductive numbers during the initial period of the outbreak when the outbreak is growing exponentially provide an estimate of the basic reproductive number.

White and Pagano[4] provide another approach to estimating R_0 using data from the epidemic curve during the exponential growth phase of the outbreak to estimate the basic reproductive number R_0. If the serial interval is known, the estimate is:

$$\hat{R}_0 = \frac{\sum_{t=1}^{t^*} N_t}{\sum_{t=1}^{t^*} \sum_{j=1}^{\min(k,t)} q_j N_{t-j}}$$

where q_i is the probability of a serial interval of length i and t^* is the length of the exponential growth period of the outbreak. White and Pagano further explain how to estimate the serial interval if it is unknown and only data on the epidemic curve are available.[4]

The R package EpiEstim has been developed to implement these and other methods.

Interval estimation

In addition to factors associated with greater susceptibility to illness and the average number of secondary cases caused by infectious individuals, estimating the time between successive cases of disease is also of interest, including multiple types of intervals (see ➲ Chapter 1):

- Serial interval—the time between clinical disease in a primary and secondary case.
- Generation interval—the time between infection between a primary and secondary case.
- Incubation period—time between infection and onset of symptoms.
- Latent period: time between infection and infectiousness.

The serial interval has the advantage of being entirely observable, while the other intervals are more challenging to observe, as they require knowledge of the time of infection, which is seldom known.

An understanding of these intervals is critical to understanding the speed at which an outbreak will unfold. For example, the mean serial interval for influenza is estimated to be between 2 and 3 days, while the serial interval for SARS is approximately 8–10 days, which is one factor that made the SARS pandemic much easier to control and contain than an influenza pandemic. Clearly, there is potential for substantial variability in the individual values of these intervals, so it is often helpful to think of these intervals in terms of the distribution of the values that they can attain, rather than a single numeric estimate of the mean.

Estimation of these intervals is not straightforward. For example, to estimate the serial interval might involve following individuals in households with a single infected index case and observing serial intervals as household members become ill. It might be tempting to assume that the best estimate of the serial interval is the mean of these observed intervals, but an estimate of the standard deviation (SD) of these data would give a sense of the variability of the serial interval. However, this approach fails to estimate the potential variation in serial intervals and omits consideration of some important issues in the observed data.

The distribution of the interval to be estimated can be described in a more general way by expressing the interval through a parametric distribution such as a lognormal, gamma, or Weibull distribution. These distributions are described by two parameters and only assume positive values. They tend to be skewed, which is similar to observed intervals. Estimates of the parametric distribution can be obtained by using a method of moments approach, in which the mean and SD of the observed intervals are set equal to the estimates of the mean and SD in terms of the parameters that describe them. For example, the lognormal distribution is characterized by the parameters μ and σ, with the mean given by:

$$exp\{\mu + \sigma^2 / 2\}$$

and the variance given by:

$$\left(exp\left\{\sigma^2\right\}-1\right)exp\left\{2\mu+\sigma^2\right\}$$

Setting the mean and variance in the observed data equal to these quantities means that estimates of parameters μ and σ can be obtained and the serial interval distribution can be described by a lognormal distribution with the estimated parameters. Figure 13.1 shows actual serial interval data from the 2009 H1N1 influenza pandemic, overlaid by estimates for three parametric distributions using this approach.

However, this estimator overlooks three important considerations. Firstly, observations of the serial interval are often discrete, rather than continuous, estimating these intervals in days, rather than some more precise time measure. This is often the best we can do, as we do not know the instant when an individual becomes ill or infected. The parametric distributions described are continuous, so some adjustments must be made to the estimation approach to avoid bias in the estimated interval. One such approach for estimation of the serial interval during the SARS outbreak of 2003 is described by Donnelly *et al.*[5]

Secondly, infected individuals in household contact studies are typically enrolled after they have been sick for some time. This means that

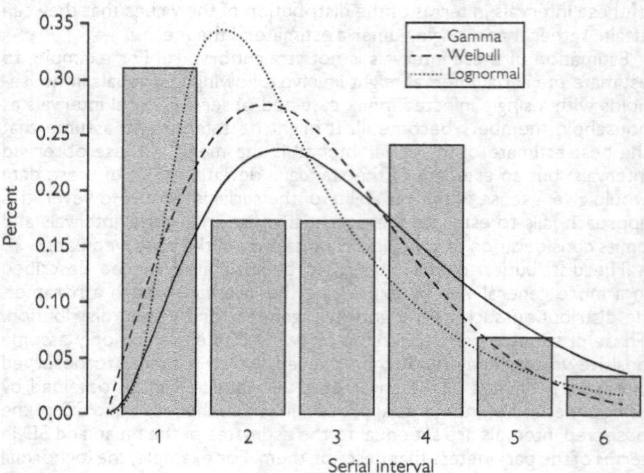

Figure 13.1 Serial interval data from the 2009 H1N1 influenza pandemic overlaid with estimates for three parametric distributions.

Source: data from Archer BN *et al.*, Reproductive number and serial interval of the first wave of influenza A(H1N1)pdm09 virus in South Africa, *PLoS One*, Volume 7, Issue 11, e49482.

all observed intervals have a lower bound—an issue called truncation. Estimations of the parametric distribution can adjust for truncation using an approach described by Cowling *et al.*[6]

Finally, the time that a household contact has a positive test for disease is often used as the point of illness onset; however, infection and symptom onset occur prior to the positive test. In general, this leads to censoring where the onset of disease cannot be estimated accurately. Methods for handling censored observations can also be incorporated into the estimation procedure.[6]

Estimates of severity

Often we wish to estimate the severity of a particular outbreak and/or pathogen through the case fatality ratio (or rate) (CFR) and attack rate (AR). The basic formulae for these are relatively simple and, in theory, should be easy to implement (Table 13.2).

In a small-scale outbreak where the entire exposed population and all the cases and their eventual outcomes can be determined, these are very simple calculations. For instance, the AR of a food-borne outbreak at a one-time event with a complete listing of all participants could be assessed by considering the number diseased divided by the total number of who ate food and likely were exposed. This quantity can further subdivided to get ARs for each type of food consumed. The CFR can be estimated by considering the number who died divided by the total number diseased. Assuming there is not an overwhelming number of individuals to interview and track, this is feasible.

Symptomatic case fatality ratio

In many cases, the number of individuals who are exposed to the pathogen and the number infected are not known, so it is quite common for these numbers to be much more challenging to calculate. Furthermore, fatalities may be missed due to incorrect ascertainment of the cause of death. A common example of this arises from influenza, as many individuals who are infected with influenza never seek care and thus are not recorded. Mortality is often recorded as some other cause, most commonly pneumonia. This leads to uncertainty in both the numerator and denominator of both quantities.

One proposed approach to this problem is to estimate the symptomatic CFR (sCFR). As the name implies, this only considers individuals who actually have symptoms, excluding asymptomatic individuals from the calculation. Estimation of the quantity is based on the use of a pyramid that describes how data might appear. Figure 13.2 shows an example of this type of pyramid; variations specific to the reporting and progression of a particular disease can be created. If the probability of progression to state j from state i is denoted as $P(j/i)$, the sCFR can be calculated as $sCFR = P(\text{D/H}) \times P(\text{H/M}) \times P(\text{M/S})$.[7] The challenge comes in obtaining estimates of these probabilities. Typically, practitioners use

Table 13.2 Basic estimates of severity

Statistic	Estimator
AR	(number diseased/number exposed)
CFR	(number dead/number diseased)
sCFR	(number symptomatic who die/number infected and diseased)

AR, attack rate; CFR, case fatality ratio; sCFR, symptomatic case fatality ratio.

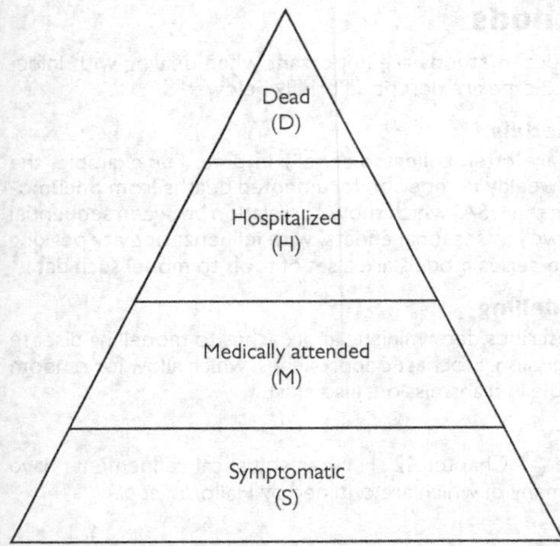

Figure 13.2 Pyramid illustrating the distribution of symptomatic, medically attended, hospitalized, and dead patients.

information from surveillance systems to estimate these parameters. For example, in the H1N1 pandemic of 2009, Presanis *et al.*[8] used disparate pieces of information collected from New York and Milwaukee, data from telephone surveys, and case reports in a complex Bayesian algorithm to infer the probabilities in the pyramid and ultimately estimate the sCFR.

Other methods

Many more statistical methods are important when dealing with infectious disease data. Some are described briefly below.

Time-series models

Surveillance data are often collected serially in time. For example, the CDC gathers the weekly number of documented deaths from pneumonia and influenza in the USA, which show correlation between sequential values in time, as well as seasonal effects, with influenza activity peaking every winter. Time-series models are a set of tools to model such data.[9]

Stochastic modelling

➲ Chapter 16 describes deterministic approaches to modelling disease spread and transmission. Stochastic approaches, which allow for random chance to play a role in transmission, also exist.[10]

Vaccine efficacy

VE is discussed in ➲ Chapter 12. Further statistical refinements have been developed, many of which are outlined by Halloran *et al.*[11]

References

1. Vittinghoff E, Glidden DV, Shioboski SC, McCulloch CE (2012). *Regression methods in biostatistics: linear, logistic, survival, and repeated measures models*, 2nd edn. Springer, New York.
2. Fitzmaurice GM, Laird NM, Ware JH (2011). *Applied longitudinal analysis*, 2nd edn. Wiley, Hoboken.
3. Wallinga J, Teunis P (2004). Differential epidemic curves for severe acute respiratory syndrome reveal similar impacts of control measures. *Am J Epidemiol*, **160**, 509–16.
4. White LF, Pagano M (2008). A likelihood based methods for real-time estimation of the serial interval and reproductive number of an epidemic. *Stat Med*, **27**, 2999–3016.
5. Donnelly CA, Finelli L, Cauchemez S, *et al.* (2011). Serial intervals and the temporal distribution of secondary infections within households of 2009 pandemic influenza A (H1N1): implications for influenza control recommendations. *Clin Infect Dis*, **52**(Suppl 1), S123–30.
6. Cowling BJ, Fang VJ, Riley S, Malik Peiris JS, Leung GM (2009). Estimation of the serial interval of influenza. *Epidemiology*, **20**, 344–7.
7. Pelat C, Ferguson NM, White PJ, *et al.* (2014). Optimizing the precision of case fatality ratio estimates under the surveillance pyramid approach, *Am J Epidemiol*, **180**, 1036–46.
8. Presanis AM, De Angelis D, New York City Swine Flu Investigation Team, *et al.* (2009). The severity of pandemic H1N1 influenza in the United States, from April to July 2009: a Bayesian analysis. *PloS Med*, **6**, e1000207.
9. Brockwell PJ, Davis RA (2010). *Introduction to times series and forecasting*, 2nd edn. Springer, New York.
10. Becker NG (1989). *Analysis of infectious disease data*. Chapman & Hall/CRC Press, Boca Raton.
11. Halloran ME, Longini IM, Struchiner CJ (2009). *Design and analysis of vaccine studies*. Springer, New York.

Further reading

Pagano M, Gauvreau K (2000). *Principles of biostatistics*, 2nd edn. Duxbury Press, Pacific Grove.

Spatial epidemiology

Tom A. Yates, Alexandre Blake, and Frank Tanser

Introduction to spatial epidemiology

Health protection practitioners have long used informal observations about the spatial patterning of diseases to inform their work. Spatial data are often used in a purely descriptive way that can inform resource allocation and generate hypotheses. However, rigorous spatial and spatio-temporal methods are now increasingly being used.

The location of a susceptible person in relation to sources of infection, such as infectious cases, is an important determinant of transmission for most pathogens. Recent developments in statistics and computing have allowed sophisticated analyses of such spatial phenomena and will increasingly contribute to our understanding of infectious disease epidemiology and control.

This chapter aims to introduce key concepts in spatial epidemiology and to point readers towards sources of more detailed information.

Spatial data

Types of spatial data

Point pattern data

The geographical positions of events in a defined region are a spatial point pattern. Such data are often used to represent the locations of cases and non-cases of a given disease.

Areal data

When attributes—non-spatial characteristics associated with locations—are assigned to areas, not points, this is termed areal data. Examples of areal units include local municipalities and clinic catchment areas.

Vector and raster data

Spatial data can be encoded and represented in two primary ways:

- In vector-based systems, each component has a precise location; components (Figure 14.1) can include:
  - points, e.g. homes of cases and controls (spatial point pattern data)
  - lines, e.g. rivers or roads
  - polygons, e.g. administrative areas.
- In raster-based systems, space is divided into a regular grid of cells. Attributes, such as average rainfall or whether there have been cases of a certain disease in that grid square, are then assigned to each cell. Raster-based systems are commonly used to represent environmental measurements.

Coordinate systems

Because the Earth is spherical, mapping locations on a flat surface requires subtle modifications, and various coordinate systems exist. World Geodesic System 1984 (WGS84) is standard for global positioning systems (GPS). Different coordinate systems may be better adapted for particular locations or analyses.

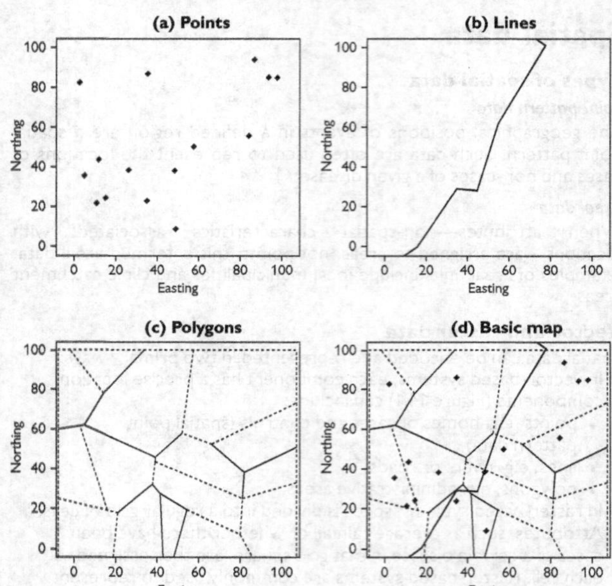

Figure 14.1 Independent display of points (a), lines (b), and polygons (c). The three vector datasets (a–c) are combined to create a basic map (d).

Visual display of spatial data

Point maps are a simple means of visualizing point data that avoid many of the pitfalls associated with more complex approaches. However, it is important to consider the need to protect confidentiality. Furthermore, when point data are crowded, interpretation is difficult.

Kernel density smoothing (a moving window method; see ➔ Characterizing first-order effects, p. 201) is a solution to these problems.

On choropleth maps, areas are given colours according to an aggregate measure, such as risk or rate. They are commonly used when only areal data are available or to protect confidentiality. There are many drawbacks to this approach:

- Large areas may dominate visually, even if they have few observations.
- The appearance can vary significantly if the observations are aggregated differently, i.e. with different placement of boundaries.
- Choices regarding cut-points (e.g. quantiles versus even steps) and colours will emphasize certain aspects of the data.
- Uncertainty, variance, and the distribution of the data within areas are not apparent.

The solutions to some of these issues are the same as those for the modifiable areal unit problem (see ➔ Modifiable areal unit problem, p. 206). Other solutions include the use of cartograms,[1] in which areas are scaled according to the data they contribute, e.g. according to population. However, scale and proportion are lost. More complex methods are also available.[2]

Concepts in spatial epidemiology

Spatial autocorrelation

Spatial data tend to be autocorrelated. This means that observed attributes that are closer to one another in space, such as the wealth of households, tend to be more similar than more distant pairs of observations. Spatial autocorrelation is also known as spatial dependency.

Many statistical techniques assume that observations are independent. Using such methods to analyse data showing spatial autocorrelation can result in optimistic claims about precision.

Albeit rarer, negative autocorrelation, in which closer observations are more likely to be different, also exists. This can occur, for example, when there is local competition for resources.

First-order effects describe overall trends, whereas second-order effects are local effects caused by spatial autocorrelation.

Complete spatial randomness

In spatial analysis, the null hypothesis is often that the observed distribution could have occurred if events were randomly positioned. This is called complete spatial randomness (CSR).

Poisson processes are used to represent CSR. Poisson processes can be homogeneous or inhomogeneous. Both assume events are independent, but inhomogeneous Poisson processes (IPP) allow for a non-constant distribution and are usually more realistic given, for example, varying population densities.

Second-order effects can be classified as attraction, which means clustering, and inhibition, which means regularity. Their presence means that CSR is absent.

With CSR, clusters of events or a degree of regularity may be observed by chance. The key difference in the presence of second-order effects is that the locations of points are influenced by the proximity of others, increasing or decreasing the likelihood of neighbouring events. Such patterns are shown in Figure 14.3.

Ecological and atomistic fallacies

In many low-income countries, urban areas, which tend to be more affluent than rural areas, have higher rates of tuberculosis (TB). However, within urban areas, poor people have higher rates of TB. This demonstrates that associations observed at one level of aggregation do not necessarily hold true at a different level. This can present a problem in spatial analyses if, for example, conclusions at an individual level are required but only areal data are available.

This is an example of the ecological fallacy, which is described in ➲ Chapter 4. The atomistic fallacy—erroneously assuming that a correlation will be observed in aggregated data because it is observed at an individual level—can also present problems in spatial analysis.

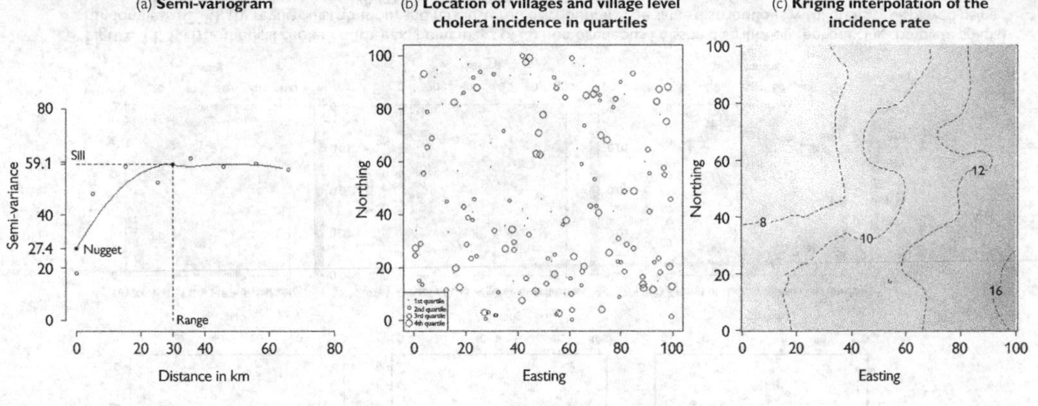

Figure 14.2 Hypothetical cholera outbreak: incidence rates by village, displayed in a semi-variogram (a), described using a quartile distribution on a point map (b), and mapped using ordinary kriging interpolation based on the semi-variogram (c).

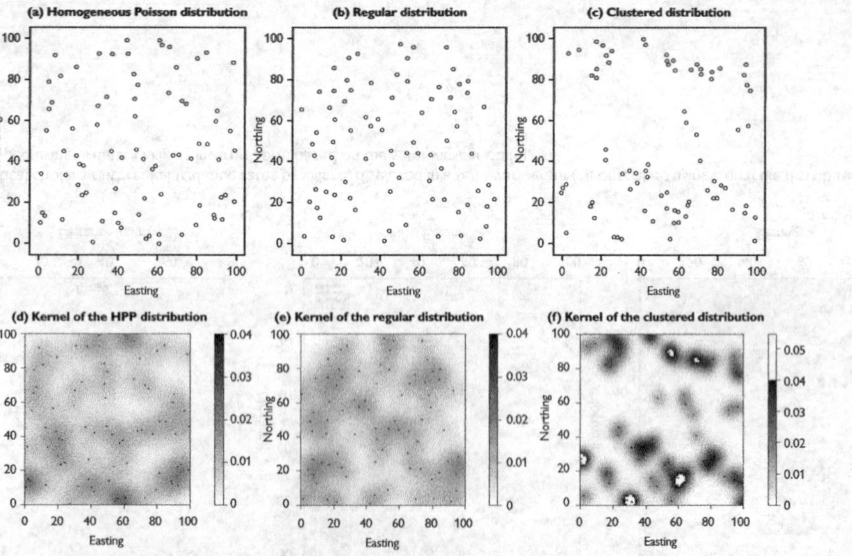

Figure 14.3 Hypothetical cholera outbreak: point maps of (a) homogeneous Poisson distribution reproducing complete spatial randomness (CSR), (b) regular distribution, and (c) clustered distribution. The same distributions with intensity displayed using kernel density smoothing (d), (e), and (f). The scale would be number of events per unit of area.

'Hot spots' and heterogeneity

Spatial heterogeneity is important in the epidemiology of many infectious diseases. For example, 'hot spots' of high-intensity transmission of malaria are thought to drive incidence in surrounding areas.[3] As such, spatial epidemiology is likely to play an increasing role informing disease control programmes for multiple pathogens.[4]

Techniques in spatial analysis

This section describes a number of core techniques used in spatial analysis.

Point pattern data

Semi-variograms

A key question in most spatial analyses is the extent to which observations that are in close proximity to each other are more similar than observations further apart. Semi-variograms (Figure 14.2a) plot the distance between pairs of observations against half of the variance of the differences between those measurements. They allow assessment of how variance differs with distance. This relationship can then be used to inform interpolation (see ➔ Interpolation). Semi-variograms assume stationarity and isotropy, although they can be adapted to release those assumptions.

Stationarity means that key statistical properties are not dependent on their exact location, i.e. the expected value and pattern of variance are the same across the area under study, and the correlation between two points depends on their relative locations.

Isotropy means that the correlation between two locations depends only on the distance between them (rather than their relative orientations).

Nugget, range, and sill are key characteristics of semi-variograms (Figure 14.2a). The nugget is the semi-variance for a null relative distance and often reflects measurement error. The range is the point at which the curve flattens out; it represents the relative distance beyond which there is no autocorrelation. The sill is the semi-variance at that point.

Interpolation

When spatial data are incomplete, interpolation techniques can be used to estimate missing values using adjacent observed data. Such techniques include inverse distance weighting and kriging. Kriging is an interpolation method that uses the semi-variogram model to provide an estimate of the uncertainty of predictions assuming that the pattern of variation is the same across the spatial surface.

Figure 14.2 shows a semi-variogram (a) and an associated point pattern (b); the increase in semi-variance with distance suggests spatial autocorrelation. Also shown is a map produced by kriging from the same data (c).

A hypothetical cholera outbreak in West Africa is used through the rest of this chapter to illustrate some of the statistical approaches described. This example assumes that data, including location, were collected on cholera cases and a representative sample of controls. Were data on the incidence of cholera available for some, but not all, villages, interpolation could be used to suggest which villages to prioritize for active case-finding.

Characterizing first-order effects

In the hypothetical cholera outbreak, the first step is to describe the spatial distribution. First-order effects are commonly described using kernel density estimation. They can also be described by noting the number of events in a set of quadrats. Both describe spatial variation in intensity.

Intensity is the term used in spatial epidemiology for density, i.e. the number of cases of a disease per square metre or kilometre.

Quadrats are areas—most often, rectangular—of identical size.

Kernel intensity smoothing methods produce continuous raster surfaces known as 'isopleth maps' from point pattern data. Kernel smoothing is a common way to display first-order effects (Figure 14.3d–f). Kernel intensity smoothing methods require the user to choose a probability distribution (e.g. normal or gamma) and a bandwidth—the scale over which smoothing occurs. If the bandwidth is too big, important variation is lost; if it is too small, patterns cannot be seen over the noise. The choice of probability distribution typically has less impact on the resulting estimates than the choice of bandwidth.

Characterizing second-order effects

Measuring autocorrelation

In the hypothetical cholera outbreak, identifying clustering of cases might indicate a local source, such as an infected well. Particular insight can be gained by observing the type of spatial clustering and the distribution of cases. The point maps in Figure 14.3 show a spatially random distribution (a), a clustered distribution (b), and a regular distribution (c). We might see (b) for the cases and (a) for the controls—we would not expect to see (c).

Sometimes, it can be difficult to differentiate between first-order effects and clustering, as aggregation of cases can occur as a result of higher population density. Ripley's K function, for example, counts the number of events at a given distance to any event. Information on the distance of aggregation gives insights on the predominant transmission route. Short distances might indicate person-to-person transmission. Comparing K functions between cases and controls is a way to check for false-positive 'clustering' induced by variation in population density.

Locating clusters

Stating a trend towards clustering is informative, but clusters must be located to enable intervention. This can be done using Kernel ratios[5] or spatial scanning statistics, as shown in Figure 14.4.

Areas with higher rates of disease can be detected by calculating odds or risk ratios (OR or RR). These compare the number of cases and non-cases within kernels of a common bandwidth. Relabelling tests, which are also used in spatial scanning statistics, allow p values to be calculated and then mapped by generating a large set of alternative spatial data sets. In these data sets, the locations remain the same, but the positions of the cases and controls are randomly reassigned. Statistical significance can then be calculated from the proportion of the alternative data sets in which the same effect or a more extreme effect is observed.

In Figure 14.4b, kernel ratio estimation detects three large zones with a high OR in the north-western corner, a band in the north extending towards the north-east, and a curved band in the central part of the map. However, there is little statistical evidence that this aggregation is more than would be expected by chance.

Spatial scan statistics can test for the presence of higher or lower numbers of events relative to expectation across space. Some can test for clustering across both space and time. These are another way to precisely identify areas with too many cases, given the number of controls. Kulldorf spatial scanning statistics[6] can be implemented in the freely available software SaTScan. A limitation of this tool is that it can only test for circular or elliptical clusters. As presented in Figure 14.4c and d, SaTScan detects potential clusters; however, there is still little evidence that these are not due to chance (i.e. p values are >0.05).

Modelling

The analyses presented so far only took location into account. A multivariable analysis that adjusts for known risk factors—classic and spatial—could be performed using a generalized additive model (GAM)[7] or other regression techniques.

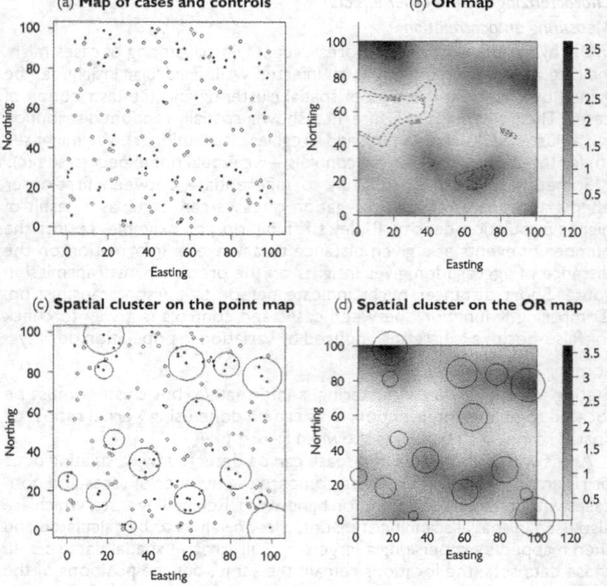

Figure 14.4 Hypothetical cholera outbreak: point maps showing cases and controls (a and c) with the corresponding odds ratio (OR) maps (b and d). Overlaid on top, a p value map derived using kernel ratios (b) and clusters identified using a Kulldorff spatial scanning statistic implemented in SaTScan (c and d).

Areal data

Characterizing first-order effects

Areal data—in the hypothetical example, data on cholera cases by clinic catchment area—can help identify areas more at risk or with a heavier burden of disease. Choropleth maps of the standardized morbidity ratio (SMR) are often used for this purpose (Figure 14.5).

Characterizing second-order effects

Spatial autocorrelation can also be seen in areal data, with neighbouring areas more or less similar than might be expected by chance.

The Global Moran's I tool can test for spatial dependence but requires the user to define a set of neighbours for each area. This can be based on contiguity or distance, depending on the hypothesis. Assumptions should be based on knowledge about the location and of the biology of the condition being studied.

The way in which neighbours are defined can have an impact on estimates of the SMR. For the cholera example, Figure 14.5 shows SMRs calculated using a Poisson gamma model then using a local Bayes'

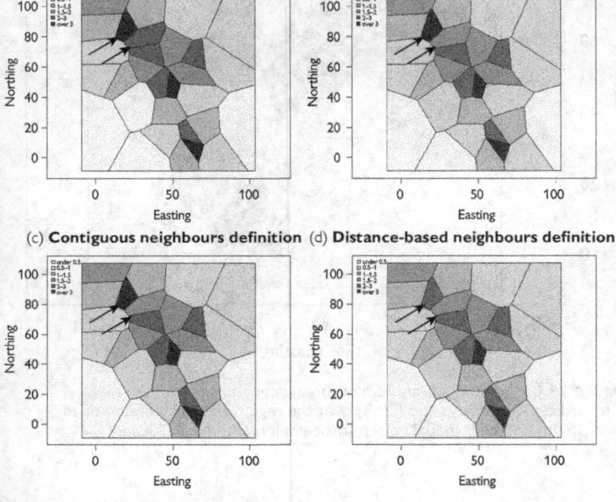

Figure 14.5 Hypothetical cholera outbreak: choropleths calculated with four different approaches: the raw standardized morbidity ratio (SMR) over the region (a), estimates using a Poisson gamma model (b), and estimates using a local empirical Bayes' estimator with two different neighbour definitions (c) and (d). Arrows indicate areas that are recategorized when different definitions are used.

estimator, with two different definitions of neighbour. Choosing different techniques or definitions of neighbours affects which SMR category two administrative areas are assigned.

It is possible to look for clustering in areal data. The spatial scan statistic approach can be applied using polygon centroids, producing good evidence for two clusters (Figure 14.6) (p<0.001). The local Moran's I test can also be used for this purpose.[8]

Modelling

Adjustment for covariates can be made using, for example, Poisson gamma models, Poisson generalized linear models, and simultaneous or conditional autoregressive models. More detailed information is available elsewhere[9] (Box 14.1).

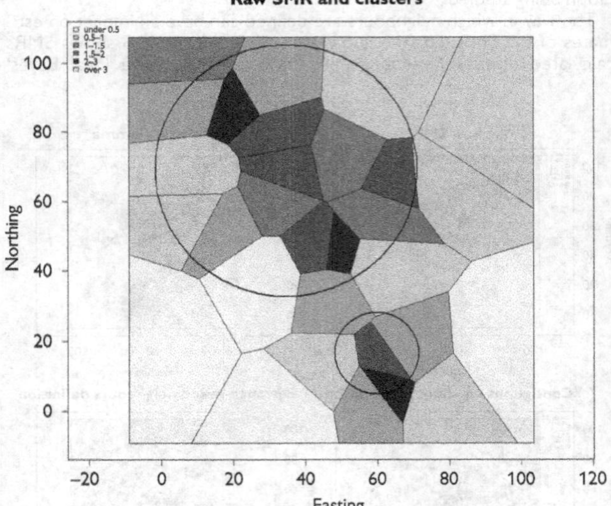

Figure 14.6 Hypothetical cholera outbreak: choropleth with the raw standardized morbidity ratio (SMR) over the region and clusters identified through the Kulldorff spatial scan statistic implemented in SaTScan.

Box 14.1 Criticisms of spatial epidemiology

Rothman[10] has prominently criticized the practice of investigating spatial clustering of disease, noting that:

- such investigations rarely lead to the discovery of previously unknown causes of disease
- the underlying population is often defined in relation to the existing cases—a phenomenon termed the 'Texas sharpshooter' procedure (in which the target is drawn once the shots have been fired!)
- publicity generated by the cluster can introduce substantial bias, particularly when interviews or questionnaires are used in the cluster investigation.

Rothman argues that location is simply another attribute, such as sex or age, and that simply noting an increase in occurrence of a disease in a certain location is rarely useful. He contends that investigation of disease clusters is likely to be most informative when cases are well defined and either the study is large or the cases within identified clusters have occurred at a rate substantially above the background rate. It is important that data on putative exposures are collected rigorously.

Source: data from Rothman KJ, A sobering start for the cluster busters' conference, *American Journal of Epidemiology*, Volume 132, Supplement 1, pp. 6–13, Copyright © 1990.

Practical problems in spatial analysis

Sampling bias

In both spatial and non-spatial epidemiology, sampling bias can affect results. For example, mapping that passively detected cases of a disease may result in a map illustrating spatial variation in access to healthcare, rather than the true distribution of disease.

Modifiable areal unit problem

Spatial data are often aggregated into areal units, such as a census tract, for logistical reasons or to preserve anonymity. Choices made about boundary placement are usually somewhat arbitrary, and different results can be often obtained when different choices are made. Avoiding such aggregation is recommended. Where unavoidable, the smallest units feasible should be chosen and, ideally, sensitivity analyses should be conducted to explore the impact of alternative boundary placements.

Scale

Ideally, measurements would be taken at a fine scale over a vast area, but this is not usually possible. Choices ideally should be informed by an understanding of the distribution of risk factors, the biology of the disease, and the extent of transmission networks.

Choosing a fine scale may result in important patterns being missed if transmission networks are large or there is insufficient variation in potential exposures of interest across the study area. Fine spatial heterogeneity may be missed if too coarse a scale is chosen.

Locating individuals in time and space

When studying the spatial epidemiology of infectious disease, choices regarding the location of individuals are critical. For example, if transmission is occurring in the workplace, analyses locating individuals to their homes will miss important patterns. In diseases with long latent periods, it may be appropriate to locate individuals to previous locations.

Emerging disciplines, such as the study of mobile phone records, and the rapidly falling costs of GPS tracking devices will allow more sophisticated spatial analyses. It may be possible to move beyond point locations to look at people's spatial networks or 'dynamic contexts'.

Edge effects and non-uniformity

Space is inherently heterogeneous. The distributions of cases of disease and the underlying population are therefore unlikely to be uniform. People living on the edge of a lake—like people living on the edge of a study area—will not have neighbours on every side.

These so-called 'edge effects' cause problems for many spatial analytical techniques, and statistical techniques exist for dealing with them in some situations. Sometimes these issues can be avoided by collecting data in marginal zones but only using these data to inform estimates in adjacent areas, leaving them out of the main analysis.

Table 14.1 Spatial statistics toolbox

Tool	Type of data	Type of presentation	Outcomes
Descriptive purpose/mapping	Point	Point map	AR
	Areal	Choropleth	SMR, assuming neighbouring effect or not or using various models (Poisson, Poisson gamma, etc.)
Interpolation	Point	Semi-variogram Kriging	Deaggregation and reaggregation techniques Multivariate areal interpolation techniques
First-order effect	Point	Intensity estimates	Kernel smoothing Parametric estimates
	Areal	Choropleth	AR SMR, assuming neighbouring effect or not
Second-order effect	Point	Trend for general clustering/ regularity	K function Difference of K function G function
		Local clustering	Kernel ratio Kulldorff spatial scan statistic SpODT
	Areal	Research of autocorrelation	Moran's I
		Clustering	SaTScan Local Moran's I
Modelling	Point		GAM Logistic regression with distance decaying function
	Areal		Poisson gamma, Poisson generalized linear model SAR CAR

AR, autoregressive; CAR, conditional autoregressive, GAM, generalized additive model; SAR, simultaneous autoregressive; SpODT, spatial oblique decision tree.

Tools and resources

Table 14.1 summarizes the key tools available for spatial statistics.

Global positioning system devices

Inexpensive GPS devices are widely available and can measure location to within 10 metres.

Sources of spatial data

Truly analytical spatial epidemiology, which requires spatial data on risk factors and outcomes, is likely to be used more often, as large geo-located data sets become increasingly available. Many are now freely available online; good sources include:

- DIVA-GIS, which maintains a list of freely available spatial data
- OpenStreetMap
- http://www.gis4biologists.info, which maintains a list of cheap or free sources of satellite images
- Gridded Population of the World (GPW) project, which provides raster data on population density
- WorldClim and the National Center for Atmospheric Research Climate Data Guide, which provide data on climate.

Software

A number of proprietary packages combine mapping and analytical capabilities. ArcGIS is used widely, but powerful open-source software offers similar functionality, including QGIS and a growing number of R packages. Free stand-alone packages to calculate spatial scanning statistics include SaTScan and FleXScan.

References

1. Worldmapper. Available at: http://www.worldmapper.org (accessed 30 January 2015).
2. Openshaw S (1983). *The modifiable areal unit problem*. Geo Books, Norwich.
3. Bousema T, Griffin JT, Sauerwein RW, *et al.* (2012). Hitting hotspots: spatial targeting of malaria for control and elimination. *PLoS Med*, **9**, e1001165.
4. Woolhouse ME, Dye C, Etard JF, *et al.* (1997). Heterogeneities in the transmission of infectious agents: implications for the design of control programs. *Proc Natl Acad Sci U S A*, **94**, 338–42.
5. Kelsall JE, Diggle PJ (1995). Non-parametric estimation of spatial variation in relative risk. *Stat Med*, **14**, 2335–42.
6. Kulldorff M, Nagarwalla N (1995). Spatial disease clusters: detection and inference. *Stat Med*, **14**, 799–810.
7. Wood SN (2006). *Generalized additive models: an introduction with R*. CRC Press, Boca Raton.
8. Anselin L (1995). Local indicators of spatial association—LISA. *Geogr Anal*, **27**, 93–115.
9. Cameron AC, Trivedi PK (1998). *Regression analysis of count data*. Cambridge University Press, Cambridge, p. 436.
10. Rothman KJ (1990). A sobering start for the cluster busters' conference. *Am J Epidemiol*, **132**(Supp1), 6–13.

Further reading

Bivand RS, Pebesma E, Gómez-Rubio V (2013). *Applied spatial data analysis with R*, 2nd edn. Springer, New York.

Gatrell AC, Bailey TC, Diggle PJ, Rowlingson BS (1996). Spatial point pattern analysis and its application in geographical epidemiology. *Trans Inst Br Geogr*; **21**, 256.

Gelfand AE, Diggle PJ, Fuentes M, Guttorp P (2010). *Handbook of spatial statistics*. CRC Press, Boca Raton.

Chapter 15

Contact studies

Ken Eames and Charlotte Jackson

Introduction to contact studies

The transmission of many infectious agents requires close proximity between an infectious individual and a susceptible individual. The precise nature of the contact necessary for transmission ('effective contact') depends on the pathogen, the characteristics of the host population (such as hand-washing behaviour), and the environment. Quantifying relevant social contacts within a population helps us to understand the likely patterns of transmission; such contact data form an important part of mathematical modelling as applied to public health problems.

Information from contact studies provides information about two distinct aspects of population behaviour. Firstly, it highlights the range of individual behaviours within a population, e.g. identifying individuals who are unusually highly socially active. Secondly, it describes the way in which population subgroups interact, e.g. the relative contact rate within and between different age groups or between individuals at high and low risk. Many applications make use of the second aspect, so this chapter focuses on studies that are capable of quantifying mixing between subgroups (noting that such studies will generally also give information about variation between individuals). Carrying out these studies is inherently challenging, as they require collection of information about study participants and about those people with whom participants interact. The field of contact studies is still in development and is likely to advance rapidly, as techniques are enhanced and technological solutions become better, cheaper, and more acceptable.

This chapter gives a brief overview of some current methods for collecting social contact information and some of the issues likely to arise when designing and carrying out contact studies. It also discusses uses for, and interpretation of, contact data.

Measuring contact patterns

Measurement of human interactions, particularly human social networks, has a long history within the social sciences. Networks are often used as a visually appealing way to display interactions within a population. However, contact studies do not need to generate networks in order to be useful.

Epidemiology is concerned with interactions that carry some relevance for the spread of infection, e.g. sexual partnerships, friendships, and close proximity. Methods to measure these interactions are summarized below.

Patterns of sexual contact

A great deal of information about patterns of sexual contact has emerged as a result of network surveys and partner notification (PN) activities, in which the current and recent sexual partners of individuals with a diagnosed sexually transmitted infection (STI) are sought for screening and treatment. This is especially useful when a high proportion of infections are likely to be asymptomatic, as it allows previously undiagnosed cases to be identified. If individuals are identified by name, good record-keeping can allow networks of sexual contacts to be constructed. Further details can provide information about settings and/or activities in which the risk of transmission is especially high. PN is particularly adept at accessing 'high-risk' parts of a network (sometimes termed core groups), in which infection is concentrated, and is therefore a useful disease control tool. However, it is less useful for generating data about the population as a whole, as attention is generally focused on infected individuals.

More commonly, sexual contacts are measured through general population surveys, in which a representative sample of the population is asked about their sexual contact behaviour, e.g. the National Survey of Sexual Attitudes and Lifestyles (NATSAL).[1] Of particular interest are factors such as the frequency of unprotected intercourse, the number and rate of change of partnerships, possible concurrency (overlap) of partners, and age differences between partners.

Sexual contact behaviour is sensitive, so those conducting studies must be aware that participants may feel uncomfortable about answering, be unwilling to answer, or unwilling to provide truthful answers to certain questions. An important advance in survey methods has been the development of computer-assisted self-interview surveys, in which participants enter data directly into a computer for all or some of the survey; this allows sensitive information to be elicited without direct involvement of an interviewer.

Good survey design and sensitive survey protocols can help reduce non-response. Response rates are likely to be higher when the scientific value of the research is made evident. A more detailed discussion of the challenges inherent in measuring sexual behaviour can be found in Fenton *et al.*[2] and Cleland *et al.*[3] and their associated references.

Social contact patterns

In comparison to sexual contacts, contacts that may allow transmission of a respiratory infection (such as influenza or measles) are difficult to define. Several studies have defined contact as a face-to-face conversation of at least three words, with or without physical contact; the extent to which such contact reflects opportunities for transmission is the subject of current research and likely depends on the organism being transmitted.

The first large-scale study of contact patterns relevant to the spread of respiratory infections (the POLYMOD study, described in Mossong *et al.*[4]) collected data in eight European countries through a prospective contact diary, in which participants recorded details about all the people with whom they had contact over the course of a day. Participants were asked to estimate the ages of the people they met, allowing the frequency of interactions between different age groups to be quantified. Additional questions about the encounter (its duration, social setting, and whether it involved any physical contact) allow the intensity of the encounter to be estimated. Adaptations of these diaries have since been used in several other studies and have also been administered retrospectively (e.g. collecting data about contacts made on the previous day).

Alternatively, data on contact patterns can be collected by asking participants about their contacts during a typical day, e.g. the number of people they would speak to during an average day or week. Similarly, questionnaires that record who participants spend most of their time with can be used to characterize networks.

Recently, contact patterns have been measured using electronic methods, such as mobile phones and electronic tags that record proximity to other participants carrying a similar device. These devices measure spatial proximity, rather than conversational contact, and can be designed to record only face-to-face interactions, e.g. by being worn on the front of the body.

Comparison of methods

Contact studies are subject to the same sources of error as any epidemiological study, including selection bias, low response rates, issues with generalizability, and recall errors (see ➲ Chapter 4). The different methods of data collection also have specific advantages and disadvantages in relation to one another. The best approach to measuring contact patterns may depend on the aims and setting of a particular study. There is no accepted 'gold standard' method, and very little work has compared different methods in the same setting.

Contact diaries can collect detailed information about participants' contact patterns, such as the age and sex of the contacted person and the location and duration of contact, which allows different types of contact to be compared as a proxy for the risk of infection. Conversational contact data have been validated against serological data and seem to be a reasonable proxy for infection risk.

A limitation of the diary method is the time and effort required from participants to report each individual with whom they make contact, which may lead to low response rates or poor completion. The difficulty in remembering brief contacts may also mean that numbers of contacts, particularly casual contacts, are underestimated. Recall errors are particularly likely if the diaries are completed retrospectively. Questionnaires that ask about 'typical' contact patterns require less effort from participants than contact diaries but may be less suited to the collection of detailed information and require participants to describe a 'typical' day accurately.

Participant burden with electronic methods is minimal, and electronic devices can be used to collect data over long time periods (e.g. weeks or months), which would be unfeasible using diaries or questionnaires. However, data can be collected only on contacts made with individuals also wearing the devices; they are therefore more useful for characterizing contact patterns in self-contained settings such as schools or hospitals than in the wider community. Although such studies can be carried out entirely anonymously, reluctance to take part in 'electronic surveillance' might discourage participation.

Practical considerations are also important when deciding on a method of data collection in contact studies. For example, the logistics of distributing (and collecting back) questionnaires or electronic devices should be considered, as well as issues such as battery life and cost. Engagement with potential participants is important, and response rates may be higher if the study can be explained face-to-face than if diaries are mailed out unsolicited.

Results of contact studies

Contact studies from several different settings have consistently found that most individuals' encounters are with people of a similar age to themselves; this is especially true for school-aged children and adults of working age. A lower intergenerational peak of interactions between children and adults is also seen, reflecting (for example) contact between children and their parents or children and their grandparents. Numbers of reported contacts are often lower during weekends than weekdays, and school holidays are associated with reductions in the number of contacts, compared to term time, particularly among children. Encounters are typically more intense (longer-lasting and more likely to involve physical contact) if they occur in the home than in schools, workplaces, or the community, although specific patterns vary by setting. Additional details can be found in ➔ Further reading, p. 221.

Some key issues

Defining contacts

Of vital concern in any contact study is the definition of a contact. Ideally, we would like to define unambiguously a contact via which infection could be transmitted and to measure these (and only these) contacts. In practice, we are seldom in this position. Sexual contacts can be more easily defined than other social contacts, but even then the risk associated with different sexual activities cannot be specified exactly. When considering contacts relevant to the transmission of respiratory infections, studies generally attempt to measure some plausible proxy—or set of proxies—in the certain knowledge that this will include some irrelevant interactions and omit some relevant interactions.

On a practical note, a balance has to be made between the data that would be collected in a perfect world and the data that feasibly can be collected with available methods; there is little point in asking an epidemiologically perfect question if no study participant can answer it.

Developments in genetic sequencing, combined with contact tracing and other detailed epidemiological investigation, will assist in defining a relevant contact for specific infections through accurate identification of chains of direct transmission (see ➲ Chapters 1 and 9). To determine the properties of contacts that are correlated with transmission for specific infections also requires knowledge of interactions that did not result in transmission, so the problem cannot be solved by sequencing alone. An alternative approach is to carry out studies that allow us to quantify multiple different types of contacts (e.g. physical contacts and encounters lasting more than 30 minutes) and to use this information in models to attempt to fit available epidemiological data (Figure 15.1) (see ➲ Chapter 16). Comparing the goodness of fit provided by different definitions of a contact gives information about which proxy measure is most suitable for that infection. The drawback of both of these approaches, although valuable, is that there is no guarantee that their conclusions will be transferable between populations or over time.

Individual behaviour versus contact patterns

As noted above, studies that generate information about the range of individual behaviours within a population are useful, but they do not give the full picture. To understand transmission of infection requires information about who mixes with whom (whether at the individual or group level). Transmission patterns in a population in which highly socially active people mix only with each other will be very different to those in a population in which socially active individuals also interact with the general population. The most useful studies will seek to find out not only how participants behave, but also whom they contact. However, our ability to quantify these patterns in practice is limited. Diary studies can measure mixing between age groups by asking participants to estimate the ages of their contacts, but little is known about the accuracy of these estimates. If we were seeking to categorize individuals using less apparent variables than age, e.g. social activity levels or vaccination status, we may well be

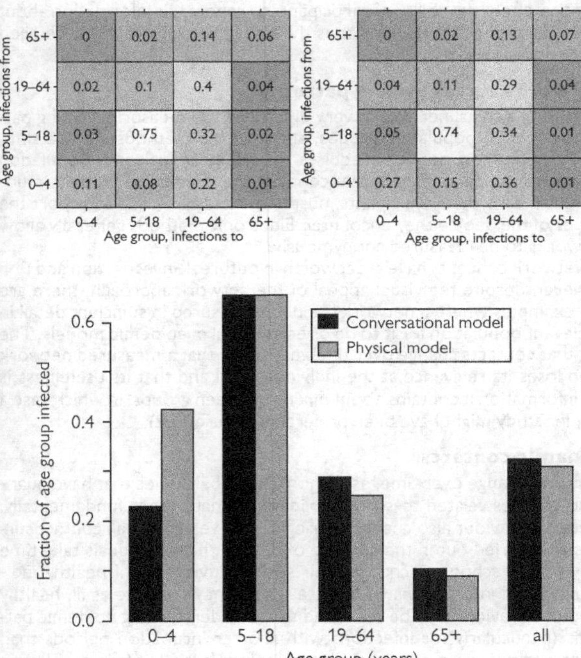

Figure 15.1 Model predictions based on different contact matrices in a population split into four age groups. $R_0 = 1.5$ throughout, but two different contact matrices are used: one based on conversational contacts (left) and one based on physical contacts (right). The different shapes of the next-generation matrices (showing the daily number of infections in each group caused by individuals in each group at the start of an outbreak) result in different distributions of infection across the population. In this case, the model using conversational contacts results in infection being shifted more towards older age groups. Information about attack rates in different groups would help determine whether conversational or physical contacts were a better proxy for the relevant contacts in this population.

Source: data from Eames KTD, *et al.*, Measured dynamic social contact patterns explain the spread of H1N1v influenza, *PLoS Computational Biology*, Volume 8, Issue 3, e1002425, Copyright © 2012 Eames KTD *et al.*

sceptical about the ability of participants to report this information about their contacts accurately and thus their ability to inform more detailed transmission models.

Networks versus mixing patterns

Measuring a social network is very different from measuring mixing patterns between population groups, although the methods may be similar. To measure a network requires that all individuals in a population of interest are sampled and that contacts are identifiable. In diary studies, this means that participants must know and be willing to report the names of the people they encounter. Electronic methods generally allow networks to be measured anonymously.

Network concepts have great worth in outbreak investigation and PN; however, despite the visual appeal of the network approach, there are few examples where a network has been measured in sufficient detail in a relevant population for it to be directly useful in epidemic models. The fact that contacts change over time may mean that a measured network soon loses its relevance at the individual level and that its usefulness is the information it contains about mixing between groups, in which case a simpler study might have been preferable (Figure 15.2).

Dynamic contacts

Contacts change over time, as demonstrated by studies that have quantified changes related to school holidays. Perhaps more fundamentally, contact behaviour also changes during illness, yet almost all contact surveys are carried out in the absence of disease. If ill individuals take time off work or school or change their social activities, or if healthy individuals avoid interactions with those whom they perceive as ill, healthy contact behaviour may be of limited use in understanding epidemic patterns (particularly for infections with shorter incubation periods than latent periods, where individuals are only infectious after developing symptoms). Studies of symptomatic individuals have shown that their contact behaviour—both in terms of the number and age distribution of contacts—is very different from their behaviour when healthy. This emphasizes the need to carry out studies in relevant settings.

Electronic methods may have a place in quantifying the dynamics of contacts. If contacts can be measured with little burden to participants, there is scope for longer-term studies to take place, which is likely to be unfeasible with self-completed contact diaries.

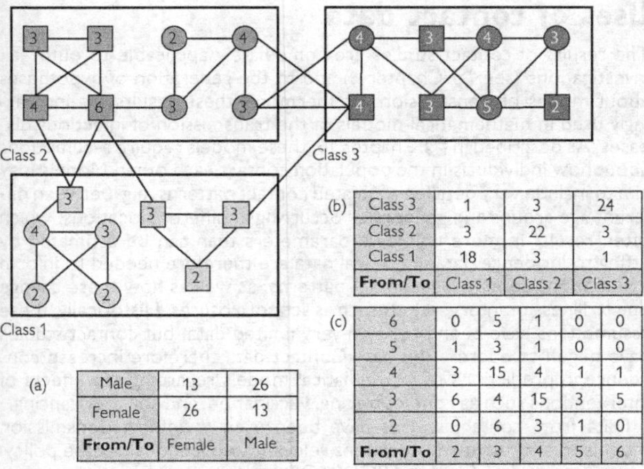

(a)

Male	13	26
Female	26	13
From/To	Female	Male

(b)

Class 3	1	3	24
Class 2	3	22	3
Class 1	18	3	1
From/To	Class 1	Class 2	Class 3

(c)

6	0	5	1	0	0
5	1	3	1	0	0
4	3	15	4	1	1
3	6	4	15	3	5
2	0	6	3	1	0
From/To	2	3	4	5	6

Figure 15.2 Contact patterns within a hypothetical population of three school classes. Information collected using a contact diary can be presented in multiple different ways. For example, the full contact network can be shown or relevant data can be extracted to quantify the amount of contact between (a) genders, (b) school classes, and (c) individuals with different degrees. The colour of the nodes indicates the school class; the shape indicates their gender (male, square; female, circle), and the nodes are labelled with their degree (number of contacts). Further categorizations are possible, e.g. by both gender and school class.

Uses of contact data

The results of contact studies are immediately applicable to outbreak investigations (see ➲ Chapter 3) and to the generation of hypotheses about modes of transmission. Furthermore, these results are increasingly used in mathematical models of the transmission of infectious diseases. As described in ➲ Chapter 16, these models require assumptions about how individuals in the population contact each other. Models may aim to include very detailed simulated contact patterns, e.g. between different age groups and genders or occurring in different locations, which often results in more unknown parameters than can be estimated by fitting to incidence data. Empirical data are therefore needed to inform assumptions about usual contact patterns, as well as how these change due to illness or interventions such as school closures. Historically, these assumptions have been based on very limited data, but contact studies have begun to address this gap. Contact data therefore increase confidence in predictions of mathematical models regarding the effects of interventions such as contact tracing, vaccination, and social distancing.

Data from contact studies have been used to inform transmission models to address many questions relevant to infectious disease policy. For example, data from the POLYMOD study have been used in models assessing the impact of extending the seasonal influenza vaccination programme in the UK to healthy children (in addition to the previously targeted clinical risk groups and people older than 65 years). The vaccine programme was modified to include healthy children in 2013, using contact studies to give detailed information about rates of contact between different age groups. Contact data from the NATSAL study have been incorporated into many models of STIs, including evaluation of the National Chlamydia Screening Programme in the UK, for which contact studies provide information about rates of contact between behavioural subgroups and the prevalence of different sexual mixing behaviours within a population. Indeed, it is common practice nowadays to use measured patterns of contacts where suitable data are available, when developing transmission-dynamic models for use in public health.

Transmission models (see ➲ Chapter 16) also provide a means to assess whether contact studies have measured the 'correct' contacts, i.e. those that are relevant to transmission. If contact data are used in a model and the model fits the data well, this implies that the measured contacts are a good proxy for transmission opportunities. As discussed above, fitting to data can be an important complement to measuring contact patterns directly, as even the best-designed contact studies are unlikely to measure those contacts that would be in place during an epidemic.

Conclusions

Studies that collect data about contacts relevant to the transmission of infection are a relatively new development, especially for respiratory infections. Carrying out and interpreting such studies is challenging:

- A suitable definition of an encounter must be determined (e.g. conversation or physical contact).
- Appropriate methods must be used (e.g. self-completed diaries or electronic tags).
- Appropriate levels of detail must be determined (e.g. range of individual behaviours, contacts between age groups, or complete networks).
- Appropriate study populations must be chosen (e.g. schools, hospitals, or the general population).
- Consideration must be given to the likelihood that the contacts, as measured, are unlikely to be the same as those that will be taking place during the transmission of infection.

Despite these challenges, data from contact studies are increasingly being used to inform models and guide decision-making. Future research will further elucidate the types of contact necessary for transmission and how the frequency of these changes with illness and interventions.

References

1. National Survey of Sexual Attitudes and Lifestyles (2014). *The National Survey of Sexual Attitudes and Lifestyles*. Available at: http://www.natsal.ac.uk (accessed 28 January 2015).
2. Fenton KA, Johnson AM, McManus S, Erens B (2001). Measuring sexual behaviour: methodological challenges in survey research. *Sex Transm Infect*, **77**, 84–92.
3. Cleland J, Boerma JT, Carael M, Weir SS (2004). Monitoring sexual behaviour in general populations: a synthesis of lessons of the past decade. *Sex Transm Infect*, **80**(Suppl 2), ii1–7.
4. Mossong J, Hens N, Jit M, *et al.* (2008). Social contacts and mixing patterns relevant to the spread of infectious diseases. *PLoS Med*, **5**, e74.

Further reading

Adams EJ, Turner KME, Edmunds WJ (2007). The cost effectiveness of opportunistic chlamydia screening in England. *Sex Transm Infect*, **83**, 267–75.

Baguelin M, Flasche S, Camacho A, *et al.* (2013). Assessing optimal target populations for influenza vaccination programmes: an evidence synthesis and modelling study. *PLoS Med*, **10**, e1001527.

Cattuto C, Van den Broeck W, Barrat A, *et al.* (2010). Dynamics of person-to-person interactions from distributed RFID sensor networks. *PLoS One*, **5**, e11596.

Eames KTD, Tilston NL, Brooks-Pollock E, Edmunds WJ (2012). Measured dynamic social contact patterns explain the spread of H1N1v influenza. *PLoS Comp Biol*, **8**, e1002425.

Jolly AM, Wylie JL (2002). Gonorrhoea and chlamydia core groups and sexual networks in Manitoba. *Sex Transm Infect*, **78**(Suppl 1), i145–51.

Melegaro A, Jit M, Gay N, Zagheni E, Edmunds WJ (2011). What types of contacts are important for the spread of infections?: using contact survey data to explore European mixing patterns. *Epidemics*, **3**(3-4), 143–51.

Read JM, Edmunds WJ, Riley S, Lessler J, Cummings DA (2012). Close encounters of the infectious kind: methods to measure social mixing behaviour. *Epidemiol Infect*, **140**, 2117–30.

Rothenberg RB, Potterat JJ, Woodhouse DE, Muth SQ, Darrow WW, Klovdahl AS (1998). Social network dynamics and HIV transmission. *AIDS*, **12**, 1529–36.

Van Kerckhove K, Hens N, Edmunds WJ, Eames KT (2013). The impact of illness on social networks: implications for transmission and control of influenza. *Am J Epidemiol*, **178**, 1655–62.

Wallinga J, Teunis P, Kretzschmar M (2006). Using data on social contacts to estimate age-specific transmission parameters for respiratory-spread infectious agents. *Am J Epidemiol*, **164**, 936–44.

Wasserman S, Faust K (1994). *Social network analysis*. Cambridge University Press, Cambridge.

Chapter 16

Transmission-dynamic models of infectious diseases

Ted Cohen and Peter White

Introduction to transmission-dynamic models of infectious diseases

Why do some pathogens fail to spread effectively in a host community, while others increase in prevalence before eventual elimination? Why do some pathogens oscillate in frequency, and how can others become stably established at relatively constant levels over long periods of time? How is it possible that interventions can perversely increase the burden of disease in the community, even as they reduce the overall prevalence of infection?

This chapter introduces transmission-dynamic epidemic models as tools to help understand the patterns that arise from these complex interactions between pathogens and hosts. Like all models, transmission-dynamic models serve as simplified representations of more complex systems, but, in contrast to purely statistical models (see ➲ Chapter 13), this chapter focuses on models that explicitly include the transmission processes of communicable diseases. These transmission-dynamic models specify how the risk of infection among susceptible hosts depends on the current (and usually time-varying) prevalence of infectious individuals (or vectors or fomites), which has consequences for the distribution of infection and the (cost-) effectiveness of interventions (see ➲ Chapter 17).

Importantly, models should not be 'black boxes' but should be clearly described, so that non-modellers are able to assess the validity of the assumptions and parameters used in the model, as well as the model itself.

Uses of transmission-dynamic models

Although transmission-dynamic models have been used for many different purposes, it is useful to classify them into two categories:

- models to study how a system behaves and responds to interventions, particularly to inform economic analysis and policy-making
- models to better understand the system itself.

Models to study how a system behaves and responds to interventions

Is the prevalence of infection expected to increase or decrease in the absence of interventions? What fraction of the population needs to be immunized in order to prevent a pathogen from causing an outbreak? If vaccine supply is limited, should elderly individuals or school-aged children be prioritized to minimize the morbidity associated with infection? Questions about how pathogen prevalence and disease burden are expected to change over time and in response to available strategies for disease control are natural applications for transmission-dynamic models.

Models to better understand the system itself

To what extent does previous infection provide protection from reinfection? How much does the incidence of infection depend on the proportion of infectious individuals who are asymptomatic? Does uncertainty about the future trajectory of an epidemic depend more on lack of a precise estimate of the probability that an individual will progress to disease after exposure or the duration of infectiousness prior to symptom onset? By fitting transmission-dynamic models to available data, it is possible to study elements of the natural history of disease that may otherwise be difficult, expensive, or unethical to study through other means. Models can also be used to prioritize which features of the system must be better understood to improve future projections and reduce uncertainty.

Defining health states and transitions

This chapter focuses on models for studying the transmission of microparasities (pathogens multiplying directly within hosts) between humans. Approaches for modelling the transmission of macroparasites (pathogens for which important reproductive stages occur outside of hosts, especially worms) or vector-borne pathogens require additional considerations and are described in greater detail elsewhere.[1]

Before constructing a transmission-dynamic model for the spread of microparasitic organisms between hosts, the host health states to represent (e.g. susceptible to infection, infectious, or recovered from a previous infection) and the transition rules that govern how hosts move between these states must be specified.

Representing health states in the model

After becoming infected, does a host rapidly become infectious to others or is there an important latent period before that host becomes infectious to others? Do individuals recover from infection? If individuals do recover, are they then immune or do they remain at risk of reinfection if exposed to the pathogen again?

The structures of transmission-dynamic models are often named according to the core health and disease states represented. For example, a 'susceptible–infectious–recovered (SIR)' model has three health states: susceptible, infectious, and recovered. An SIR structure could be chosen if hosts become infectious soon after infection and retain at least partial immunity to reinfection on recovery. In contrast, a susceptible–exposed–infectious–recovered (SEIR) model would be appropriate for a pathogen with a period of latency between time of infection and time that an infected individual becomes infectious to others (by convention, 'exposed' is commonly used, instead of 'latent'). For pathogens from which recovery from infectiousness is not associated with protection from reinfection, a susceptible–infectious–susceptible (SIS) model structure may be warranted, while a pathogen that causes a chronic infection may be represented by a susceptible–infectious (SI) structure. Box 16.1 shows the structures of several prototypical model structures and example disease prevalence trajectories associated with them (see also Figure 16.1).

Box 16.1 Structures, differential equations, and example disease prevalence trajectories associated with several prototypical model structures

Here we provide box-and-arrow diagrams and associated differential equations for simple SIS, SIR, and SEIR models in closed populations (no births or deaths). We have chosen examples in which the algebraic expression for the basic reproductive number R_0 is simple and is the same for all models. R_0 is the average number of secondary infections arising from a typical infected individual in a population where everyone is susceptible to infection, and is the ratio of the rate of transmission from an infected individual and the rate of recovery; in these models, $R_0 = \beta/\sigma$. The force of infection in these models is βI, the product of the transmission parameter and the prevalence of infectious individuals in the population; note that this changes over time as I changes. For each model, we display an example epidemic trajectory, identifying the percentage of the population in each state over time.

(a) *SIS model (susceptible–infectious–susceptible)*

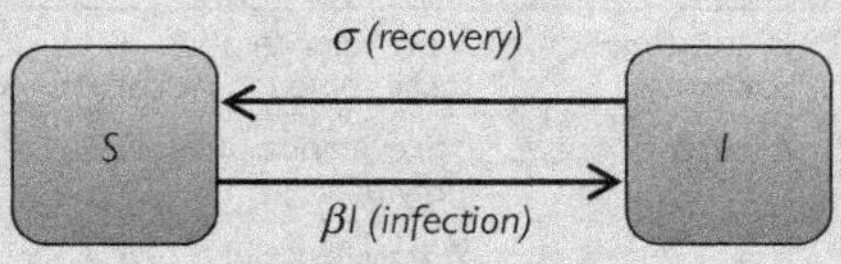

Differential equations	Parameters	Variables
$dS/dt = -\beta IS + \sigma I$	β: transmission parameter	S: prevalence of susceptible individuals
$dI/dt = \beta IS - \sigma I$	σ: recovery rate	I: prevalence of infectious individuals

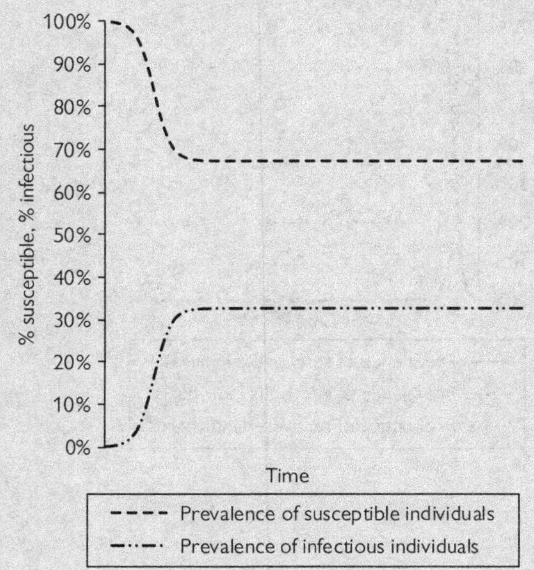

(Continued)

Box 16.1 *(Continued)*

(b) *SIR model (susceptible–infectious–recovered)*

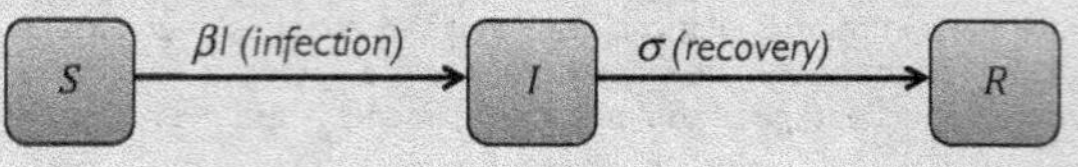

Differential equations	Parameters	Variables
$dS/dt = -\beta IS$	β: transmission parameter	S: prevalence of susceptible individuals
$dI/dt = \beta IS - \sigma I$	σ: recovery rate	I: prevalence of infectious individuals
$dR/dt = \sigma I$		*R: prevalence of recovered individuals*

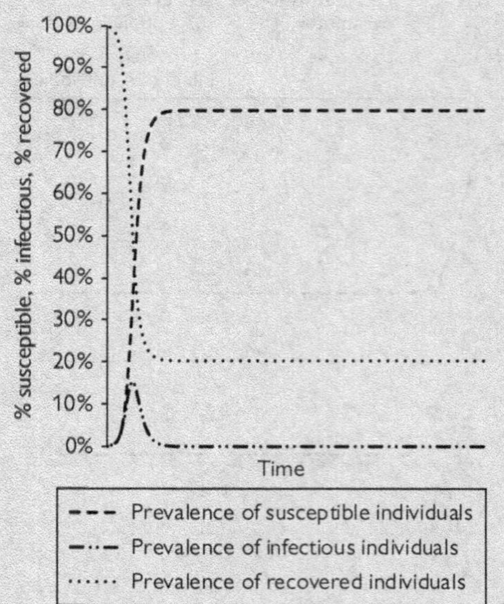

Box 16.1 *(Continued)*

(c) *SEIR model (susceptible–exposed–infectious–recovered)*

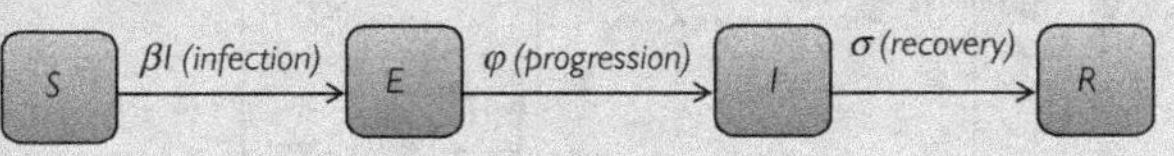

Differential equations	Parameters	Variables
$dS/dt = -\beta IS$	β: transmission parameter	*S*: prevalence of susceptible individuals
$dE/dt = \beta IS - \varphi E$	φ: progression rate	*E*: prevalence of exposed/ latent individuals
$dI/dt = \varphi E - \sigma I$	σ: recovery rate	*I*: prevalence of infectious individuals
$dR/dt = \sigma I$		*R*: prevalence of recovered individuals

E, exposed; *I*, infectious; *R*, recovered; *S*, susceptible.

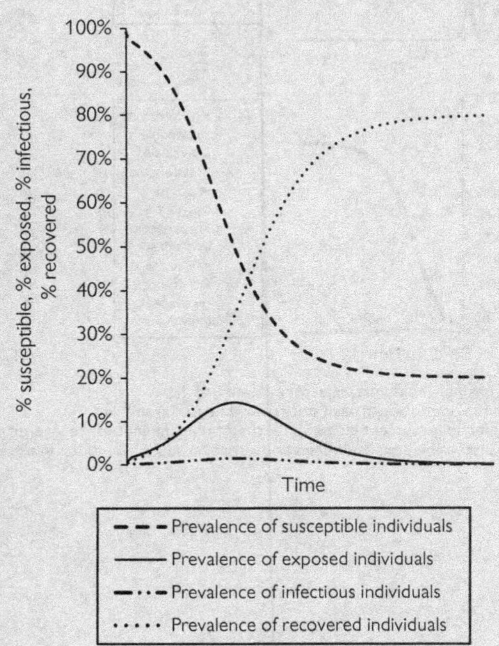

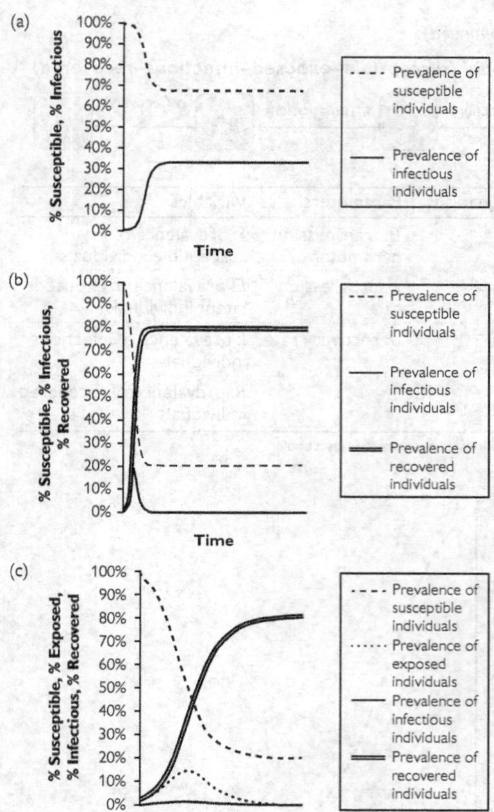

Figure 16.1 Example epidemic trajectory identifying the percentage of the population in each state over time for (a) simple susceptible–infectious–susceptible (SIS), (b) susceptible–infectious–recovered (SIR), and (c) susceptible–exposed–infectious–recovered (SEIR) models in closed populations.

Although knowledge of the natural history of the pathogen is always important, the decision about which health states should be included in the model is also strongly influenced by the question the model is being developed to address. For example, if the aim is the long-term dynamics of a disease with a short latent period, the E state could be omitted from the SEIR model. However, if understanding epidemic behaviour over a shorter period is important, exclusion of this latent period may not be reasonable.

Determining transition rules between modelled health states

After determining which health states should be represented, the rules by which hosts transition between these states must be determined. For example, in an SIR model structure, how hosts enter and exit each of these health states must be specified.

An example of a simple transition is that between the infectious and recovered states, which may be governed in some models by a single time-invariant parameter (that is, the parameter that defines the rate of recovery from infectiousness). In contrast, the transition rule that governs the process of becoming infected—the transition between the susceptible and infectious states—will usually be more complicated, because the risk of a susceptible person becoming infected per unit time (the 'force of infection') depends on the prevalence of infectious individuals (or vectors/fomites), which typically varies with time.

Building a transmission-dynamic model

Two distinct approaches can be used to translate health states and transition rules into an operable transmission-dynamic model. These approaches differ in the manner in which host populations are represented and have various attributes and limitations, as described below.

Models in which hosts are aggregated by health state

Most transmission-dynamic models consider populations of hosts aggregated by health state (e.g. susceptible, infectious, and recovered), such that, at any time, the model tracks the number or fraction of the population occupying each health state but does not track each individual independently. These models are often referred to as 'compartmental' models, because the population is divided into compartments representing aggregated groups of individuals sharing a health state (Box 16.1).

Compartmental models are encoded as systems of difference (discrete time-steps) or differential (continuous time) equations. The equations comprise parameters and variables. Variables 'keep track' of the numbers of individuals in each compartment, which can change over time. Parameters specify the *per-capita* rates of movement from one health state to another (except for the process of acquiring infection) and are usually time-invariant.

At the population level, the number of individuals flowing from one health state to another is determined by the *per-capita* rate (specified by the parameter) and the number of individuals subject to that process (specified by the variable). Changes in flow rates over time occur as a consequence of changes in the variables, not the parameters.

Importantly, the force of infection is a **variable**—it changes dynamically in response to changes in the number of infectious individuals. This means that the numbers of individuals becoming infected over time depends on both the number who are infectious and the number who are susceptible. The 'transmission term' also contains a parameter that specifies the rate of contact between individuals in the population and the probability of transmission occurring when a susceptible and infectious individual make contact.

One important attribute of compartmental models is that they can often be analysed mathematically. Simple, analytically tractable compartmental models of epidemics have facilitated fundamental insights into the dynamics and control of infectious diseases (Box 16.2), while more complicated models, which usually require numerical analysis, have also played an important role in advancing the understanding of epidemics. Other key attributes of compartmental models are that they are easy to communicate and to replicate or modify by others, as they can be written down as a series of equations that fully specify the system.

Models in which hosts are considered as individuals

Individual-based models (IBMs) are models in which individuals are tracked through health states over time. These models can generate similar output to compartment models by reporting the number or fraction of hosts in each health state over time.

Box 16.2 Dynamics of simple epidemics: model-based insights

For a perfectly immunizing acute viral pathogen, such as the measles virus, a simple susceptible–infectious–recovered (SIR) structure may suffice for capturing key dynamic behaviours. Here we illustrate two elementary insights derived from consideration of the dynamic behaviour of an SIR-type model. The first insight is generated from a closed-population model without births or deaths:

$$dS/dt = -\beta IS$$

$$dI/dt = \beta IS - \sigma I$$

$$dR/dt = \sigma I$$

Why do epidemics recede?

An epidemic can occur when the basic reproductive number (β/σ) is >1; as the epidemic progresses in the population, the pool of available susceptible individuals is depleted. The effect of depletion of susceptible individuals on transmission can be quantified by following the effective reproductive number ($R_{effective}$: the realized reproductive number which accounts for the fraction of the population that remains susceptible). As $R_{effective}$, $(\beta/\sigma) \times [S/(S + I + R)]$, falls below 1, the epidemic recedes.

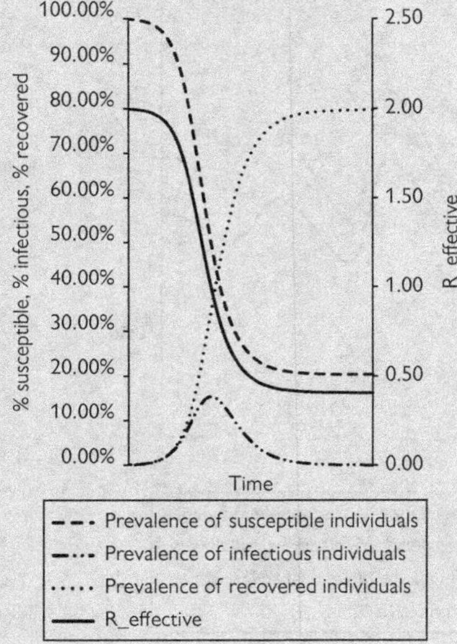

Why do we observe oscillations of some immunizing diseases in populations?

For some pathogens, we may observe repeated epidemics over time because of seasonal forcing of transmission (some pathogens may be more easily transmitted during specific times of year). But even in the absence of seasonal forcing, oscillations of disease may occur in populations if the pool of available susceptible individuals is depleted during an epidemic and later replenished by births. New epidemic waves occur, as replenishment causes the effective reproductive number to increase above 1, allowing infection to be amplified once more. We adapt the SIR model in Box 16.1 to incorporate births and deaths, and we set the per-capita rate of births and deaths to be the same (μ), such that the population size remains constant (as the modelled infection does not cause mortality):

$$dS/dt = \mu(S + I + R) - \beta IS - \mu S$$
$$dI/dt = \beta IS - \sigma I - \mu I$$
$$dR/dt = \sigma I - \mu R$$

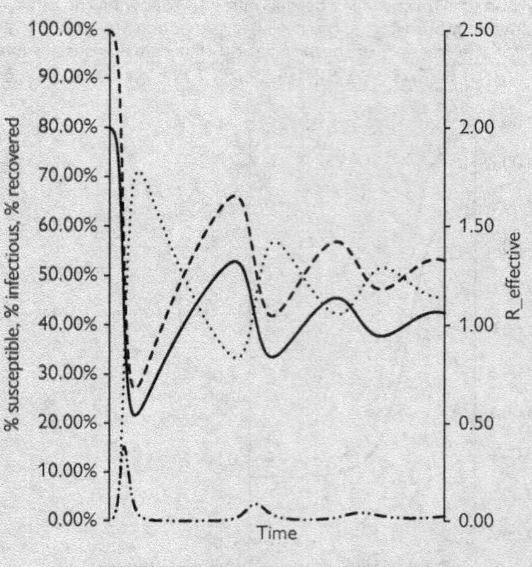

The IBMs are encoded as rules in programming languages and are implemented on computers.

Because these models follow individual hosts through their transitions between health states, they may be preferred over compartmental models for questions that require that the individual history of each host to be tracked through time. For example, an IBM might be needed if the specific contact patterns for individuals are important for the question under study (see ➔ Chapter 15) or if continuously variable host factors need to be recorded. The increased capacity of IBMs to track individual history comes at the cost of analytic tractability and usually results in diminished transparency and ease of communication, compared with compartmental models. They also typically are demanding computationally, which can limit the extent of analysis performed.

Determinism and stochasticity in models

Models can be either 'deterministic' (they omit the effects of randomness, so repeated simulations of the model with unchanged parameter values are identical) or 'stochastic' (they include the effects of randomness, so there is variation between repeated simulations, even when parameters are not changed). For questions about the expected long-term trends of pathogens circulating in large host populations, deterministic models often provide sufficient insight. However, consideration of stochastic behaviour of mathematical models is important for studying the dynamics of rare infections (e.g. when the pathogen is first introduced into a community, when a drug-resistant strain first appears through genetic change and is initially present in only one host, and when a pathogen is on the verge of local eradication) and when host population size is restricted (e.g. when modelling the spread HAIs).

Deterministic and stochastic versions of compartmental models and IBMs can be implemented, but, in practice, almost all IBMs are stochastic, as this feature is natural to include when programming the transition rules within an IBM framework.

Adding complexity: considering host heterogeneities

To address all but the simplest questions, models usually require the inclusion of additional complexity to reflect important heterogeneities between hosts.

Age and sex of hosts

Age- or sex-structured transmission-dynamic models are used when there are different age- or sex-specific natural histories of disease (e.g. when natural history varies by sex or when morbidity is associated with age at infection; Box 16.3) and when there are differences in contact patterns between hosts of different ages or sexes (see ➲ Chapter 15).

Behavioural risk patterns

For specific types of transmission, host behaviour has an immense effect on individual risk of exposure. For example, for STIs and infections transmitted through well-defined risk behaviours, such as intravenous drug use, the risk of infection can vary by orders of magnitude between individual hosts in the same community, based on behavioural risk factors. Accordingly, models of these pathogens incorporate such behavioural heterogeneity by allowing hosts to differ by risk group or by explicitly modelling the relevant contact patterns for individuals in the population.

Box 16.3 Age-structured models

For some infectious diseases, the morbidity associated with disease is associated with the age at infection. For example, the rubella virus causes little morbidity when it infects an individual at a young age, but, when it infects a woman who is pregnant, her fetus may suffer devastating abnormalities (congenital rubella syndrome, CRS). In settings where the force of infection with rubella is intense, the average age of infection is well below the reproductive age, such that few cases of CRS are expected. However, if the force of infection is reduced, but not eliminated, perhaps through vaccine campaigns with inadequate coverage, the average age of infection may increase into this dangerous age range, and the number of cases of CRS may spike. This perverse effect of imperfect vaccine campaigns was predicted in modelling papers.[2,3] Unfortunately, these predictions were realized in Greece over a decade later where a lax vaccine strategy led to a higher age of infection with rubella and a dramatic increase in the number of CRS cases.[4]

Model calibration and sensitivity/ uncertainty analyses

Once a model is built, the values for parameters governing the transition rules between health states must be specified, and the model will often be calibrated so that its behaviour fits observed data from a specific epidemic scenario. From which data sources can we estimate the model parameter values and calibrate epidemic behaviour?

Specifying model parameter values

Observational, and occasionally experimental, studies provide the commonest sources of data from which to estimate parameters governing the natural history of infection. Numerous challenges related to the use of such data sources for making inference on these fundamental parameters are worth considering. For example, as it is often difficult to identify the time that an exposed individual is infected with a pathogen, determining the rate of progression from infection to infectiousness can be challenging. For diseases for which treatments are available, studies to estimate the average duration of infectiousness for untreated disease are not ethical, so studies often rely on data gathered in an era before treatment was available. Although these data may exist, their relevance for the duration of infectiousness at other times or in different settings may be limited. In addition, there is often substantial between-host heterogeneity in the values of these natural history parameters, and understanding the importance of this variance for the behaviour of pathogen dynamics is an area of substantial current research interest.

The most difficult model parameter to measure directly is the transmission parameter, defined earlier as the product of the probability of infection conditional on contact between an infectious and a susceptible individual and the rate of contacts between individuals in the population. In most modelling studies, this parameter must be estimated by fitting models to available data on the burden of disease in the community.

Specifying epidemiological measures of disease burden over time

Data informing the burden of disease in communities over time include cross-sectional sources (e.g. seroprevalence surveys) and time-series sources (e.g. notifications data, incidence, prevalence, and disease trends). Availability of these types of data allows models to be calibrated against observed or estimated trends in disease burden such as infections, disease, mortality, case notifications, and hospitalizations.

In using such data to calibrate models, it is important to consider how observable measures may be biased representations of underlying disease trends and may thus challenge the validity of model-fitting exercises. For example, if the probability of a patient seeking care or the probability that a physician will report or notify the occurrence of an additional case changes over the course of an epidemic, notification data may be an a unreliable metric of the actual trend in incidence.

There may also be underlying bias related to the selection of which epidemics are recognized and used to calibrate models. If only large outbreaks of a novel pathogen are recognized (smaller, stuttering outbreaks that fail to propagate successfu ly will be more difficult to detect), models fit to these data will systematically overestimate the reproductive number, which is a key measure of how effectively the pathogen spreads.

Sensitivity and uncertainty analyses

Many methods are used to calibrate models to existing data on disease trends; although the technical details of such methods are beyond the scope of this chapter, these fitting methods aim to minimize the difference between modelled and observed trajectories given information on the credible values (or ranges of values) for prespecified model parameters.

The relationship between parameter values and the behaviour of models may be investigated in at least two ways.

- Sensitivity analyses can be performed, in which the behaviour of the model is evaluated as single or multiple parameters which are varied from baseline values. Accordingly, the sensitivity of the model behaviour to changes in specific parameters can be evaluated and compared. Identifying the parameters to which the model behaviour is most sensitive can provide insight into the role that these parameters play in determining the epidemic trajectory.
- Uncertainty analyses can be undertaken, in which selected outcomes of the model are evaluated across plausible or credible ranges of input parameters. Uncertainty analyses provide insight into the variability of outcomes that may arise from a model conditional on the precision (or lack thereof) in estimated model parameters. By identifying parameters that drive uncertainty in models, it is possible to prioritize future studies that, by increasing precision of relevant parameter estimates, would best reduce uncertainty in the model's behaviour and better inform public health policy.

Examples of insights from transmission-dynamic modelling

Several examples of phenomena that are well explained, even by the simplest models, are used to illustrate the types of insights made possible by transmission-dynamic models.

Vaccination coverage and herd immunity

Herd immunity is a property of communities that contain sufficient numbers of immune individuals to provide protection for individuals that are not immune (see ➲ Chapter 12). From a mechanistic perspective, the presence of immune individuals effectively 'blocks' the transmission of pathogens and thus prevents the sustained transmission of a pathogen that would otherwise lead to epidemic spread.

Simple models provide insight into the fraction of the population that must be immune to generate such herd immunity. The **effective** reproductive number ($R_{effective}$) is defined as the number of expected secondary infections attributable to a single infectious individual in the population (see ➲ Chapters 1 and 13). The presence of individuals with immunity limits transmission. When there are no immune individuals in the population, $R_{effective}$ is equal to the **basic** reproductive number R_0 (Box 16.1). Assuming homogeneous mixing of individuals, the general relationship is $R_{effective} = R_0 \times$ (1 − the fraction of the population that is immune). Algebraic manipulation of the relationship provides insight that epidemics are not expected to occur when the fraction of the population that is immune exceeds the quantity $1 - (1/R_0)$. Thus, $1 - (1/R_0)$ defines the critical fraction of the population to immunize to prevent an epidemic. For example, if $R_0 = 3$, at least two-thirds of the population must be immune to guard against epidemic spread. For pathogens with higher R_0, a larger fraction of the population must be successfully immunized to prevent such epidemics; importantly, if a vaccine is not 100% protective (see ➲ Chapter 12), it may not be feasible to deliver the vaccine to enough individuals to provide herd immunity.

Controllability of infections and contribution of transmission from asymptomatic cases

The simplest models predict that if $R_{effective}$ of a pathogen can be reduced to <1, the pathogen will eventually be eliminated from the host population. Calculations of R_0 and $R_{effective}$ for directly transmitted pathogens depend directly on the duration of infectiousness; for otherwise identical pathogens, one with twice the duration of infectiousness will also be expected to produce twice the number of secondary cases in an exponentially growing epidemic.

Accordingly, reducing the average duration of infectiousness may allow for effective control of an emerging pathogen by lowering $R_{effective}$ below this critical threshold. From a practical perspective, reductions in the duration of infectiousness usually require an infectious individual effectively to be removed from the population, so they do not further expose susceptible individuals; this may be achieved through treatment or isolation. However, in most cases, early identification of these infectious cases requires that symptom onset either precedes or is synchronous with the onset of infectiousness (see ➔ Chapter 1). If infectiousness precedes the onset of symptoms (or asymptomatic infections are infectious), as is the case for many important pathogens, the feasibility and degree to which the average duration of potential transmission may be reduced are themselves reduced.

Simple models provide insight into how transmission from asymptomatic cases would make control of infections impossible through earlier detection of symptomatic cases. Using the notation of Fraser *et al.*[5], if θ = the proportion of transmission that occurs before the onset of symptoms, then when $\theta > 1/R_0$, it is not feasible to control an epidemic by early identification of symptomatic individuals. This insight follows from the fact that, under the optimistic assumption of immediate detection and removal of symptomatic cases, R_0 can be reduced to $\theta \times R_0$, and when the value of this product is <1, epidemic spread is obstructed. Algebraic manipulation reveals that when $\theta > 1/R_0$, it is not possible to bring the reproductive number below 1 in the absence of additional public health measures.

Future directions

New sources of data about host and pathogen population structure and dynamics improve the structure and parameterization of transmission-dynamic models and expand the types of questions that may be answered by these models.

New technologies for measuring an individual's location, such as mobile phones equipped with GPS trackers and sensors for measuring proximity and contacts between individuals in a community, offer opportunities for more detailed monitoring of contact networks in populations. These tools are increasingly important for pathogens, for which such detailed accounting of host contact patterns is most important for explaining existing epidemiological patterns or predicting future disease trajectories.

Molecular epidemiological tools for identification of pathogens have advanced our ability to identify linkages between infected hosts and thus to make inferences on which disease events are related through possible transmission. Such data have been used routinely to inform the structure and parameterization of dynamic mathematical models. The rapidly expanding access to technologies for WGS of pathogens has greatly increased the resolution of such approaches and offers new hope for clarifying and determining directionality of transmission between individuals and resolving clear chains of transmission within clusters of cases. Many current developments within the field of transmission-dynamic modelling are focused around the opportunities and challenges associated with use of the increasing volumes of genomic data to inform the development of new models, particularly individual-based models.

Novel approaches and expanding use of existing methods to inform the selection of model structures (i.e. which health states are included and how transition rules link these states) and to understand the contribution of model structural uncertainty to overall uncertainty are likely to play a larger role in future modelling studies.

Conclusions

Transmission-dynamic models are powerful tools that, when properly developed and analysed, can provide important insights into the complex behaviour of pathogens, as they spread through a host population. In all cases, such models formalize decisions about which details of the complicated systems of relationships between hosts in a population and of pathogens with hosts can be greatly simplified or completely ignored. Well-informed decisions about which details can be 'stripped away' from the system provide opportunities to understand better the fundamental relationships within that system and to predict how it will change over time or in response to external perturbations. This is the aim of a transmission-dynamic modeller.

At the same time, judgements that inform the development of dynamic epidemiological models are often based on incomplete (and potentially erroneous) understanding of the natural history of disease or the behaviours of host populations. In the best of cases, such uncertainty will be made explicit in the model and incorporated through sensitivity and uncertainty analyses. However, in other cases, deficiencies in the understanding of the system may not be recognized and ultimately may undermine the usefulness of the model. An attribute of a transmission-dynamic model is that it requires explicit identification of key assumptions within the model equations or code, and best practices dictate that the researcher must highlight such key assumptions when communicating the model-based findings.

The discipline of transmission-dynamic modelling is young but rapidly maturing. Transmission-dynamic models are increasingly linked with economic analysis (see ➲ Chapter 17) and are being used to inform policy and to help design and analyse studies. Improving modelling methods, coupled with increasing computing power, better sources of data with which to calibrate models, and sober consideration of the particular strengths and challenges associated with the use of such models, will ensure that these tools will continue to be used to improve insight into the behaviour of epidemics.

References

1. Anderson RM, May RM (1991). *Infectious diseases of humans: dynamics and control*. Oxford University Press, Oxford.
2. Knox EG (1980). Strategy for rubella vaccination. *Int J Epidemiol*, **9**, 13–23.
3. Anderson RM, May RM (1983). Vaccination against rubella and measles: quantitative investigations of different policies. *J Hyg (Lond)*, **90**, 259–325.
4. Panagiotopoulos T, Antoniadou I, Valassi-Adam E (1999). Increase in congenital rubella occurrence after immunisation in Greece: retrospective survey and systematic review. *BMJ*, **319**, 1462–7.
5. Fraser C, Riley S, Anderson RM, Ferguson NM (2004). Factors that make an infectious disease outbreak controllable. *Proc Natl Acad Sci U S A*, **101**, 6146–51.

Chapter 17

Economic analysis of interventions against infectious diseases

Mark Jit and Peter White

What is health economics?

Healthcare resources, such as money, staff time, and hospital beds, are **scarce**—their supply is limited and insufficient to meet all possible needs for healthcare. Any particular use of healthcare resources inevitably involves giving up other possible uses of those resources. If we assume that the health budget is fixed, purchasing a vaccine for a national programme ultimately means a smaller budget to build hospitals or purchase drugs—or even to build schools or airports if vaccination is funded from a wider budget. If healthcare is funded through social or private insurance, a decision to reimburse vaccinations will result in less money for other reimbursements—or higher premiums. These choices are most apparent in resource-poor settings, but choices are inevitable, even in high-income countries, if often less explicit. As spending on infectious diseases is usually allocated from a general healthcare budget, decisions about resource allocation for infectious disease interventions usually follow the same broad principles as those for other healthcare decisions, except for special considerations to account for the unique nature of infectious diseases[1,2] (see ➲ Chapters 1 and 16).

The aim of health economics is not necessarily to save money, but to make the best use of scarce resources. Some sort of priority-setting (or **rationing**) process is inevitable, as demand exceeds supply. Historically, various mechanisms have been used, ranging from ad hoc non-explicit criteria through to free markets (rationing by willingness to pay) to waiting lists (rationing by willingness to wait). Another approach is to make these decisions through a technical process of determining the allocation of resources that would maximize some explicit criteria such as the total health of the population or the distribution of that health. One tool to aid such decisions is a **health economic evaluation**.

Health economic evaluation

An economic evaluation is a comparison of the costs and consequences of two or more options to find the option that achieves the best outcome based on specified criteria. The objective may be to maximize health in a population using a fixed quantity of resource. Economic evaluation in healthcare has increased rapidly since the 1990s, particularly for infectious diseases,[1] and economic evaluations now play a key role in many infectious disease-related decisions. For example, the UK Joint Committee on Vaccination and Immunisation (JCVI) has a statutory duty to consider cost-effectiveness when making recommendations.[3] Donor organizations, such as the WHO and GAVI, the Vaccine Alliance, also recommend consideration of value for money before health interventions are implemented. Economic modelling has informed international guidelines on infectious disease interventions such as treatment for HIV.[4] In turn, international consortia have produced guidelines for the development of economic models for such interventions.[5,6]

Several types of economic evaluations are used in healthcare.[7] A **cost-effectiveness analysis** estimates the ratio of the incremental cost of an intervention, compared to the incremental health effects—the **incremental cost-effectiveness ratio** (ICER). Note that both costs and health effects are calculated **incrementally**, i.e. they are compared to an alternative use of healthcare resources such as continuing with the present care regimen without any changes. A preventive intervention like vaccination or screening may incur costs due to the intervention, but it may also save costs as a result of needing to spend less on treatment due to illness being averted.

Costs should ideally be measured using an **ingredients approach**, which involves counting the units of input (such as medicines, hours of staff time, or occupied hospital beds) and multiplying this by the unit cost (or value) of each input. Health effects can be measured in a variety of ways such as numbers of episodes of disease, hospitalizations, or deaths prevented. Methods to estimate these outcomes are discussed in ➔ Chapter 4. However, these measures lack comparability across diseases, as duration and severity of disease will vary by infection. **Life-years gained** is a more informative measure than deaths averted. Furthermore, a major component of disease burden can be **morbidity**, rather than **mortality**.

Economic evaluations are most useful when they enable comparisons across diseases, as the same budget may be used to fund both influenza vaccination and screening for cervical cancer. This requires a trade-off between preventing influenza-related hospitalizations and deaths, primarily in young children and elderly people, and preventing cases of cervical cancer and consequent deaths in middle-aged women. One approach is to use a generic measure of health-related quality of life such as the **quality-adjusted life-year** (QALY) or **disability-adjusted life-year** (DALY). These aim to capture both the number of life-years lost due to ill health and the loss of quality of life of the years lived; maximizing QALYs thus has the aim of 'adding years to life and life to years'. A **cost–utility**

analysis is a special cost-effectiveness analysis in which the denominator is a generic quality of life measure such as a QALY.

A QALY is calculated by multiplying the amount of time someone spends in a particular health state with a weight representing the quality of life related to that state. This weight normally ranges between 1 (perfect health) and 0 (death), with more severe disease states being associated with lower weights. Various valuation techniques and survey instruments have been developed to elicit weights for different health states.[8]

The DALY is similar to the QALY in that disease states are given a weight between 0 and 1. The difference is that the best state (no disability) is weighted 0 and death is weighted 1. A beneficial intervention thus is said to gain QALYs but avert DALYs.

The DALY is used by international organizations, such as the WHO and Institute for Health Metrics and Evaluation,[9] while QALYs are used mainly in high-income countries. Although costs need to be adjusted for inflation, which means the year, as well as the currency, should be specified (e.g. '2011 USD'), the DALY or QALY associated with disease does not normally change over time.

Even broader comparisons can be made using a **cost–benefit analysis,** in which all the consequences (costs and benefits) of different options are converted into monetary units. The aim is to compare options for allocating resources to health with other uses. The difficulty is the methodological (and some would argue ethical) challenges of converting health into equivalent monetary terms.

Normative considerations in economic evaluations

Some considerations when conducting an economic evaluation are based on value judgements, rather than empirical findings. These are called **normative considerations**.

The economic perspective of the analysis

A **healthcare provider's** or **payer's** perspective only considers costs that accrue to the health sector (whether it is the state, national insurance, or private provider). A wider **societal** perspective considers other costs, such as travel expenses that patients and their families pay to access care, as well as the value of any work lost as a result of sickness. This perspective can make a large difference to the result of an economic evaluation for diseases, such as seasonal influenza, which are usually self-limiting but are responsible for work absenteeism. In some settings, out-of-pocket medical costs and lost earnings may be so catastrophic that families have to fall into debt or sell their assets.[10]

Yet even a societal perspective may be too limited if it only considers healthcare and productivity costs in patients. Such analyses implicitly assume that a person becoming ill has little effect on the wider macroeconomy—the supply of, and demand for, goods, services, and jobs in the economy. In practice, infectious diseases, such as cholera and influenza, can cause large disruptions to the economy when they occur in epidemics or even pandemics.[11]

Discounting

In general, people value having benefits sooner rather than later and would rather pay costs (or have harms) later rather than sooner. Economists call this change in value over time **discounting**. This is implemented in analyses by reducing the incremental costs and benefits of an intervention by a fixed proportion for each year in the future that they occur. The National Institute for Health and Care Excellence (NICE) in the UK recommends discounting both costs and benefits by 3.5% a year, while the WHO uses a rate of 3%.[9] Some countries adopt different rates for discounting costs and benefits. For example, the Netherlands uses a rate of 4% for costs and 1.5% for benefits.

Discounting is particularly important in the evaluation of preventive interventions for which the costs are borne years, or even decades, before the benefits. Vaccination and screening for HBV and HPV are two examples of interventions that look substantially less cost-effective as a result of discounting. Some economists have recommended 'slow' or **hyperbolic** discounting, in which the discount rate decreases over time, so that costs and benefits that occur decades into the future are less severely diminished.[2]

Time horizon of the analysis

This is the period of time over which the costs and effects of the intervention are considered. With non-communicable diseases, the lifetime of the patient is usually an uncontroversial time horizon, as any intervention on a patient is unlikely to have effects that persist beyond the life of the patient. However, with infectious diseases, the indirect consequences of the intervention (such as continuing chains of transmission) may outlive the patient. Indeed, the cost-effectiveness of chickenpox and shingles vaccination is influenced by effects that may accrue a century after the start of vaccination.[12] The potential for global eradication (e.g. smallpox in humans and rinderpest in cattle)—a concept unique to infectious diseases—offers economic benefits that stretch indefinitely into the future, and so vaccination has tremendous value. However, when resources must be apportioned rationally among competing health priorities, it is important not to overvalue these benefits. Unless a finite time horizon and/or non-zero discount rate is used, the benefits of eradicating one disease will always seem to be greater than the benefits from any health intervention that does not result in disease eradication.

Analytical approaches

Economic evaluation can be conducted as part of a clinical trial by incorporating economic outcomes (costs and patient-reported quality-of-life measures) alongside clinical outcomes (see ➲ Chapter 5). However, trials are usually designed to measure effects in individuals, rather than populations. Effects, such as herd immunity (see ➲ Chapter 12), serotype replacement, and the spread of antimicrobial resistance, can only be captured with special designs, such as household or cluster randomized trials, which add costs and limit the external validity. Furthermore, infectious disease interventions, such as vaccination and screening, often have long time lags before their benefits are apparent. Although trials can measure precursors or surrogate markers of the events of interest (such as markers of infection or precancerous cervical lesions), these need to be 'translated' into human and economic benefits.

An alternative (or complementary) method is to use mathematical models to extrapolate the costs and outcomes of an infectious disease intervention. The traditional toolkit of health economic evaluation consists of models, such as decision trees and Markov models,[13] which consider events and health states that represent the natural history of disease and the effects of interventions (Figure 17.1). These are 'static' models, which assume that an individual's risk of acquiring infection is unrelated to the status of other people in the same population. However, **transmission-dynamic** effects mean that intervening in the course of an infection affects not only the recipient of the intervention, but also other people who may potentially contract the infection from that person through indirect population-level ('herd') effects (see ➲ Chapters 12 and 16). This is not relevant when the cases prevented are not infectious and are not relevant for transmission, e.g. tetanus in humans (see ➲ Chapter 12).

Population-level effects can be the **major component** of the benefit of interventions against infectious diseases. In an empirical demonstration of these effects, paediatric vaccination against *Streptococcus pneumoniae* reduced the incidence of disease in older people.[14] However, indirect effects can also be **detrimental**, such as type replacement, and increase in the age of infection which, for some pathogens, is associated with worse outcomes (see ➲ Chapter 12).

Despite the importance of these indirect population-level effects, static models are often used **inappropriately** to model infectious disease interventions. For example, the vast majority of economic evaluations of paediatric influenza and pneumococcal conjugate vaccination used static models.[15,16] One reason for the unpopularity of transmission-dynamic models is that they have substantially greater requirements in terms of expertise, computing power, and data. Transmission-dynamic models generally require information not only on the usual cost and health-related utility implications of a disease, but also the way transmission events occur in a population. As it is usually almost impossible to observe these events directly, models have to be informed by data on contacts relevant to the spread of infectious disease in a population, as well as the relationship between markers of infection history (such as antibodies)

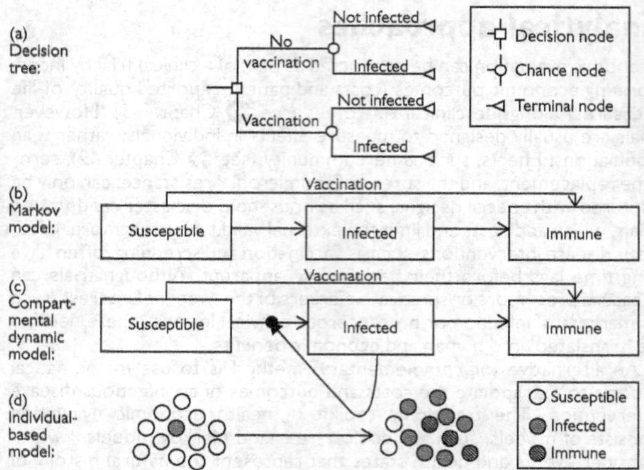

Figure 17.1 Four kinds of models to represent transmission of, and vaccination against, an infection. (a) Decision tree: a cohort of individuals enters the tree, with the flow dividing at decision nodes (based on decisions like whether or not to vaccinate) and chance nodes (based on chance events like whether or not infection occurs), until a terminal node, representing the ultimate outcome, is reached. Note that time is not explicitly represented. (b) Markov model: a cohort of individuals occupies a range of health states, and, through time, there is movement between the states at rates determined by parameters, so that the distribution changes over time. (c) Compartmental (or 'systems dynamics') transmission-dynamic model: similar in structure to Markov models, with the crucial difference that the per-capita rate of infection occurring depends upon the proportion of the population that is infectious and can change over time, as this proportion changes. (d) Individual-based model: individuals in the population are represented as individuals, rather than in aggregate (as in the other models), and individuals transition between different states with probabilities specified by parameters. This type of model might be transmission-dynamic (if the probability of an individual acquiring infection depends upon the number of infectious individuals in the population with whom the person makes contact). The illustration shows the state of the population at two time-points: when one individual is infected in an otherwise naive population, and later when infection has spread to others and some have recovered to immunity.

and disease. They also require complex computational and statistical techniques to estimate parameters from data on these indirect markers.

There are occasions when static models can be applied to infectious diseases. For example, if a static analysis finds that an intervention is incrementally cost-effective, compared to no intervention, with transmission effects, population-level effects that are ignored by the model will be beneficial—so cost-effectiveness is underestimated—and the categorization as cost-effective will be robust (e.g. active case-finding and enhanced patient management for TB).[17] However, transmission-dynamic modelling is still preferable, as subtle effects might not be anticipated. (Clearly, if a static analysis finds that an intervention is not cost-effective, a transmission-dynamic analysis should be performed to avoid concluding wrongly that the intervention is not cost-effective.) Several authors have proposed algorithms that can be used to decide whether a transmission-dynamic model would be more appropriate.[1,2]

Presenting the results of a cost-effectiveness analysis

To be meaningful, the results of cost-effectiveness analyses (e.g. 'adding a vaccine against influenza to the current schedule costs £10 000 per QALY gained') needs to refer to some indication of what ICER would be considered cost-effective. Many countries have an explicit or implicit threshold against which an ICER can be compared; an ICER falling below this threshold would indicate an intervention that is cost-effective. In the UK, NICE has a threshold of £20 000–£30 000 per QALY gained.[18] The WHO has proposed a threshold of the gross domestic product (GDP) per capita in the country of interest for an intervention to be considered 'very cost-effective' and three times the GDP per capita for an intervention to be 'cost-effective'.[9]

Cost-effectiveness analyses should take into account uncertainty in measured parameters and understanding of disease, as reflected in the model's structure. One method for capturing this uncertainty is **probabilistic sensitivity analysis.** This involves taking multiple samples from probability distributions representing uncertainty in the input parameters and then calculating the corresponding ICER for each set of parameter values. The resulting uncertainty can be represented as a 'cloud' of ICERs on a **cost-effectiveness plane** or as a cost-effectiveness acceptability curve (Figure 17.2).

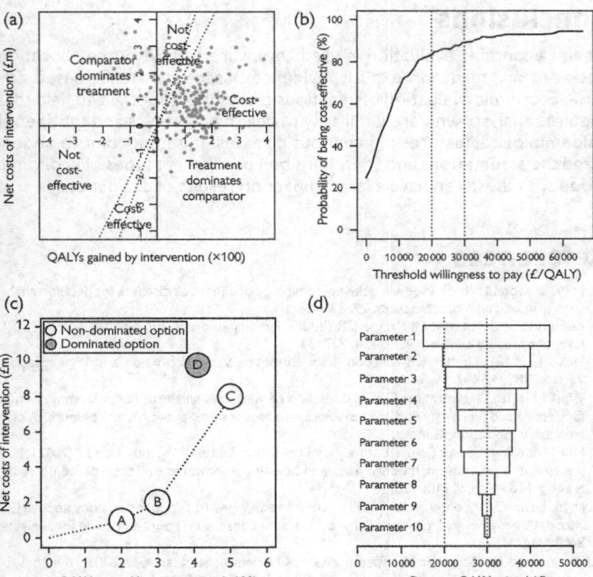

Figure 17.2 Ways to present results of a cost-effectiveness analysis and its associated uncertainty. (a) Cost-effectiveness plane (with cloud of uncertainty): the two axes representing the incremental cost (numerator, vertical axis) and incremental health effects (denominator, horizontal axis) of the ICER, respectively. Points closer to the bottom right of the plane represent choices that are incrementally less expensive but more health-gaining, and hence more likely to be cost-effective. The two dotted lines have gradients corresponding to thresholds defined by policy-makers (e.g. £20 000/QALY gained and £30 000/QALY gained) at which an intervention becomes cost-effective. (b) Cost-effectiveness acceptability curve: this curve represents the proportion of points in the cloud of uncertainty in Figure 17.2(a) that lie below a given threshold (represented by the dotted lines), i.e. the proportion of ICER values that represent a cost-effective choice. As the threshold increases, the probability that the choice will be considered cost-effective also increases. (c) Cost-effectiveness frontier: here a number of options with different costs and health effects are shown on the cost-effectiveness plane. The dominated option is not considered, because it is both more costly and less effective than some combination of the non-dominated options. (d) Tornado plot: illustration of univariate sensitivity analysis, showing which parameters are most influential on the ICER. The bars illustrate how much the estimated ICER changes as each parameter is varied across its defined range.

Conclusions

Health economic evaluation is used to ensure that resource allocation decisions are made on explicit, evidence-based, and needs-based criteria. Economic evaluation of infectious diseases is a specialized field that requires analysts who are familiar with health economics and the special epidemiological features of infectious diseases. It is important to understand the assumptions and limitations behind different types of economic models, as these can have a large impact on results of evaluations.

References

1. Jit M, Brisson M (2011). Modelling the epidemiology of infectious diseases for decision analysis: a primer. *Pharmacoeconomics*, **29**, 371–86.
2. Beutels P, Scuffham PA, MacIntyre CR (2008). Funding of drugs: do vaccines warrant a different approach? *Lancet Infect Dis*, **8**, 727–33.
3. Hall AJ (2010). The United Kingdom Joint Committee on Vaccination and Immunisation. *Vaccine*, **28S**, A54–7.
4. World Health Organization (2013). *Consolidated guidelines on the use of antiretroviral drugs for treating and preventing HIV infection. Recommendations for a public health approach*. World Health Organization, Geneva.
5. HIV Modelling Consortium Treatment as Prevention Editorial Writing Group (2012). HIV treatment as prevention: models, data, and questions—towards evidence-based decision-making. *PLoS Med*, **9**, e1001259.
6. Jit M, Levin C, Brison M, *et al.* (2013). Economic analyses to support decisions about HPV vaccination in low- and middle-income countries: a consensus report and guide for analysts. *BMC Med*, **11**, 23.
7. Drummond MF, Sculpher MJ, Torrance GW, O'Brien BJ, Stoddart GL (2005). *Methods for the economic evaluation of health care programmes*, 3rd edn. Oxford University Press, Oxford.
8. Green C, Brazier J, Deverill M (2000). Valuing health-related quality of life. *Pharmacoeconomics*, **17**, 151–65.
9. Tan-Torres Edejer T, Baltussen R, Adam T, *et al.* (2003). *Making choices in health: WHO guide to cost-effectiveness analysis*. World Health Organization, Geneva.
10. Kruk ME, Goldmann E, Galea S (2009). Borrowing and selling to pay for health care in low- and middle-income countries. *Health Affairs*, **28**, 1056–66.
11. Keogh-Brown M (2014). Macroeconomic effect of infectious disease outbreaks. In: Culyer AJ (ed). *Encyclopedia of health economics*. Elsevier, San Diego, pp. 177–80.
12. Van Hoek AJ, Melegaro A, Gay N, Bilcke J, Edmunds WJ (2012). The cost-effectiveness of varicella and combined varicella and herpes zoster vaccination programmes in the United Kingdom. *Vaccine*, **30**, 1225–34.
13. Barton P, Bryan S, Robinson S (2004). Modelling in the economic evaluation of health care: selecting the appropriate approach. *J Health Services Res*, **9**, 110–18.
14. Lexau CA, Lynfield R, Danila R, *et al.*; Active Bacterial Core Surveillance Team (2005). Changing epidemiology of invasive pneumococcal disease among older adults in the era of pediatric pneumococcal conjugate vaccine. *JAMA*, **294**, 2043–51.
15. Newall AT, Jit M, Beutels P (2012). Economic evaluations of childhood influenza vaccination: a critical review. *Pharmacoeconomics*, **30**, 647–60.
16. Beutels P, Thiry N, Van Damme P (2007). Convincing or confusing? Economic evaluations of childhood pneumococcal conjugate vaccination—a review (2002–2006). *Vaccine*, **25**, 1355–67.

17. Jit M, Stagg HR, Aldridge RW, White PJ, Abubakar I (2011). A dedicated outreach service to hard-to-reach tuberculosis patients in London: observational study and economic evaluation. *BMJ*, **343**, d5376.
18. National Institute for Health and Care Excellence (NICE) (2012). Assessing cost effectiveness. In: *The guidelines manual. NICE article (PMG6)*. Available at: ↗ https://www.nice.org.uk/article/pmg6/chapter/7-assessing-cost-effectiveness (accessed Feb 2015).

Further reading

World Health Organization (2008). *WHO guide for standardization of economic evaluation of immunization programmes*. World Health Organization, Geneva.

Section 2

Epidemiology of Selected Major Diseases

Chapter 18

Respiratory infections

Mary Cooke and John M. Watson

Introduction to respiratory infections

A wide range of infectious organisms, including viruses, bacteria, mycobacteria, and fungi, are responsible for communicable diseases of the respiratory tract. The clinical manifestations of disease vary considerably from mild, self-limiting illness, such as the common cold, to severe infections resulting in pneumonia or acute respiratory distress syndrome. The public health impact of communicable respiratory disease is substantial—coughs and colds are responsible for much sickness absence; lower respiratory tract infections (LRTIs) are the most important cause of global disease burden after ischaemic heart disease, and influenza epidemics and pandemics cause unpredictable and major morbidity and mortality worldwide.[1]

Clinical features

Most communicable diseases of the respiratory tract are the result of upper respiratory tract infections (URTI), LRTIs, or both,[2,3] Many viral infections, such as rhinoviruses and some coronaviruses, result in common colds and coughs affecting the upper respiratory tract.[4] RSV commonly affects the lower respiratory tract, causing, for example, bronchiolitis in infants.[2] Influenza virus infections may cause upper or lower respiratory tract illness, including bronchitis and viral pneumonia.[5]

Bacterial and fungal infections may also affect the upper respiratory tract, causing illnesses such as tonsillitis, but they are more often diagnosed in association with lower respiratory tract illnesses such as bronchitis and pneumonia. TB, a mycobacterial infection, may involve any part of the body but commonly involves the lungs and is transmitted through the respiratory route (Table 18.1).

Respiratory viral infections typically have a short incubation period—up to a few days—and are transmissible to others from around the onset of illness to when symptoms begin to subside. It should be noted that some infections may transmit before symptom onset (see ➔ Chapter 1), e.g. influenza, which presents challenges for their control. Important exceptions to this, such as SARS and MERS-CoV infections, may have longer incubation periods and, in the case of SARS, are infectious predominantly in the period when symptoms are most severe, making control efforts easier.

Bacterial respiratory infections often have longer incubation periods—from a few days to 1 or 2 weeks—but are less easily transmitted. TB may have an incubation period from a few weeks to decades but is usually only transmitted from individuals with pulmonary disease and the organism detectable in sputum.

Table 18.1 Aetiological agents and characteristics of viral and bacterial respiratory infections

Disease agent	Disease/key symptoms	Principal site(s) of disease	Incubation period	Vaccine-preventable
Viruses				
Rhinoviruses	Rhinitis (common cold) Pharyngitis Tonsillitis	Upper respiratory tract	10–48 hours	No
Parainfluenza viruses (I, II, II, and IV)	Rhinorrhoea Cough Pharyngitis Tonsillitis Epiglottitis Laryngitis Bronchitis Bronchiolitis Pneumonia	Upper respiratory tract Lower respiratory tract	2–4 days	No
Coronaviruses	Rhinitis (common cold) Pharyngitis Tonsillitis Cough Myalgia Pneumonia (SARS)	Upper respiratory tract Lower respiratory tract	2–5 days 2–12 days (SARS)	In development (SARS)

Adenoviruses	Rhinitis (common cold) Pharyngitis Tonsillitis Bronchitis Bronchiolitis Pneumonia	Upper respiratory tract Lower respiratory tract	4–8 days	Yes (types 4 and 7 only)
Respiratory syncytial viruses	Rhinitis (common cold) Epiglottitis Laryngitis Bronchitis Bronchiolitis	Upper respiratory tract Lower respiratory tract	3–7 days	In development
Influenza viruses	Rhinitis (common cold) Influenza-like illness Pneumonia	Upper respiratory tract Lower respiratory tract	1–4 days	Yes
Coxsackie virus (group B)	Pharyngitis Tonsillitis	Upper respiratory tract	4 days	No
Epstein–Barr virus	Pharyngitis Tonsillitis	Upper respiratory tract	33–49 days	In development
Herpes simplex virus	Rhinitis (common cold) Pharyngitis Tonsillitis Bronchitis Bronchiolitis Pneumonia	Upper respiratory tract Lower respiratory tract	4–6 days	In development

(Continued)

Table 18.1 (*Contd.*)

Disease agent	Disease/key symptoms	Principal site(s) of disease	Incubation period	Vaccine-preventable
Varicella-zoster virus	Pneumonia	Lower respiratory tract	14–16 days	Yes
Measles virus	Pneumonia	Lower respiratory tract	8–14 days	Yes
Cytomegalovirus	Pneumonia	Lower respiratory tract	4–12 weeks	In development
Hantavirus	Pneumonia	Lower respiratory tract	9–33 days	In development
Bacteria				
Haemophilus influenzae type B	Epiglottitis Laryngitis Bronchitis Bronchiolitis Pneumonia Meningitis Joint infection Cellulitis	Lower respiratory tract	Uncertain	Yes
Corynebacterium diphtheriae	Pharyngitis Tonsillitis Epiglottitis Laryngitis	Upper respiratory tract	2–5 days	Yes
Streptococcus pneumoniae	Bronchitis Bronchiolitis Pneumonia	Lower respiratory tract	Uncertain	Yes

Streptococcus pyogenes	Pneumonia Haemorrhagic pneumonitis Empyema	Lower respiratory tract	2–4 days	In development
Staphylococcus aureus	Pneumonia	Lower respiratory tract	Uncertain	In development
Klebsiella pneumoniae	Pneumonia	Lower respiratory tract	Uncertain	In development
Mycoplasma pneumoniae	Pharyngitis, Tonsillitis Bronchitis, Bronchiolitis Pneumonia	Upper respiratory tract Lower respiratory tract	1–3 weeks	No
Pseudomonas aeruginosa	Pneumonia	Lower respiratory tract	Uncertain	In development
Mycoplasma hominis	Pharyngitis Tonsillitis	Upper respiratory tract	Uncertain	No
Group A β-haemolytic *Streptococcus*	Pharyngitis Tonsillitis	Upper respiratory tract	1–3 days	No
Mycobacterium tuberculosis	Pneumonia	Lower respiratory tract	1–5 years	Yes
Coxiella burnetii	Pneumonia	Lower respiratory tract	1–3 weeks	Yes
Chlamydia psittaci	Pneumonia	Lower respiratory tract	5–14 days	No
Chlamydia pneumoniae	Pneumonia	Lower respiratory tract	7–21 days	No
Legionella spp.	Pneumonia	Lower respiratory tract	2–14 days	No

Source: data from Singh SK. 2014[4]; Sethi S. 2009[5]; Harris JM, Gwaltney JM. 1996[6]; Vainionpää R, Hyypiä T. 1994[7]; Lessler J, Reich NG *et al.* 2009[8]; Meltzer MI. 2004[9]; Tracy S *et al.* 2008[10]; Odumade OA *et al.* 2011[11]; Whitley RJ. 1996[12]; Young JC *et al.* 2000[13]; Bonnet JM and Begg NT. 1999[14]; Twisselmann B. 2009[15]; Kashyap S and Sarkar M. 2010[16]; Choby BA. 2009[17]; Borgdorff MW *et al.* 2011[18]; Maurin M and Raoult D. 1992[19]; Public Health England. 2013[20]; Centres for Disease Control. 2015[21].

Diagnosis

Most communicable respiratory infections require collection of specimens from the upper or lower respiratory tract and/or blood or serum to make a diagnosis.

Point-of-care (POC) tests are not used widely for respiratory diseases in the UK. POC tests for influenza, legionella, RSV, and other infections of the respiratory tract have been developed but are limited by their diagnostic validity (the ability of a test to avoid false-positive or false-negative results; see ➲ Chapter 8) and their clinical practicability.

Laboratory diagnosis varies by infection and may be based on microscopic identification of the organism, other methods to detect the infecting organism directly (such as immunofluorescence), culture of the organism from respiratory specimens or blood, and detection of infection-specific antibodies in serum. Molecular methods, such as PCR, are now used extensively to identify specific infections, and genetic sequencing of the genome of the infecting organism is becoming established for diagnostic, as well as other, purposes[2] (see ➲ Chapters 9 and 10).

Transmission

The commonest routes of transmission are:

- droplets
- droplet nuclei
- direct contact and fomites.

Droplets and droplet nuclei carrying organisms can be expelled via talking, singing, sneezing, coughing, and breathing. The size of the droplet is dependent on environmental conditions, the origin of the droplet and whether it is artificially induced, and individual variability. Droplets >5 micrometres are expelled and tend to fall quickly; thus, infections transmitted in this way, such as influenza, require physical proximity. Smaller droplets, called droplet nuclei, stay airborne for longer and potentially represent a greater transmission risk, e.g. transmission of TB.

Some respiratory viral infections may be transmitted by direct contact through contamination of hands with respiratory secretions, e.g. rhinoviruses are commonly transmitted in this way. Fomites, surfaces that can carry microorganisms, can aid the transmission of respiratory viruses. In certain environmental conditions, some pathogens, such as rhinoviruses, can survive in the environment for a considerable period and infect other individuals, gaining entry through the mouth, nasopharynx, and eyes.

Most people are susceptible to communicable respiratory infections, but previous exposure to some of these infections—and immunization—may protect against infection. Some individuals are at particular risk of severe manifestations of infection such as bronchiolitis in infants, complications of infection resulting in bacterial superinfection (such as bacterial pneumonia that may follow an influenza infection), and exacerbation of underlying chronic illness (such as asthma, chronic bronchitis, diabetes, and ischaemic heart disease).

Some population subgroups are at increased risk as a result of greater likelihood of exposure to infection (such as TB among individuals from parts of the world with high incidence). Immunosuppresion due to illness (such as HIV infection and some cancers) or treatment (such as chemotherapy for cancer) may also render an individual at greater risk of infection.

Many types of respiratory infection represent a challenge when tracking transmission routes in the human population. In some cases, such as TB, the development of molecular typing tools is increasingly helping researchers and public health officials to identify clusters of cases with organisms with similar genetic characteristics and potentially track an infection back to a probable source (see ➔ Chapter 10).

Prevention and control measures

As many communicable respiratory infections are transmitted by respiratory droplets or direct or indirect contact, general respiratory hygiene (covering coughs and sneezes, using tissues, and frequent hand-washing) is an important infection control measure that should be recommended for all members of the population.

Within healthcare settings, good respiratory hygiene may need to be accompanied by a range of specific measures to reduce the risk of infection of other patients, staff, and visitors, depending on the transmission characteristics of the infection and the likely severity of the illness if transmitted (see ➲ Chapter 7). These include adequate ventilation, use of masks or respirators, wearing other elements of personal protective equipment such as masks and gowns, and use of negative pressure ventilation.

In outbreaks of respiratory disease, additional measures may be considered in both the healthcare setting and the community (see ➲ Chapters 3 and 7). In hospitals and other residential settings, patients may need to be 'isolated' (separating those with and without evidence of infection) to reduce the likelihood of further spread of infection. In potential population-wide outbreaks, such as pandemic influenza or the SARS outbreak of 2003, community measures, such as voluntary isolation of people who are ill, school closures, and reduction in mass gatherings, may be recommended, although the extent of the effectiveness of these measures in reducing transmission will vary.

For TB, early identification of active cases and initiating treatment are effective at reducing transmission. In addition, contacts of cases who have been infected but have no evidence of active disease can be identified by testing and offered treatment for their 'latent' infection.

Immunization forms an important part of the prevention of respiratory infections, although vaccines have not yet been developed for some important respiratory pathogens (Table 18.1).

Reporting of microbiologically confirmed diagnoses of respiratory infections provides the backbone of surveillance of these infections. However, many patients with respiratory infections do not present to medical care, and, even if they do, they are not investigated microbiologically. Sentinel surveillance, based on consultation with healthcare providers and defined clinical syndromes, is used to augment microbiological surveillance. Collection of clinical, epidemiological, and microbiological data on reported cases enables investigation of the occurrence of, and risk factors for, respiratory communicable disease in the population. Molecular typing and genomic sequencing of the infecting organisms increasingly contribute to the investigation of transmission of these diseases (see ➲ Chapter 10).

References

1. Murray CJ, Vos T, Lozano R, *et al.* (2012). Disability-adjusted life years (DALYs) for 291 diseases and injuries in 21 regions, 1990–2010: a systematic analysis for the Global Burden of Disease Study 2010. *Lancet*, **380**, 2197–223.
2. Pavia AT (2011). Viral infections of the lower respiratory tract: old viruses, new viruses, and the role of diagnosis. *Clin Infect Dis*, **52**(Suppl 4), S284–9.
3. Annesi-Maesano I, Lundbäck B, Viegi G (eds) (2009). *Respiratory epidemiology.* European Respiratory Society Publications, Sheffield.
4. Singh SK (2014). *Human respiratory viral infections.* Taylor & Francis, Bosa Roca.
5. Sethi S (2009). *Respiratory infections*. Taylor & Francis, New York.
6. Harris JM, Gwaltney JM (1996). Incubation periods of experimental rhinovirus infection and illness. *Clin Infect Dis*, **23**(6), 1287–90.
7. Vainionpää R, Hyypiä T (1994). Biology of parainfluenza viruses. *Clin Microbiol Rev*, **7**(2):265.
8. Lessler J, Reich NG, Brookmeyer R, Perl TM, Nelson KE, Cummings DAT (2009). Incubation periods of acute respiratory viral infections: a systematic review. *Lancet Infect Dis*, **9**(5), 291–300.
9. Meltzer MI (2004). Multiple contact dates and SARS incubation periods. *Emerg Infect Dis*, **10**(2), 207–9. Epub 2004/03/20.
10. Tracy S, Oberste S, Drescher KM (2008). *Group B Coxsackieviruses*. Springer, New York.
11. Odumade OA, Hogquist KA, Balfour HH (2011). Progress and problems in understanding and managing primary Epstein-Barr virus infections. *Clin Microbiol Rev*, **24**(1), 193–209. doi:10.1128/CMR.00044-10.
12. Whitley RJ (1996). Herpesviruses. In: Baron S (ed.), *Medical microbiology.* The University of Texas Medical Branch at Galveston.
13. Young JC, Hansen GR, Graves TK, Deasy MP, Humphreys JG, *et al.* (2000). The incubation period of hantavirus pulmonary syndrome. *Am J Trop Med Hyg*, **62**(6), 714–17.
14. Bonnet JM, Begg NT (1999). Control of diphtheria: guidance for consultants in communicable disease control. World Health Organization. *Commun Dis Public Health*, **2**(4), 242–9.
15. Twisselmann B (2000). Epidemiology, treatment, and control of infection with Streptococcus pyogenes in Germany. *Euro Surveill*, **4**(46), 1490.
16. Kashyap S, Sarkar M (2010). Mycoplasma pneumonia: Clinical features and management. *Lung India*, **27**(2), 75–85.
17. Choby BA (2009). Diagnosis and treatment of streptococcal pharyngitis. *Am Fam Physician*, **79**(5), 383–90. Epub 2009/03/12.
18. Borgdorff MW, Sebek M, Geskus RB, Kremer K, Kalisvaart N, van Soolingen D (2011). The incubation period distribution of tuberculosis estimated with a molecular epidemiological approach. *Int J Epidemiol*, **40**(4), 964–70. Epub 2011/03/29.
19. Maurin M, Raoult D (1992). Q fever. *Clin Microbiol Rev*, **12**(4), 518–53. Epub 1999/10/09.
20. Public Health England. Immunisation against infectious disease: the Green Book. July 2013.
21. Centres for Disease Control (2015). *Vaccine Information Statements*. Available at: ☞ http://www.cdc.gov/vaccines/hcp/vis/index.html (accessed 27 April 2015).

References

Chapter 19

Faeco–oral infections

Emma Meader and Paul Hunter

Introduction to faeco–oral infections

Acute diarrhoea can be defined as the passage of three or more loose stools per day—or more than is normal for the individual—preceded by a symptom-free period of at least 3 weeks. Diarrhoea is regarded as persistent if it lasts longer than 14 days, and as chronic if it lasts longer than 30 days. Many episodes of gastroenteritis are short-lived and self-resolving, which means that patients often do not seek medical attention, so estimates of burden based on cases presenting to health services are underestimates. Studies assessing the true incidence and consequences of infectious diarrhoea by calculating disability-adjusted life-years (DALYs) for each pathogen, which takes into account the short- and long-term consequences of the infection, allow comparability between other causes of morbidity and mortality (see ➲ Chapter 17). Collectively, diarrhoeal diseases account for an annual 89.5 million DALYs across the world, and they remain one of the leading causes of infant mortality.

Besides gastrointestinal infection, diarrhoea is a common symptom of both infectious and non-infectious processes and may also result from disturbances of the normal enteric flora. Routine microbiological analysis will not encompass all possible causes of infectious diarrhoea, and it is important to describe the clinical presentation, with onset dates and risk factors, on test request forms to enable appropriate test selection. The symptoms, patient demographics, and estimated incubation periods can sometimes indicate which pathogen may be implicated (Tables 19.1, 19.2, and 19.3; Figure 19.1).

Table 19.1 Common bacterial pathogens

Organism	Presentation	Patient groups/global burden	Vectors and seasonality	Testing	Treatment and management*
Campylobacter spp. (*C. jejuni* most common)	• Diarrhoea (1–14 days), which may turn bloody • May lead to Guillain–Barré syndrome • Relapses sometimes occur in untreated patients	• All groups • Infants more likely to be affected in developing countries • 7.5 million DALYs	• Undercooked poultry or contaminated cooked/raw products • Commoner in summer months	• Culture of stool (with or without filtration) on selective media, with Gram stain/dark field microscopy or detection by PCR	• Normally self-limiting • Patients who are very unwell may be given erythromycin, azithromycin, or ciprofloxacin
Clostridium difficile	• Normally associated with broad-spectrum antibiotic use (or other drugs/conditions that compromise normal gut flora) • Diarrhoea ensues due to action of two potent enterotoxins, lasts for days to weeks, and normally requires treatment • Relapses are common	• Patients aged >65 years and those with long history of broad-spectrum antibiotic use • Data on global burden not available, but estimated to cause one episode in every 10 000 days in hospital in Europe	• Hardy spores transmitted via faeco–oral route • Transmission readily occurs in hospitals or institutional environments	• Combination of detection of glutamate dehydrogenase, toxins, and lactoferrin (as marker of inflammation)	• Metronidazole • Vancomycin for severe or relapsed disease • Cases should be isolated

(Continued)

Table 19.1 (*Contd.*)

Organism	Presentation	Patient groups/global burden	Vectors and seasonality	Testing	Treatment and management*
Clostridium perfringens	• Diarrhoea via action of enterotoxins produced *in vivo* • Normally lasts <24 hours • May be associated with antibiotics	• All groups • Data on global burden not available, but during 2000–2012, there were, on average, seven outbreaks per year in England and Wales	• Food-borne, typically associated with stews/gravies • Inoculation via food handlers or contaminated animal products	• Detection of organism in stool (>10^6 CFU/mL) or implicated food (10^5 CFU/mL) • Detection of enterotoxin in stool	• Normally self-limiting
Enterotoxigenic Escherichia coli (ETEC)	• Watery diarrhoea via action of toxins, similar to cholera • Usually resolves within a week	• All groups of patients, especially children in developing countries and travellers to those areas • 6.8 million DALYs	• Food, water, and faeco–oral	• Not routine • Enterotoxins can be detected by immunoassay or PCR of genetic elements	• Normally self-resolving • Fluoroquinolones, azithromycin, and rifaximin can be effective for severe infections
Enterohaem-orrhagic, verotoxigenic, Shiga toxin-producing, and Shiga-like toxin-producing *Escherichia coli* (EHEC, VTEC, STEC, and SLTEC)	• Severe watery and bloody diarrhoea lasting for 1 week in adults, but up to 3 weeks in children • About 15% of infected children develop HUS, which typically affects renal function	• Most commonly children and elderly patients in developed countries • Data on global burden not available, but estimated to be 110 DALYs in Europe	• Undercooked beef mince/burgers • Contact with farm animals • Drinking/ recreational water	• Stool sample cultured on sorbitol MacConkey agar (non-fermenters) with latex agglutination • Immunoassay or PCR detection of toxin • O157:H7 is commonest serotype	• Antibiotic therapy is contraindicated • Patients should be isolated, with enteric precautions

Salmonella enterica serovars Enteritidis, and Typhimurium	• Diarrhoea, cramps, nausea, and headaches, often with fever, lasting days to weeks • Some patients may become chronic carriers	• All patient groups • 4.8 million DALYs	• Undercooked or contaminated poultry • Eggs • Person-to-person • Contact with reptiles • Commoner in summer months	• Stool culture on selective media with sugar fermentation profiles • Serotyping and phagotyping • PCR	• Normally self-limiting • Treatment with ciprofloxacin or amoxicillin for severe disease, extraintestinal symptoms, infants aged <2 years, elderly patients, and immuno-compromised patients • Resistant strains emerging
Salmonella enterica serovars Typhi and Paratyphi	• Diarrhoea, often with systemic symptoms, lasting for days to weeks • Some patients may become chronic carriers	• Patients in Asia, Africa, and South America and travellers from those areas • 12.2 million DALYs	• Faeco–oral transmission in water and food (including poultry and eggs) • Raw fruit and vegetables, milk, and shellfish are high-risk	• Stool or blood culture on selective media with sugar fermentation profiles • Serotyping and phagotyping • PCR	• Fluoroquinolones, subject to antimicrobial susceptibility testing

(*Continued*)

Table 19.1 *(Contd.)*

Organism	Presentation	Patient groups/global burden	Vectors and seasonality	Testing	Treatment and management*
Shigella sonnei	• Diarrhoea (which may be bloody) and cramps ± fever lasting for 5–7 days • High mortality in dehydrated, malnourished children	• All patient groups • Commoner in developed world • 7 million DALYs	• Food, water, and person-to-person • Very low infectious dose	• Stool culture on selective media (swiftly processed due to rapid decline in organism viability outside body) with sugar fermentation profiles • Serotyping and phagotyping • PCR	• Only treat severe infections according to local antibiotic sensitivities
Staphylococcus aureus	• Ingestion of preformed heat-stable toxin can cause diarrhoea and cramps • Upper gastrointestinal symptoms often commoner • Normally resolves within 24 hours	• All patient groups • Data on global burden not available, but estimated to be 770 DALYs in the Netherlands alone	• Organism contamination via food handlers, particularly bakery products, cheese, and meat	• Isolation of $>10^5$ organisms per gram of stool/vomitus or implicated food; however, bacteria may have been killed, leaving only the toxin	• Normally self-resolving

Vibrio cholerae O1 and O139	• Heat-labile toxin produced *in vivo* binds to enterocytes and interferes with sodium absorption and chloride secretion, causing profuse watery diarrhoea for days • Dehydration can ensue within hours	• All patient groups returning from endemic countries • 4.4 million DALYs	• Predominantly waterborne	• Stool culture on selective media • PCR detection of toxins	• Severely ill patients may be treated with tetracycline or doxycycline, guided by susceptibility test results

*In addition to rehydration and electrolyte replacement.

CFU, colony-forming unit; DALY, disability-adjusted life-year; EHEC, enterohaemorrhagic *Escherichia coli*; ETEC, enterotoxigenic *Escherichia coli*; HUS, haemolytic–uraemic syndrome; PCR, polymerase chain reaction; SLTEC, Shiga-like toxin-producing *Escherichia coli*; STEC, Shiga toxin-producing *Escherichia coli*; VTEC, verotoxigenic *Escherichia coli*.

Table 19.2 Common viral pathogens

Organism	Presentation	Patient groups (and global burden)	Vectors and seasonality	Test	Treatment and management*
Adenovirus	• Diarrhoea for up to 2 weeks • May be severe enough to require hospitalization	• Children • Data on global burden not available	• Faeco–oral transmission • Common in winter months	• Antigen detection in stool by immunoassay or PCR	• Normally self-limiting
Rotavirus	• Severe diarrhoea lasting up to 2 weeks • Immunization now in childhood vaccination schedule in the UK	• Children older than 3 months • Elderly people • Immunocompromised patients • 18.7 million DALYs	• Faeco–oral transmission	• Stool sample • Antigen detection by immunoassay or PCR	• No specific treatment • Cases should be isolated on paediatric or geriatric wards
Norovirus/ SRVSV	• Sudden vomiting and/or diarrhoea with nausea and aches • Resolves within 48 hours	• All patient groups • Commonest cause of viral diarrhoea in adults • Data on global burden not available, but estimated to be 1480 DALYs in the Netherlands alone	• Faeco–oral transmission	• PCR detection from stool/rectal swabs	• Normally self-limiting • Cases should be isolated

*In addition to rehydration and electrolyte replacement.

DALY, disability-adjusted life-year; PCR, polymerase chain reaction; SRVSV, small, round-structured virus.

Table 19.3 Common parasitic pathogens

Organism	Presentation	Patient groups (and global burden)	Vectors and seasonality	Test	Treatment and management*
Cryptosporidium parvum	• Persistent watery diarrhoea, which can last for months	• All groups • 8.3 million DALYs	• Faeco–oral • Drinking/ recreational water	• Antigen detection in stool by immunoassay or PCR detection • Faecal microscopy ± stain	• Normally self-limiting
Giardia lamblia	• Diarrhoea, bloating, and nausea • Usually resolves within a few days but can become chronic	• All groups, mainly adults • Data on global burden not available, but estimated to be 162 DALYs in the Netherlands alone	• Faeco–oral • Drinking/ recreational water • Commoner in summer and autumn	• Antigen detection in stool by immunoassay or PCR detection • Faecal microscopy ± stain	• Metronidazole or tinidazole

*In addition to rehydration and electrolyte replacement.

DALY, disability-adjusted life-year; PCR, polymerase chain reaction.

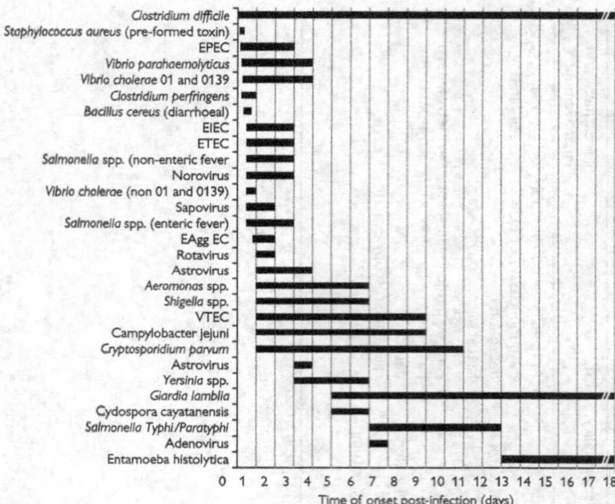

Figure 19.1 Incubation periods for faeco–oral pathogens.

Modes of transmission

Person-to-person

Person-to-person transmission of gastrointestinal pathogens is via the faeco–oral route. Faeces containing the infective agent can contaminate improperly washed hands after toileting or handling contaminated material, which can then transfer to inanimate objects or surfaces such as door handles. Viable pathogens can be picked up by others and then ingested via hand-to-mouth contact. This pathway is a significant route of transmission for all enteric pathogens, especially norovirus, and spread is hard to control when sanitation standards are poor.

Food

Food-borne transmission can occur via ingestion of raw/undercooked produce that is intrinsically contaminated with a pathogen such as *Salmonella* spp. and *Campylobacter* spp. in poultry, *Escherichia coli* in beefburgers, and norovirus via filter-feeding shellfish. Products can also be contaminated by food handlers, e.g. salad prepared by someone infected with norovirus who has not washed their hands adequately. Washing food products in untreated water can also lead to contamination. Improper storage of products contaminated by food handlers can give rise to growth of pathogen and production of toxins such as *Staphylococcus aureus* in fresh cream.

Water

Waterborne transmission is the primary route for *Vibrio cholerae*, and outbreaks are common in the developing world. Human and/or animal faecal contamination of untreated water supplies can serve as an efficient vector for any enteric pathogen. Parasitic infections are particularly common, even in treated water supplies, as *Cryptococcus parvum* and *Giardia lamblia* are resistant to chlorine disinfection and can be difficult to eradicate.

Zoonotic

Zoonotic infections, which arise from contact with colonized/infected animals, have been known to occur for *E. coli*, *Salmonella* spp., *Campylobacter* spp., *G. lamblia*, and *C. parvum*. Outbreaks of verotoxigenic *E. coli* (VTEC) have been well described in children who have visited petting farms/zoos.

Boxes 19.1 and 19.2 describe two examples of faeco–oral infections in two different settings.

Box 19.1 Outbreak in a nursing home

An elderly resident in a nursing home presented with sudden-onset vomiting and diarrhoea with stomach cramps. The residents have separate rooms but eat their meals and spend most of the day in communal areas. The following day, two more residents presented with the same symptoms, and two members of staff phoned in sick, complaining of vomiting and/or diarrhoea. The cases were nursed in their rooms after they became unwell, and a clinical clean was undertaken in the communal areas at this time. On day 4, another two residents developed diarrhoea. Communal areas were clinically cleaned again. No further cases presented after day 4. The symptoms in each case lasted for no longer than 24 hours.

What is the likely causative agent?

Norovirus is the most likely candidate due to the sudden-onset diarrhoea and/or vomiting, the short-lived symptoms, and the fact that it affected both elderly residents and healthy adults. As the symptoms were short-lived and cases presented within a short time frame, person-to-person transmission may have been occurring with an incubation period as short as 12 hours.

What is the best specimen for diagnosis?

A faecal sample or rectal swab from symptomatic cases submitted for polymerase chain reaction (PCR).

Should cases be treated?

There is no treatment, so management is purely supportive. Infections in healthy adults should resolve uneventfully. The very young and very old, as well as immunosuppressed patients and those with comorbidities, should be reviewed by a doctor for evidence of dehydration and malnutrition.

What infection control precautions and interventions are indicated for this kind of outbreak?

Due to the highly infectious nature of norovirus, cases should be isolated in separate rooms with enteric precautions. In institutional environments, cases and recovered cases from the same outbreak can be cohort-nursed. Cases are considered infectious for 48 hours after the symptoms have resolved. Notify suspected outbreaks and confirmed cases to the local health protection authority.

Cleaning of areas potentially contaminated with norovirus should comprise a detergent-based clean to remove protein matter, followed by cleaning with bleach to inactivate the viral particles. All floors, surfaces, and equipment should be cleaned, paying particular attention to hand rails, light switches, and door handles.

Box 19.2 Outbreak in children

A 4-year-old child was taken to the general practitioner with diarrhoea, vomiting, and abdominal pains. The child's 3-year-old friend also had symptoms of diarrhoea, as well as a fever. The parents and an older sibling did not have any symptoms. Three days earlier, the family had visited a petting farm, with cattle, goats, poultry, and rabbits. The child's symptoms did not improve, and the diarrhoea became bloody. The child was admitted to hospital on day 4 after the onset of symptoms. On day 13 after symptom onset, the child developed evidence of renal insufficiency.

What is the likely cause?

The symptoms and patient demographics, with a recent history of contact with cattle and other farm animals, are highly indicative of verotoxigenic *Escherichia coli* (VTEC).

What is the best specimen for diagnosis?

As VTEC is a hazard group 3 pathogen, a stool sample from the child should be sent to the laboratory, clearly noting the suspicion of VTEC to ensure that correct containment is employed during sample processing.

Should cases be treated?

Antimicrobials are contraindicated, and treatment is purely supportive.

What infection control precautions and interventions are indicated for this kind of outbreak?

General practitioners are responsible for notifying cases of bloody diarrhoea or suspected VTEC to the health protection authorities. Confirmed cases should be notified by the testing laboratory. These actions help to ensure that control measures can be put in place to prevent any further infections such as temporary closure of any implicated facilities. Cases must be isolated, with enteric precautions to prevent person-to-person spread, and any close contacts and other possible cases should be tested.

Prevention

Water treatment

The provision of effective, well-maintained water treatment facilities is the single greatest way of reducing cases of infectious diarrhoea. In areas where this has not yet been introduced, water filtration (with the smallest pore size possible) and/or boiling (for at least 1 minute, but longer at high altitudes) can reduce the number of, and inactivate, enteric pathogens. Chlorine- or iodine-based treatments can also be effective, as long as turbidity has been reduced as much as possible (by filtration or sedimentation) and adequate contact times are adhered to in line with recommendations.

Good standards of toileting and hand-washing facilities

By providing and maintaining contained latrines or toilets, contamination of the surrounding environmental and water supplies can be greatly reduced. This should also be accompanied by provision of hand-washing facilities and educating communities about how these resources can reduce the transmission of enteric pathogens.

Food hygiene

Food handlers must be educated about how infectious diarrhoea is transmitted and fully trained to implement the control measures required to prevent it. This includes good standards of hygiene, especially hand hygiene, at all times. Any wounds or infective lesions should be cleansed and covered, and fingernails should be kept clean and short. Long hair should be tied back.

Sourcing produce from certified and well-maintained premises, using thermometers to ensure food has reached the required cooking temperature, dividing up large batches for rapid chilling after cooking, and storing food in suitable refrigerators (with regular temperature checks) will all help to minimize the risks of transmitting enteric pathogens. If food handlers suffer from gastroenteritis, they must be excluded from work until at least 48 hours after their symptoms have resolved, and diagnostic specimens should be taken if a bacterial or parasitic cause is suspected. It is also important to educate communities about safe handling of food to help reduce the frequency of infectious diarrhoea in the home and transmission to close contacts.

Vaccination

Vaccinations are available for some pathogens and may be of particular benefit to travellers in endemic regions and to help contain spread in outbreak situations. A single-dose vaccine (based on the Vi capsular polysaccharide) is available to protect against *Salmonella enterica* serovar Typhimurium; it is sometimes combined with hepatitis A immunization.

A vaccination for *V. cholerae* (01 serogroup only), available as a two- to three-dose schedule, with doses given 6 weeks apart, is based on killed whole cells with a recombinant B subunit of the cholera toxin. It is up to 85% efficacious, but this depends on the nutritional and immunological status of the host and the nature of the exposures. Protection lasts about 2 years, but booster doses may be given. It also provides some cross-protection against the effects of enterotoxigenic *E. coli* (ETEC).

Two rotavirus vaccinations are available: monovalent Rotarix and pentavalent RotaTeq. A two-dose schedule is now part of the routine childhood immunization programmes in the USA and UK, and this has had a considerable impact in terms of reducing the number of consultations, hospitalizations, and complications due to rotavirus infection in children.

In China only, a bivalent *Shigella flexneri* and *Shigella sonnei* vaccination is licensed. Vaccine development is problematic due to the abundance of different serotypes of *Shigella* spp.

Vaccination of animals can also be considered to help reduce contamination of meat products such as immunization of chicken flocks against *Salmonella* spp.

Surveillance and screening

In the UK, 25% of the population is estimated to develop infectious gastroenteritis every year, and about 2% of these patients will seek medical attention, some of whom also submit specimens for investigation. Significant results from clinical diagnostic laboratories are sent to local health protection teams for the purpose of surveillance, but about 147 other cases are estimated to exist in the community for every one that is notified.

Suspicious clinical presentations, such as haemolytic–uraemic syndrome (HUS) or bloody diarrhoea, and suspected cases of food poisoning are also notified by GPs. This helps to highlight clusters of cases early and initiates investigation of possible sources and preventative measures. An alternative approach to surveillance is via sales figures of antidiarrhoeal medications, as is the case in France. However, this method is subject to many confounding variables, including advertising.

In some cases, screening may serve as an effective preventative strategy, e.g. screening of patients for the presence of *Clostridium difficile* via glutamate dehydrogenase to assess their risk of developing the infection, which allows appropriate selection of antimicrobial therapy. Screening hospital environments for *C. difficile* and norovirus, to ensure adequate cleaning of patient areas, can also be useful (see ➲ Chapter 7). Screening water supplies for *Cryptosporidium parvum* can also help to highlight problems early and prevent outbreaks.

Diagnosis and treatment

Diagnosis of the cause of acute diarrhoea is based on laboratory examination of stool, rather than clinical grounds, due to the similarities of the clinical features.

Antimicrobial therapy for most infectious agents is not normally indicated, but there are some exceptions (Tables 19.1 and 19.3). Rehydration and electrolyte replacement are indicated in all cases of infectious diarrhoea, the method of which depends on the severity of the symptoms and should be subject to medical assessment. Elemental zinc supplements are sometimes recommended for children after episodes of severe diarrhoea.

Further reading

Bouza E (2012). Consequences of *Clostridium difficile* infection: understanding the healthcare burden. *Clin Microbiol Infect*, **18**, 5–12.

Centers for Disease Control and Prevention (2015). *Diseases and conditions*. Available at: ℜ http://www.cdc.gov/DiseasesConditions/ (accessed 4 April 2014).

Havelaar AH, Haagsma JA, Mangen MJJ, *et al.* (2012). Disease burden of foodborne pathogens in the Netherlands, 2009. *Int J Food Microbiol*, **156**, 231–8.

Heyman D (2008). *Control of communicable diseases manual*, 19th edn. American Public Health Association, Washington, DC.

Mandell GL, Bennett JE, Dolne R (2009). *Mandell, Douglas, and Bennett's principles and practice of infectious diseases*, 7th edn. Churchill Livingstone, London.

Mangen MJJ, Plass D, Havelaar AH, *et al.* (2013). The pathogen- and incidence-based DALY approach: an appropriated methodology for estimating the burden of infectious diseases. *PLoS One*, **8**, e79740.

Murray C, Vos T, Lozano R, *et al.* (2012). Disability-adjusted life years (DALYs) for 291 diseases and injuries in 21 regions, 1990–2010: a systematic analysis for the Global Burden of Disease Study 2010. *Lancet*, **380**, 2197–223.

Nataro JP, Kaper JB (1998). Diarrheagenic *Escherichia coli*. *Clin Microbiol Rev*, **11**, 142–201.

Patel M, Steele D, Gentsch JR, Wecker J, Glass RI, Parashar UD (2011). Real world impact of rotavirus vaccination. *Pediatr Infect Dis J*, **30**(Suppl), S1–S5.

Poitrineau P, Forestier C, Meyer M, *et al.* (1995). Retrospective case-control study of diffusely adhering *Escherichia coli* and clinical features in children with diarrhea. *J Clin Micro*, **33**, 1961–2.

Public Health England. *Infectious diseases*. Available at: ℜ https://www.gov.uk/health-protection/infectious-diseases (accessed 4 April 2014).

Tam CC, Rodrigues LC, Viviani L, *et al.* (2012). Longitudinal study of infectious intestinal disease in the UK (IID2 study): incidence in the community and presenting to general practice. *Gut*, **61**, 69–77.

van Lier EA, Havelaar AH, Nanda A (2007). The burden of infectious diseases in Europe: a pilot study. *Euro Surveill*, **12**, E3–4.

Vila J, Ruiz J, Gallardo F, *et al.* (2003). *Aeromonas* spp. and travelers' diarrhoea: clinical features and antimicrobial resistance. *Emerg Infect Dis*, **9**, 552–5.

Wilcox MH, Cook AM, Eley A, Spencer RC (1992). *Aeromonas* spp. as a potential cause of diarrhoea in children. *J Clin Pathol*, **45**, 959–63.

Chapter 20

Vector-borne infections

Maria Gloria Teixeira

Introduction to vector-borne infections

Through human history, vector-borne diseases (VBDs) have been a major cause of morbidity and mortality. VBDs are caused by parasites, viruses, and bacteria transmitted to humans by arthropods, usually blood-sucking insects. In the first half of the 20th century, the discovery of the epidemiological chain man–mosquito–man for malaria enabled disease control through strategies which interrupted the transmission cycle through the elimination of vectors.[1] Several of these pathogens have re-emerged as important public health problems. Estimates suggest that 17% of the current burden of infectious diseases[2] is due to VBDs. This chapter discusses six VBDs of global public health importance: malaria, dengue, visceral leishmaniasis, Chagas' disease, sleeping sickness, and yellow fever (Tables 20.1 and 20.2).

Table 20.1 Characteristics of vector-borne diseases of greatest epidemiological importance in the world

Disease/agents	Main vectors	Incubation periods	Reservoirs	Main diagnostic tests	Treatment
Malaria *Plasmodium falciparum* *P. vivax* *P. malariae* *P. ovale*	• *Anopheles darling* • *A. aquasalis* • *A. gambiae* • *A. albitarsis* • *A. cruzii* • *A. belator*	• 7–30 days (depending on which *Plasmodium* spp.)	• Man	• Parasitological • Thick drop • Smear • RDT	• Chloroquine • Artemisinin • Primaquine, etc.
Dengue DENV 1, 2, 3, and 4	• *Aedes aegypti* • *A. albopictus*	• 3–15 days	• Man and mosquitoes	• NS1 MAC-ELISA (IgM) • Dose-matched IgG • PCR • Cell culture	• No specific treatment • Antipyretic/analgesic • Fluid replacement
Visceral leishmaniasis (kala-azar) *Leishmania chagasi* *L. infantum* *L .tropica* *L .donovani*	• Sandflies • *Phlebotomus argentipes* and *P. orientalis* • *P. martini* and *P. celiae*	• Ranges from weeks to months	• Dogs, marsupials, and foxes	• Parasitological • Serological	• Antimonate *N*-methyl-glucamine (first choice) • Amphotericin B

(*Continued*)

Table 20.1 (*Contd.*)

Disease/agents	Main vectors	Incubation periods	Reservoirs	Main diagnostic tests	Treatment

Chagas' disease/ American trypanosomiasis
Trypanosoma cruzi
	• Triatomine bugs:
	  • *Triatoma infestans*
	  • *Rhodinus prolixus*
	  • *Panstrongylus megistus*
		• Vector: 4–15 days
		• Blood transfusion: 30–40 days
		• Vertical: any time during pregnancy or delivery
		• Oral: 3–22 days
		• Accidental: about 20 days
			• Man and >150 species of wild and domestic mammals	• Parasitological
				• Serological
					• Acute form: benznidazole, nifurtimox
					• Chronic form: no specific treatment

African trypanosomiasis/ sleeping sickness *Trypanosoma brucei gambiense* *T. b. rhodesiense*	• Tsetse fly • *Glossina* genus	• Months to years • 3 days to some weeks	• Cattle and other wild and domestic animals	• Parasitological • Serological	• First stage: pentamidine (*T. b. gambiense*), suramin (*T. b. rhodesiense*) • Second stage: eflornithine (*T. b. gambiense*); nifurtimox–eflornithine (*T. b. gambiense*)
Yellow fever Yellow fever virus	• *Aedes aegypti* (urban) • Different species of *Haemogogus* (wild)	• 3–6 days	• Monkeys	• MAC-ELISA (IgM) • Dose-matched IgG ELISA • RT-PCR • Cell culture • Tissue samples immunohistochemistry	• No specific treatment other than supportive care

DENV, dengue virus; ELISA, enzyme-linked immunosorbent assay; MAC-ELISA, M antibody capture enzyme-linked immunosorbent assay; NS1, non-structural protein 1; PCR, polymerase chain reaction; RDT, rapid detection test; RT-PCR, reverse transcription polymerase chain reaction.

Table 20.2 Burden, prevention, and control of vector-borne diseases of greatest epidemiological importance in the world

Disease/agents	Regions/countries most affected	Estimates of cases and deaths	Prevention and control
Malaria *Plasmodium falciparum* *P. vivax* *P. malariae* *P. ovale*	• 97 countries worldwide • Africa: 95% of all cases • South Africa more affected • South America and South Asia	• 207 million cases • 627 000 deaths • 3.7 billion at risk	• Environmental management strategies to eliminate vectors • Personal protective measures (repellents and mosquito nets) • Control blood products • Early diagnosis and treatment • Chemoprophylaxis (sulfadoxine–pyrimethamine)
Dengue • DENV 1, 2, 3, and 4	• >100 countries in Americas, South East Asia and Western Pacific	• 100 million cases • 500 000 severe forms • 12 500 deaths • 2.4 billion at risk	• Environmental management strategies to eliminate vectors • Personal protective measures (repellents, mosquito nets) • Early diagnosis and treatment
Visceral leishmaniasis (kala-azar) *Leishmania chagasi* *L. infantum* *L .tropica* *L .donovani*	• Bangladesh, Brazil, Ethiopia, India, South Sudan, and Sudan represent 80% of cases	• 300 000 cases • 30 000 deaths	• Environmental management strategies to eliminate vectors • Control of reservoir hosts (mainly infected dogs) • Personal protective measures (repellents and mosquito nets) • Early diagnosis and treatment

(Continued)

Table 20.2 (*Contd.*)

Disease/agents	Regions/countries most affected	Estimates of cases and deaths	Prevention and control
Chagas' disease/ American trypanosomiasis • *Trypanosoma cruzi*	• America: Mexico to southern Argentina	• 10 million cases	• Environmental management strategies to eliminate vectors • Control plant foods in endemic areas • Control blood products
African trypanosomiasis/ sleeping sickness *Trypanosoma brucei gambiense* • *T. b. rhodesiense*	• 36 countries in sub-Saharan Africa	• 70 million at risk • 20 billion cases • 7216 notifications in 2012 • 6314 notifications in 2013	• Human treatment • Vector control • Control of infection in the animal reservoir
Yellow fever • Yellow fever virus	• About 32 countries in sub-Saharan Africa and ten countries in South and Central Americas	• 200 000 cases and 30 000 deaths	• Yellow fever vaccine

DENV, dengue virus.

Malaria

The symptomatic phase of malaria (**infection period**) manifests with malaise, fatigue, myalgia, and fever, followed by characteristic paroxysmal attacks involving fever (which can reach 41°C) and chills, accompanied by generalized tremors lasting 15–60 minutes, then intense sweating. The temperature then declines (**remission period**), with the patient feeling an improvement. New episodes of paroxysmal attacks occur at varied intervals (hours to some days), with a state of intermittent fever. Without appropriate and timely specific treatment, the signs and symptoms may evolve to serious and complicated forms (**toxaemic period**), depending on the immune response, increase in parasitaemia, and species of *Plasmodium* involved. Signs of severe and complicated malaria are hyperpyrexia (temperature >41°C), convulsions, hyperparasitism (>200 000/mm^3), repeated vomiting, oliguria, dyspnoea, severe anaemia, jaundice, bleeding, and hypotension, and, with *P. falciparum*, potentially altered consciousness, delirium, coma, and death.[3]

Dengue

Dengue fever (DF) is an acute febrile disease. Most cases are benign and self-limited, but some cases evolve to severe, highly lethal forms (dengue haemorrhagic fever (DHF)/dengue shock syndrome (DSS)).

DF begins with a high fever (39–40°C), followed by a headache, myalgia, prostration, arthralgia, anorexia, asthenia, and retro-orbital pain. Nausea, vomiting, skin rash (40% of cases), and hepatomegaly can also occur. At the end of the febrile period, which lasts 5–7 days, a few haemorrhagic manifestations (petechiae, epistaxis, gingival bleeding, and menorrhagia) may occur, more often among adults. Convalescence is accompanied by physical weakness that lasts for several weeks.

On day 3 or 4, however, some cases of DF exhibit signs and symptoms that indicate the development of DHF—sudden disappearance of fever, abdominal pain, persistent vomiting, hypotension, and major bleeding—due to increased vascular permeability, followed by extraordinary plasma leakage shown by haemoconcentration, effusions, hypoalbuminaemia, and circulatory failure. Some cases of DHF develop into DSS, which usually is expressed by cold extremities, cyanosis, rapid and weak pulse, agitation, lethargy, hypovolaemia, hypothermia, and respiratory distress. The duration of DHF is short, and death can occur within 12–24 hours. Serial tests of haematocrit, platelet count, and measurement of albumin are required to determine the severity of the condition and to monitor patients with the warning symptoms of evolution to DHF.[4]

Chikungunya

Chikungunya is an emergent disease characterized by abrupt onset of high fever (39–40°C) and joint pain, accompanied by headache, rash, muscle pain, and fatigue. Frequently, the joint pain is very severe, symmetrical, over a group of joints, and accompanied by oedema (no redness or heat), stiffness, and debilitation. It can last for a few days or for weeks and so cause acute, subacute, or chronic disease. After the acute phase, some patients present with fatigue, lasting several weeks. Comorbidities, such as hypertension, diabetes, or heart disease, are risk factors for chronic chikungunya and poor outcomes, mainly in older individuals. Transmission during birth can result in severe neonatal disease. Deaths from chikungunya are rare.

In the acute phase, the clinical signs of chikungunya can be misdiagnosed as dengue in areas where dengue is endemic-epidemic.

Visceral leishmaniasis

In endemic areas, some cases of visceral leishmaniasis (VL) have discrete clinical symptoms, including fever of short duration of about 15 days (**initial period**), which evolves into spontaneous healing (oligosymptomatic). However, VL is most often characterized by irregular fever of long duration, mucocutaneous pallor, hepatosplenomegaly, weight loss, and progressive impairment of the patient's general status (**state period**).

Without specific treatment, the disease progresses to the **final period**, with continuous fever and intense impairment of general health. Patients develop malnutrition (with brittle hair, dry skin, and elongated eyelashes), lower limb oedema, which can progress to anasarca, bleeding (epistaxis, gingival bleeding, and petechiae), jaundice, and ascites. Death usually results from associated bacterial infections that progress to sepsis and/or bleeding, most commonly epistaxis and gingival bleeding secondary to thrombocytopenia. Jaundice and gastrointestinal bleeding, when present, indicate severe disease.

From the onset of disease, laboratory tests reveal pancytopenia, hypergammaglobulinaemia, and increased erythrocyte sedimentation rate. Immunosuppression caused by HIV (see ➲ Chapter 25) modifies the progression of VL, with frequent involvement of organs outside the mononuclear phagocyte system and post-treatment relapse of VL.

Parasitological diagnosis is based on investigations for amastigote forms of the parasite in specimens obtained from the bone marrow, lymph node, or spleen. In East Africa and India, a macular, papular, or nodular rash or skin lesions (on the face, upper arms, and trunk, etc.) often appear 6 months, or even years, after apparent cure of the disease. This indicates post-kala-azar dermal leishmaniasis (PKDL). These lesions are very rich in parasites, are an important source of infection, and are difficult to treat.[5]

Chagas' disease

The point of entry of *Trypanosoma cruzi* to the human body is marked by a 'chagoma' (skin lesion) or 'Romana sign' (palbebral oedema). The acute phase (**initial phase**) is characterized by prolonged fever (lasting up to 12 weeks), with a large number of parasites found in the bloodstream. Signs and symptoms may disappear spontaneously or progress to severe forms with acute myocarditis and/or meningoencephalitis, which, if left untreated, can lead to death.

After many years without symptoms (**indeterminate phase**), trypanosomiasis can progress to a chronic phase, in which parasites in the bloodstream are rare. About 30% of infections progress to dilated cardiomyopathy and congestive heart failure (CHF), the main cause of mortality in patients with Chagas' disease. About 10% develop a digestive form, characterized by the presence of mega-oesophagus and/or megacolon. These two forms may occur concomitantly.[6]

Sleeping sickness

After a bite from an infected fly, the *Trypanosoma brucei* spp. parasite multiplies locally for about 3 days; it may cause a red sore (a 'chancre') lasting up to 3 weeks. About half of infections caused by *T. b. rhodesiense* have a chancre, but few of those caused *by T. b. gambiense*.

Parasites multiply in the lymph and blood; at this early stage, patients may have no clinical symptoms or present with headache, fever, weakness, arthralgia, enlarged lymph nodes, and irritability. Subsequently, the parasite crosses the cerebrospinal barrier, penetrating the central nervous system and causing neurological disorders (psychiatric disorders, changes in the sleep cycle, confusion, chills, changes in gait and speech, seizures, and coma), which can lead to death when untreated. Although infections caused by *T. b. rhodesiense* (2% of cases) manifest as acute illness that lasts for a few weeks or months, *T. b. gambiense* (98% of cases) produces chronic disease that usually lasts several years with or without clinical manifestations.[7,8]

Yellow fever

The characteristic clinical features of yellow fever—urban or wild—are fever (usually biphasic), with its sudden onset accompanied by chills, headaches, back pain, generalized myalgia, prostration, nausea, and vomiting (**prodromal period**).

In general, after 3 days, there is a decline in temperature and remission of symptoms, causing a sense of improvement in the patient. This remission lasts a few hours or 1–2 days at most, and symptoms soon reappear in the form of fever, diarrhoea, and vomiting, with the appearance of coffee grounds (**toxaemic period**), hepatorenal failure (evidenced by jaundice, oliguria, anuria, and albuminuria), haemorrhagic manifestations (gum bleeding, nosebleeds, otorragias, haematemesis, melaena, haematuria, and bleeding at venepuncture sites), severe prostration, and sensory impairment with mental obtundation and stupor. The pulse becomes slower, despite the high temperature (Faget sign). More than 50% of clinical cases of yellow fever progress to coma and death.[9]

Global burden

Annually, more than one billion people are infected with VBDs. Tropical and subtropical areas of the world are disproportionately affected, which have about 80% of cases (Table 20.1) and deaths from VBDs (Figure 20.1).[10] This distribution is partly due to climatic conditions in this part of the globe, which favour the proliferation of mosquito vectors, making them more receptive to the establishment of transmission cycles. The transmission-dynamics of VBDs in human populations is particularly complex, because each of the agents involved live in very different ecological niches. For example, yellow fever has two transmission cycles, wild and urban, each with specific mosquitoes, although the yellow fever virus is the same.

The WHO estimates that malaria is the VBD with the highest incidence and mortality, while DF is the fastest growing VBD, with a 30-fold increase in incidence in the past 50 years.[10] Leishmaniasis is considered among the most neglected diseases, affecting mainly people living below the poverty line in Africa. Despite the availability of safe and efficacious vaccines, yellow fever continues to cause about 30 000 deaths each year. The vectorial transmission of Chagas' disease was interrupted in some Latin American countries, but the severity of the chronic disease it produces and the number of individuals infected in the past still means a very high burden of this disease.

From 2012, Zika virus (ZIKV) emerged from Africa producing epidemics in the South Pacific islands (Yap, French Polynesia), and in 2014, in several cities in north-eastern Brazil. This arbovirus, also transmitted by Aedes aegypti, has similar clinical manifestations to Dengue and Chikungunya. It has triggered a major public health emergency because it has become apparent that it is associated with Guillain-Barré syndrome and potentially related to a severe microcephaly epidemic (with nearly 6000 notified cases by February 2016) in newborns to mothers resident in Brazilian cities where this flavivirus has circulated in large numbers.

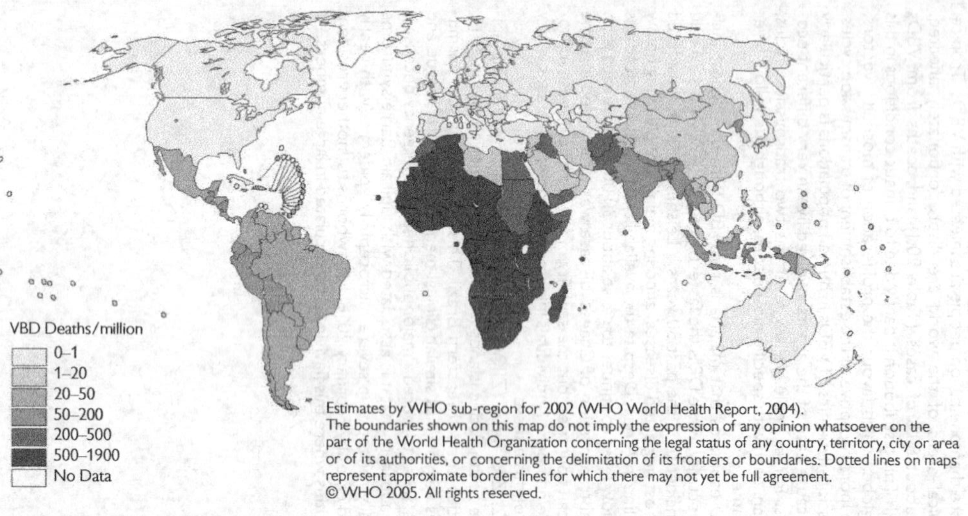

VBD Deaths/million
0–1
1–20
20–50
50–200
200–500
500–1900
No Data
Estimates by WHO sub-region for 2002 (WHO World Health Report, 2004).
The boundaries shown on this map do not imply the expression of any opinion whatsoever on the part of the World Health Organization concerning the legal status of any country, territory, city or area or of its authorities, or concerning the delimitation of its frontiers or boundaries. Dotted lines on maps represent approximate border lines for which there may not yet be full agreement.
© WHO 2005. All rights reserved.

Figure 20.1 Deaths from vector-borne disease.

Reproduced with permission from World Health Organization (WHO), *Priority risks maps: Vector-borne disease*, Copyright © WHO 2005, available from http://www.who.int/heli/risks/risksmaps/en/index1.html.

Surveillance and epidemiological investigation

Surveillance of VBDs should be made via case reporting (national information systems) and monitoring, with a view to eliminating the vectors and animal reservoirs in environments populated by people (see ➲ Chapter 2). Field epidemiological investigations are essential when cases are suspected in non-endemic areas and for outbreaks in endemic areas in order to adopt prompt and appropriate vector control interventions, help patients, prevent occurrence of new cases, and reduce the transmission threshold of the agent.[10,11]

International travel and vector-borne disease

Visitors to areas with high incidence of VBDs should take precautions to protect their health, which will vary according to the circulating pathogen. These precautions may include personal protection against insects, malaria chemoprophylaxis, considering the safety of different environmental settings, choosing to stay in places with reduced environmental risk, etc. Vaccination for yellow fever is mandatory for patients visiting countries where it is present. Travellers who develop fever should seek immediate medical attention for treatment and to prevent progression.

Challenges and prospects

The emergence and re-emergence of some VBDs in countries outside of the tropical and subtropical areas, combined with maintenance of high rates of transmission and mortality in historically affected countries, present a challenge. Although climate change is highlighted as a determining factor in this expansion, many of the key factors behind this phenomenon were anthropogenic, related to the rapid flow of human populations, animals, and goods between countries and continents and lifestyles in large urban centres, among other reasons.[1,2] The emergence of West Nile virus and DF in the USA is evidence of the geographical spread of vectors and pathogens[1] formerly confined to the tropics. The lack of vaccines for most VBDs and the failure of previous control programmes indicate that it will be very difficult to reduce the burden of these diseases and control the geographic expansion process in the short or medium term. Reversing this trend is one of the main challenges for public health in the 21st century.

References

1. Gubler DJ (1998). Resurgent vector-borne diseases as a global health problem. *Emerg Infect Dis*, **4**, 442–50.
2. World Health Organization (2014). *About vector-borne diseases*. Available at: http://www.who.int/campaigns/world-health-day/2014/vector-borne-diseases/en/ (accessed 30 January 2015).
3. Trampuz A, Jereb M, Muzlovic I, Prabhu RM (2003). Clinical review: severe malaria. *Crit Care*, **7**, 315–23.
4. Teixeira MG, Barreto ML (2009). Diagnosis and management of dengue. *BMJ*, **339**, b4338.
5. Chappuis F, Sundar S, Hailu A, *et al.* (2007). Visceral leishmaniasis: what are the needs for diagnosis, treatment and control? *Nat Rev Microbiol*, **5**, 873–82.
6. Prata A (2001). Clinical and epidemiological aspects of Chagas disease. *Lancet Infect Dis*, **1**, 92–100.
7. World Health Organization (>2015). *Human African trypanosomiasis: symptoms, diagnosis and treatment*. Available at: http://www.who.int/trypanosomiasis_african/diagnosis/en/ (accessed on 30 January 2015).
8. Fèvre EM, Wissmann BV, Welburn SC, Lutumba P (2008). The burden of human African trypanosomiasis. *PLoS Negl Trop Dis*, **12**, e333.
9. Monath TP (2001). Yellow fever: an update. *Lancet Infect Dis*, **1**, 11–20.
10. World Health Organization. *A global brief on vector-borne diseases*. Available at: http://apps.who.int/iris/bitstream/10665/111008/1/WHO_DCO_WHD_2014.1_eng.pdf (accessed 30 January 2015).
11. Rozendaal JA (1997). *Vector control: methods for use by individuals and communities*. World Health Organization, Geneva.

Further reading

Institute of Medicine (2008). *Vector-borne diseases: understanding the environmental, human health, and ecological connections*. National Academies Press, Washington, DC.

World Health Organization (2014). *A global brief on vector-borne diseases*. Available at: http://apps.who.int/iris/bitstream/10665/111008/1/WHO_DCO_WHD_2014.1_eng.pdf (accessed 30 January 2015).

Chapter 21

Healthcare-associated infections

David J. Weber, Emily E. Sickbert-Bennett, and William A. Rutala

Definition and impact

Healthcare-associated infections (HAIs) are generally defined as infections that were not present or incubating at the time of admission to hospital. They are major causes of morbidity and mortality in the USA and around the world. The WHO reported in 2014 that the frequency of HAIs per 100 hospitalized patients was at least seven in high-income, and ten in low- or middle-income, countries. Among critically ill and vulnerable patients in intensive care units, the frequency rises to around 30 per 100.[1] A recently published point-prevalence survey in the USA estimated that more than 700 000 HAIs occur each year (Table 21.1).[2] This survey found that about one in 25 hospital patients has at least one HAI on any given day. The CDC has estimated that about 75 000 hospital patients in the USA with an HAI die each year during their hospitalization.

Using 2012 US $, Zimlichman and colleagues estimated that the most costly HAI was central line bloodstream infections (CLA-BSIs) at $45 814 per episode, followed by ventilator-associated pneumonia (VAP) at $40 144, surgical site infections (SSIs) at $20 785, *Clostridium difficile* infections (CDIs) at $11 285, and catheter-associated urinary tract infections (CA-UTIs) at $896.[3] The total annual costs for the five major HAIs were $9.8 billion, with SSIs contributing most to the overall costs (33.7%) followed by VAP (31.6%), CLA-BSIs (18.9%), CDIs (15.4%), and CA-UTIs (<1%).

Several factors increase the risk of HAIs in countries with limited resources, including poor hygiene and waste disposal, inadequate infrastructure and equipment, understaffing, overcrowding, lack of infection control knowledge and implementation, unsafe procedures, and a lack of guidance and policies.[4]

Table 21.1 Estimated numbers of major types of healthcare-associated infections occurring in acute care hospitals in the United States of America, 2011

Major site of infection	Estimated number of infections in the United States
Pneumonia	157 500
Surgical site infections	157 500
Gastrointestinal illness	12 300
Urinary tract infections	93 300
Primary bloodstream infections	71 900
Other types of infections	118 500
Estimated total number of infections in hospitals	721 800

Source: data from Centers for Disease Control and Prevention, *Healthcare-associated pathogens (HAI)*, available from http://www.cdc.gov/hai/index.html; and Magill SS *et al.*, Multistate point-prevalence survey of health care-associated infections. *New England Journal of Medicine*, Volume 370, Number 13, pp. 1198–208,

Surveillance

Surveillance of HAIs is a key component of infection control. Surveillance allows feedback of HAI rates to healthcare providers and hospital administrators, allows tracking over time to identify the magnitude of the impact of HAIs (incidence, pathogens, and outcomes), provides a baseline for detection of outbreaks (i.e. episodes with a greater than expected number of cases), allows assessment of the impact of interventions to control HAIs, and allows prioritization of resources based on hospital sites and patient populations with the highest incidence of HAIs.

In the USA, the premier HAI surveillance is the CDC's National Healthcare Safety Network (NHSN). The advantages of this surveillance system are the use of standard definitions of HAIs, the large number of participating hospitals (4444 in 2012), determination of the incidence of HAIs risk-adjusted by hospital location and the use of invasive devices (e.g. central line catheters, ventilators, and urinary catheters), some patient-level risk adjustment (e.g. by neonatal birthweight and by several risk factors for SSIs), and periodic publication of the data.[5] Limitations of NHSN include that: longitudinal comparisons of rates are not possible, as it is not strictly a cohort and surveillance definitions have changed over time; surveillance is limited to device-related infections (i.e. CLA-BSIs, VAP, and CA-UTIs) and surgical site infections; there is only limited risk adjustment, impairing comparisons between hospitals with disparate patient populations; and the validity of reported data is not uniformly assessed.[6] Surveillance systems (see ➲ Chapter 2) for HAIs worldwide—the NHSN, International Nosocomial Infection Control Consortium (INICC), ECDC, WHO—have been reviewed, including their advantages and disadvantages, by El Saed *et al.*[6]

Some of the key findings in the recent surveillance of HAIs in the USA include that >50% of HAIs are not device-associated,[2,7] >50% of HAIs occur outside intensive care units,[2,8] and dramatic decreases in the incidence of device-associated infections have occurred over time.[7] Decreased incidence of some HAIs has been reported in many other countries.

Pathogens

The commonest pathogens causing HAIs include Gram-positive cocci (e.g. *Staphylococcus aureus*, *Enterococcus* spp., coagulase-negative staphylococci, and *Streptococcus* spp.), enteric Gram-negative bacilli (e.g. *Klebsiella* spp., *Escherichia coli*, and *Enterobacter* spp.), non-enteric Gram-negative bacilli (e.g. *Pseudomonas aeruginosa*, *Acinetobacer baumannii*, and *Stenotrophomonas maltophilia*), and *Candida* spp. (Box 21.1).[2] Although the relative rankings of the top 25 pathogens vary among different sites of infection (i.e. pneumonia, SSIs, urinary tract infections (UTIs), and bloodstream infections (BSIs)), almost all HAIs are caused by these 25.[2] Importantly, in the USA, *C. difficile* is now the most commonly reported healthcare-associated pathogen.

Multidrug-resistant pathogens are a growing problem as aetiologic agents of HAIs. In the USA, data from the NHSN from 2009–2010 showed that nearly 20% of pathogens from all HAIs were drug-resistant phenotypes: MRSA (8.5%); vancomycin-resistant *Enterococcus* spp. (VRE) (3%); extended-spectrum cephalosporin-resistant *Klebsiella pneumoniae* and *K. oxytoca* (2%), *E. coli* (2%), and *Enterobacter* spp. (2%); carbapenem-resistant *P. aeruginosa* (2%), *K. pneumoniae*/*K. oxytoca* (<1%), and *Enterobacter* spp. (<1%).[9] A recent report from the WHO noted very high rates of resistance in bacteria that cause common healthcare-associated and community-acquired infections in all of the organization's regions.[10] Furthermore, the report assessed the scientific literature and noted a higher 30-day mortality and bacterium-attributable mortality for third-generation cephalosporin-resistant *E. coli* and *K. pneumoniae* and MRSA.

Box 21.1 Commonest pathogens associated with healthcare-associated infections

1. *Clostridium difficile* (12.1%)
2. *Staphylococcus aureus* (10.7%)
3. *Klebsiella* spp. (9.9%)
4. *Escherichia coli* (9.3%)
5. *Enterococcus* spp. (8.7%)
6. *Pseudomonas aeruginosa* (7.1%)
7. *Candida* spp. (6.3%)
8. Streptococcal spp. (5.0%)
9. Coagulase-negative staphylococci (4.8%)
10. *Enterobacter* spp. (3.2%)
11. *Acinetobacter baumannii* (1.6%)
12. *Proteus mirabilis* (1.6%)
13. Yeast, unspecified (1.6%)
14. *Stenotrophomonas maltophilia* (1.6%)
15. Other (17.5%)

Source: data from Magill SS *et al.*, Multistate point-prevalence survey of health care-associated infections. *New England Journal of Medicine*, Volume 370, Number 13, pp. 1198–208,

Risk factors for healthcare-associated infections

Determining the risk factors for specific HAIs is crucial to developing strategies to prevent HAIs.[12–15] Risk factors may be categorized as intrinsic (i.e. patient-related) or extrinsic (i.e. procedure-related), and modifiable (e.g. duration of invasive medical device or failure to use aseptic technique when inserting or manipulating an indwelling device) or non-modifiable (e.g. older age or comorbidities) (Table 21.2).

Table 21.2 Risk factors for selected healthcare-associated infections in adults

Infection	Risk factor
Central line-associated bloodstream infection	• Duration of central line use • Prolonged hospitalization before catheterization • Heavy microbial colonization at insertion site • Heavy microbial colonization of catheter hub • Internal jugular catheterization • Femoral vein catheterization • Neutropenia • Prematurity • Total parenteral nutrition • Substandard care of catheter • Failure to insert catheter using maximum barrier precautions • Failure to access catheter using aseptic technique
Ventilator-associated pneumonia	• Duration of mechanical ventilation • Extremes of age • Enteral feeding • Nasotracheal intubation • Witnessed aspiration • Use of paralytic agents • Gastric acid-suppressive therapy • Emergent intubation • Comorbidities • Supine position
Catheter-associated urinary tract infection	• Duration of urinary catheterization • Female sex • Older age • Failure to maintain closed urinary drainage system

(*Continued*)

Table 21.2 (*Contd.*)

Infection	Risk factor
Surgical site infection	• Older age • History of radiation • History of skin and soft tissue infections • Elevated glucose • Obesity • Smoking • Immunosuppression • Hypoalbuminaemia • Preoperative infections • Improper antimicrobial prophylaxis timing • Excessive operative time • Failure to adhere to strict aseptic technique • Poor surgical skill
Clostridium difficile infection	• Colonization with toxin-producing *C. difficile* • Antibiotic use • Older age • Gastric acid suppression • Admission to room that previously housed patient with *C. difficile* infection • Shared electronic thermometers

Source: data from Anderson *et al.* 2014[11]; Lo E *et al.* 2014[12]; Dubberke *et al.* 2014[13]; Coffin *et al.* 2008[14]; and Marschall *et al.* 2008[15]

Prevention and control

The key methods of preventing person-to-person transmission of pathogens in hospital settings include hand hygiene, prompt institution of isolation precautions for patients with communicable diseases, immunization of healthcare personnel (HCP) with recommended vaccines for vaccine-preventable diseases, appropriate disinfection of the surface environment, and adherence to recommended methods for disinfecting and sterilizing medical devices. The CDC provides guidance on prevention of HAIs in other settings, including outpatient medical facilities, nursing homes and assisted living facilities, dialysis facilities, and dental offices.[16]

Hand hygiene is considered to play a vital role in protecting patients from acquiring HAIs. The WHO recommends that HCPs perform hand hygiene before touching a patient, before clean and aseptic procedures (e.g. inserting devices such as intravenous catheters), after contact with body fluids, after touching a patient, and after touching patients' surroundings.[1] Hand hygiene may be performed by using an alcohol-based rub or by washing with soap and water (or an antiseptic). The latter should be used when hands are visibly dirty and should be strongly considered when managing patients with pathogens that are relatively non-susceptible to alcohol such as norovirus and *C. difficile*.

As noted above, prompt institution of isolation precautions is a key measure in preventing person-to-person transmission of communicable diseases in hospitals.[17] Standard precautions are used with **all** patients, because it is assumed that every person is potentially infected or colonized with an organism that could be transmitted in the healthcare setting. Standard precautions include the appropriate use of hand hygiene plus gloves whenever it can be reasonably anticipated that contact would occur with blood or body fluids (i.e. any bodily excretion or secretion, with the exception of sweat). Gowns are used if clothes could become contaminated, and face protection (e.g. face shield) is used if contamination of mucous membranes could occur. Contact precautions are used for pathogens (e.g. MRSA, VRE, norovirus, and *C. difficile*) that could be transmitted via direct contact (i.e. touching a patient) or indirect contact (i.e. touching the area around the patient). Droplet precautions are used for pathogens transmitted by respiratory droplets that travel a maximum of 3–6 ft (e.g. *Bordetella pertussis* and influenza) and consist of placing the patient in a single room and donning a surgical mask prior to room entry. Airborne precautions are used for pathogens transmitted by respiratory droplets that travel substantial distances (e.g. varicella and TB) and consist of placing the patient in an airborne infection isolation room (i.e. >12 air exchanges per hour, direct-out exhausted air, and negative pressure) and donning an N95 respirator prior to room entry.

All HCPs should be immune to mumps, measles, rubella, varicella, pertussis, and influenza,[18] and HCPs reasonably anticipated to have contact with blood or contaminated body fluids should be immune to hepatitis B. Immunity can always be documented by receipt of the appropriate immunization (written proof required), positive serology (mumps, measles, rubella, varicella, and hepatitis B after ≥3 doses of vaccine), or a history of disease diagnosed by a physician with (measles and mumps) or without (varicella) laboratory confirmation.

It is critical to clean and then disinfect or sterilize medical devices prior to use. More than 45 years ago, Earle Spaulding devised a rational approach to disinfection and sterilization of medical devices and equipment that still provides the basis for current recommendations.[19] Critical items that contact sterile tissue or the vascular system (e.g. surgical instruments and implants) confer a high risk of infection if they are contaminated, and so they should be sterilized. Importantly, surgical instruments contaminated with prions (e.g. Creutzfeldt–Jacob disease agent) need to undergo special prion reprocessing.[20] Semi-critical items that contact mucous membranes or non-intact skin (e.g. vaginal specula and endoscopes) should undergo high-level disinfection that eliminates all microbial agents, except high numbers of spores. Non-critical items that contact intact skin (e.g. blood pressure cuffs) should undergo low-level disinfection.

Contaminated environmental surfaces have been linked to patient-to-patient transmission of important hospital pathogens, including MRSA, VRE, norovirus, and *C. difficile*.[16] Hospitals should adhere to current guidelines for routine cleaning and disinfection of hospital rooms, as well as proper disinfection of terminal rooms.[19,21]

Excellent published guidelines recommend interventions to prevent specific HAIs, based on eliminating or minimizing the known risk factors for those HAIs.[12–15]

Future research needs

Hospital epidemiologists have been very successful in lowering the incidence of HAIs in recent years. However, efforts should continue to develop scientifically demonstrated reduction strategies, focusing on improved surveillance methods and methods to improve HCP behaviour (e.g. increased compliance with hand hygiene), reduce device-facilitated infections, reduce infections in high-risk groups of patients (e.g. immunocompromised patients), improve environmental and device disinfection, and develop endoscopes that can be steam-sterilized.

References

1. World Health Organization (2014). *Good hand hygiene by health workers protects patients from drug resistant pathogens*. Available at: http://www.who.int/mediacentre/news/releases/2014/hand-hygiene/en/ (accessed 26 May 2014).
2. Magill SS, Edwards JR, Bamberg W, *et al.* (2014). Multistate point-prevalence survey of health care-associated infections. *N Engl J Med*, **370**, 1198–208.
3. Zimlichman E, Henderson D, Tamir O, et *al.* (2013). Health care-associated infections: a meta-analysis of costs and financial impact on the US health care system. *JAMA Intern Med*, **173**, 2039–46.
4. World Health Organization (2010). *Health care-associated infections more common in developing countries*. Available at: http://www.who.int/mediacentre/news/notes/2010/infections_20101210/en/# (accessed 26 May 2014).
5. Dudeck MA, Weiner LM, Allen-Bridson K, *et al.* (2013). National Healthcare Safety Network (NHSN) report, data summary for 2012, device-associated module. *Am J Infect Control*, **41**, 1148–66.
6. El-Saed A, Balkhy HH, Weber DJ (2013). Benchmarking local healthcare-associated infections: available benchmarks and interpretation challenges. *J Infect Public Health*, **6**, 323–30.
7. DiBiase LM, Weber DJ, Sickbert-Bennett EE, Anderson DJ, Rutala WA (2014). The growing importance of non-device-associated healthcare-associated infections: a relative proportion and incidence study at an academic medical center, 2008–2012. *Infect Control Hosp Epidemiol*, **35**, 200–2.
8. Weber DJ, Sickbert-Bennett EE, Brown V, Rutala WA (2007). Comparison of hospitalwide-surveillance and targeted intensive care surveillance of healthcare-associated infections. *Infect Control Hosp Epidemiol*, **28**, 1361–6.
9. Sievert DM, Ricks P, Edwards JR, et *al.* (2013). Antimicrobial-resistant pathogens associated with healthcare-associated infections: summary of data reported to the National Healthcare Safety Network at the Centers for Disease Control and Prevention, 2009–2010. *Infect Control Hosp Epidemiol*, **34**, 1–14.
10. World Health Organization (2014). *Antimicrobial resistance: global report on surveillance 2014*. Available at: http://www.who.int/drugresistance/documents/surveillancereport/en/ (accessed 26 May 2014).
11. Anderson DJ, Podgorny K, Berrios-Torres SI, *et al.* (2014). Strategies to prevent surgical site infections in acute care hospitals: 2014 update. *Infect Control Hosp Epidemiol*, **35**, 605–27.
12. Lo E, Nicolle LE, Coffin SE, *et al.* (2014). Strategies to prevent catheter-associated urinary tract infections in acute care hospitals: 2014 update. *Infect Control Hosp Epidemiol*, **35**, 464–79.
13. Dubberke ER, Carling P, Carrico R, *et al.* (2014). Strategies to prevent *Clostridium difficile* infections in acute care hospitals: 2014 update. *Infect Control Hosp Epidemiol*, **35**, 628–45.
14. Coffin SE, Klompas M, Classen D, *et al.* (2008). Strategies to prevent ventilator-associated pneumonia in acute care hospitals. *Infect Control Hosp Epidemiol*, **29**(Suppl 1), S31–40.
15. Marschall J, Mermel LA, Classen D, *et al.* (2008). Strategies to prevent central line-associated bloodstream infections in acute care hospitals. *Infect Control Hosp Epidemiol*, **29**(Suppl 1), S22–30.

16. Centers for Disease Control and Prevention. *Healthcare-associated infections (HAI)*. Available at: http://www.cdc.gov/hai/index.html (accessed 26 May 2014).
17. Siegel JD, Rhinehart E, Jackson M, Chiarello L (2007). 2007 guideline for isolation precautions: preventing transmission of infectious agents in healthcare settings. Available at: http://www.cdc.gov/ncidod/dhqp/pdf/isolation2007.pdf (accessed 26 May 2014).
18. Centers for Disease Control and Prevention (2011). Immunization of health-care personnel: recommendations of the Advisory Committee on Immunization Practices (ACIP). *MMWR Recomm Rep*, 60(RR–7), 1–45.
19. Rutala WA, Weber DJ (2008). *Guideline for disinfection and sterilization in healthcare facilities, 2008*. Available at: http://www.cdc.gov/hicpac/pubs.html (accessed 26 May 2014).
20. Belay ED, Blasé J, Schulster LM, Maddox RA, Schonberger LB (2013). Management of neurosurgical instruments and patients exposed to Creutfeldt-Jakob disease. *Infect Control Hosp Epidemiol*, **34**, 1272–80.
21. Weber DJ, Anderson D, Rutala WA (2013). The role of the surface environment in healthcare-associated infections. *Curr Opin Infect Dis*, **26**, 338–44.

Chapter 22

Hepatitis B and C

Sema Mandal and Koye Balogun

Introduction to hepatitis B and C

Hepatitis B and C (HBV, HCV) are blood-borne viruses that cause acute and chronic infections that can result in chronic liver disease, cirrhosis, and hepatocellular carcinoma (HCC)[1,2] (Tables 22.1 and 22.2). They are both major global public health problems.

The WHO estimates the prevalence of chronic HBV infection to be 240–350 million people globally and chronic HCV infection 130–150 million, and annual deaths due to HBV about 600 000 and HCV 350 000–500 000. Figures 22.1 and 22.2 show the global geographical distribution of the prevalence of chronic HBV and HCV infection, respectively.

Vaccines against HBV have been available since 1982. They are safe and highly effective (95% effective in preventing chronic infection).[3] The combined efforts of immunization and effective treatments make elimination plausible. The WHO recommends universal HBV immunization of infants and/or adolescents. By 2012, 179 countries had the vaccine in their national immunization programmes,[4,5] and many have seen a decrease in the incidence of infection in infants, children, and adolescents.[6] Antiviral therapy is the only way to reduce the morbidity and mortality in those already chronically infected.

There is currently no vaccine for HCV;[7] however, it is treatable and, unlike HBV, potentially curable. Novel highly effective directly acting antiviral (DAA) drugs promise increased cure rates,[8,9] but affordability and access to these new therapies are a major challenge.[2]

Hepatitis B

There are eight HBV genotypes (A to H), with distinct geographical distributions.[10] The incubation period ranges from 40 to 160 days, with an average of 90 days. HBV is highly resistant to extreme temperatures and humidity.

Acute hepatitis B

Most cases of acute HBV are asymptomatic or subclinical, but outcomes are age-dependent. Symptoms—insidious onset of anorexia, abdominal pain, nausea, vomiting, and jaundice—occur in 5–15% of children aged 1–5 years and 33–50% of older children and adults, but rarely in newborns.[11] Less than 1% of cases have fulminant hepatic failure, which has high mortality (40%).[12] Acute infection resolves in 4–12 weeks in most immunocompetent adults. Individuals who spontaneously clear the virus have natural acquired immunity.

Chronic persistent hepatitis B

Chronic persistent HBV is defined as the presence of HBsAg in the serum for >6 months. The risk of chronicity varies with age: up to 90% for infants who are infected perinatally, 25–50% for children infected at 1–5 years, and <10% of older children and adults.[11]

Overall, 15–25% of people with chronic HBV progress to cirrhosis or HCC over decades.[13] HCC develops in up to 9% of those with HBV-associated cirrhosis but can occur in the absence of cirrhosis.[14]

Table 22.1 Occurrence and transmission of hepatitis B and C

Infectious agent	Occurrence	Global burden	Incubation period	Reservoir	Mode of transmission
Hepatitis B virus	• Worldwide • Endemic in parts of Africa, South East Asia, Amazon basin, and Arctic rim	• Worldwide: • Estimated 240–350 million people chronically infected • Up to 1 million related deaths annually	• Range: 45–180 days • Average: 60–90 days	• Humans	• Percutaneous and mucocutaneous exposure to infectious blood • Perinatal, horizontal, and sexual transmission are common • Parenteral transmission—transfusion of unscreened blood and blood products
Hepatitis C virus	• Worldwide • Central and East Asia and North Africa	• Worldwide: • Estimated 130–150 million people chronically infected • Up to 500 000 related deaths annually	• Range: 2 weeks to 6 months • Average: 6–9 weeks	• Humans	• Percutaneous exposure to infectious blood • Parenteral transmission—transfusion of unscreened blood and blood products • Contaminated needles and syringes are important vehicles of transmission among people who inject drugs

Source: data from Cindy M. Weinbaum *et al.*, 'Recommendations for Identification and Public Health Management of Persons with Chronic Hepatitis B Virus Infection', *Morbidity and Mortality Weekly Report*, Volume 57, No. RR-8, pp. 1–20, Sept 19, 2008, available from http://www.cdc.gov/mmwr/pdf/rr/rr5708.pdf.

Table 22.2 Prevention, diagnosis, and treatment of individual patients

Infectious agent	Laboratory diagnosis	Long-term complications	Prevention and treatment

Hepatitis B virus	• Serological assays to detect virus-induced host antibodies and viral antigens
	• PCR and NAAT to detect viral nucleic acid
		• Cirrhosis
		• HCC
			• Prevention:
			  • Vaccines
			• Treatment:
			  • Antivirals
			  • Immunomodulator therapy

Hepatitis C virus	• Serological assays to detect virus-induced host antibodies and viral antigens
	• PCR and NAAT to detect viral nucleic acid
		• Cirrhosis
		• HCC
			• Prevention:
			  • Harm minimization counselling and practices
			• Treatment:
			  • Antivirals
			  • Immunomodulator therapy
			  • DAAs

DAA, directly acting antiviral; HCC, hepatocellular carcinoma; NAAT, nucleic acid amplification test; PCR, polymerase chain reaction.

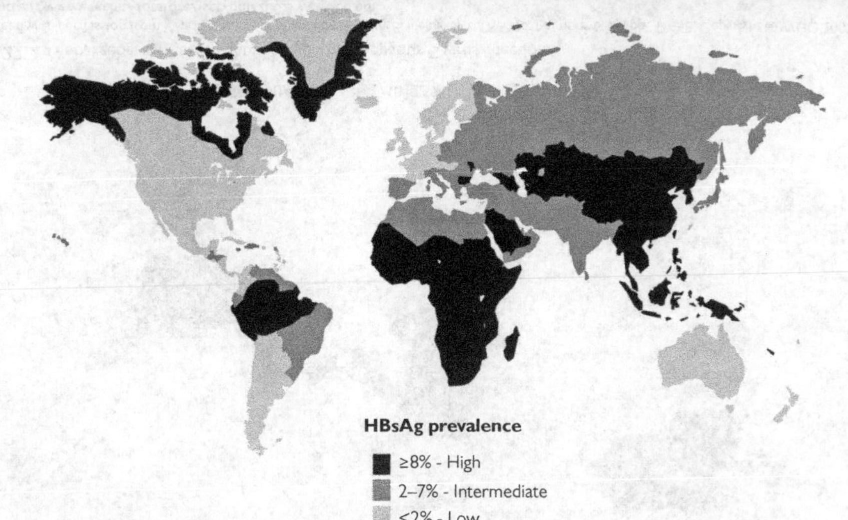

Figure 22.1 Global geographical distribution of chronic hepatitis B infection.

Reproduced with permission from Cindy M. Weinbaum *et al.*, 'Recommendations for Identification and Public Health Management of Persons with Chronic Hepatitis B Virus Infection', *Morbidity and Mortality Weekly Report*, Volume 57, No. RR-8, pp. 1–20, Sept 19, 2008, available from ℜ http://www.cdc.gov/mmwr/pdf/rr/rr5708.pdf.

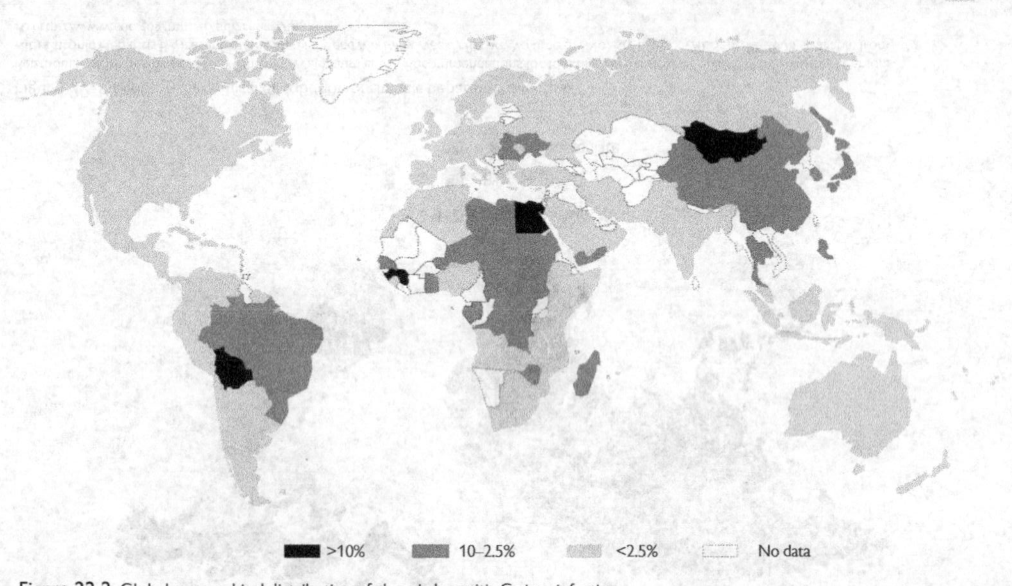

Figure 22.2 Global geographical distribution of chronic hepatitis C virus infection.

Reproduced with permission from World Health Organization, *Weekly Epidemiological Record*, Number 6, 77, pp. 41–48, Copyright © WHO 2002, available from http://www.who.int/docstore/wer/pdf/2002/wer7706.pdf.

Hepatitis C

There are six major HCV genotypes and numerous subtypes.[15] The average time from exposure to seroconversion (anti-HCV) is 8–9 weeks. Anti-HCV can be detected in >97% of people by 6 months after exposure.

Acute hepatitis C

Most people with acute HCV infection are asymptomatic, but some may experience fatigue and jaundice. About a fifth of adults with acute HCV infections will spontaneously clear the virus; the remainder go on to develop chronic HCV infection.[16]

Chronic persistent hepatitis C

Chronic HCV is defined as persistent if HCV RNA is detectable in serum for longer than 6 months. It is usually asymptomatic for many years, and any symptoms tend to be variable and non-specific such as fatigue, malaise, nausea, and abdominal discomfort. About 30% of those with chronic hepatitis C progress to liver cirrhosis. A small proportion develop HCC over 20–30 years. People who have cleared the virus spontaneously or through treatment are susceptible to reinfection.

Modes of transmission

Modes of transmission for HBV and HCV are parenteral, sexual, and from mother to child (perinatal, mainly during delivery).

Hepatitis B is mainly transmitted perinatally, or by close contact (via percutaneous and mucosal exposure) with an infected person in early childhood in high endemicity countries. In countries with lower endemicity, sexual transmission and injecting drug use are the major routes of infection.

HCV is primarily transmitted parenterally among people who inject drugs (PWIDs) after sharing injecting equipment, transfusion of blood and blood products from unscreened donors and donations, transfusion of blood products that have not undergone viral inactivation, the use of contaminated or inadequately sterilized instruments and needles in medical and dental procedures, tattooing and piercing, and other activities that break the skin. Compared to HBV, transmission by perinatal and sexual exposure is less efficient.

The risk of perinatal transmission is greater with HBV (up to 90%) than with HCV (up to 10%). Perinatal transmission is increased (>10%) in mothers co-infected with HCV and HIV.

Diagnosis and treatment

The clinical symptoms of the viral hepatitides are indistinguishable, so definitive diagnosis is dependent on serological testing (see ➲ Chapter 11).

Correct interpretation of these markers allows the determination of the individual's infection status.

Hepatitis B

Acute hepatitis B

Characterized by HBsAg in serum and the presence of IgM class antibody to the hepatitis B core antigen (anti-HBc IgM). Anti-HBc IgM is the standard diagnostic marker of acute HBV infection; however, its presence has to be interpreted correctly, as it can also be detected in an acute flare in an individual who is chronically infected. Total anti-HBc indicates current or past infection. The hepatitis B e antigen (HBeAg) may also be detected during acute infection.

Recovery from infection

HBsAg and HBeAg are cleared and replaced by antibodies to HBsAg (anti-HBs) and HBeAg (anti-HBe), respectively. Anti-HBs is a protective antibody that indicates immunity to reinfection. The presence of anti-HBc IgG indicates past exposure to the virus.

Chronic persistent HBV infection

In chronic infection, HBsAg remains detectable, indicating infectiousness. HBeAg may be present, indicating a high level of viral replication and high infectiousness (Figure 22.3). Exceptions to these general principles can occur. For example, anti-HBc IgM can be found in those with chronic infection during reactivation (an acute flare), making it difficult to distinguish from acute infection.

Active immunization

The presence of anti-HBs >10 IU/mL only in serum indicates successful active immunization against HBV.

Treatment of hepatitis B

The standard of care is treatment with immunomodulator drugs (e.g. pegylated interferon (IFN)) and antiviral therapies (e.g. nucleoside and nucleotide analogues). The aim of treatment is to suppress the viral DNA and induce HBeAg seroconversion to limit progression of liver disease, although loss of HBsAg does occur and may become the goal of future therapies.

The decision to start treatment is based on the virological, histological, and serological profile of a patient. Monitoring for increases in viral load during treatment is important, as antiviral drug resistance is an emerging problem in the management of chronic hepatitis B (Figure 22.3).

Hepatitis C

The primary screening test is for antibodies to HCV. If this is positive, a PCR test for HCV RNA is undertaken.

Early acute infection

Anti-HCV-negative, HCV RNA-positive: An antibody test result may not be present in early seroconversion and may not be reliable in

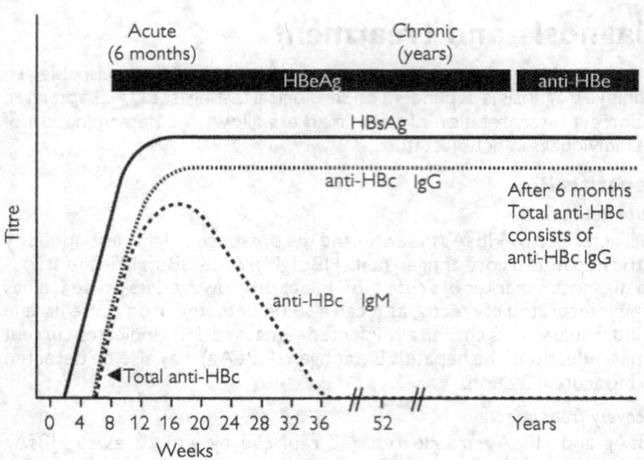

Figure 22.3 Progression to chronic persistent hepatitis B virus infection: typical serological.

Adapted from Centre for Disease Control (CDC), *Progression to Chronic Hepatitis B Virus Infection: Typical Serologic Course*, available from https://www.cdph.ca.gov/HealthInfo/discond/Documents/B%20%20Hepatitis%20B_lab%20graph_Chronic%20serology%20%28CDC%29.pdf.

immunosuppressed patients, so such patients found to be negative for HCV antibody should be tested for HCV RNA.

Chronic HCV infection

Anti-HCV-positive, HCV RNA-positive.

Cleared infection

Anti-HCV-positive, HCV RNA-negative: This can be achieved spontaneously or following treatment; for the latter, cleared infection means a sustained virological response (SVR), defined as two consecutive negative HCV RNA results, usually 6 months apart, after treatment.

Treatment of hepatitis C

The choice and duration of treatment depends upon many factors, including the genotype, response to previous therapy, and the patient's stage of disease and comorbidity. The standard of care for treatment of HCV has been triple therapy with DAAs, in combination with pegylated IFN and ribavirin. More effective DAAs have become available, with much higher SVRs in advanced liver disease stages and pangenotypic activity, thus offering the potential of cure in 50–90% of cases. Some DAAs have been shown to produce an SVR after 8–12 weeks of treatment, and some do not require IFN; however, these drugs are expensive, so affordability may be a barrier to uptake of treatment, although treating a patient with such drugs will prevent a more expensive liver transplant that might otherwise be needed in the future.

Prevention and control measures

Hepatitis B

- Immunization forms the backbone of global efforts at reducing the burden of HBV infection and its consequences.
  - Pre-exposure immunization strategies include universal immunization of infants and adolescents, the selective immunization of high-risk groups such as close household contacts, people with multiple sexual partners and MSM, people who inject drugs, and those travelling to endemic countries.
  - Post-exposure prophylaxis with a vaccine (with or without specific hepatitis B immunoglobulin, HBIG) includes for babies born to HBsAg-positive mothers (in many countries, including the UK, all pregnant women are screened for HBsAg), for sexual exposure to HBsAg-positive individuals, and for percutaneous or mucocutaneous exposure to HBsAg-positive blood.
- Screening of blood donors, virus inactivation, and testing of blood donations.
- Targeted testing of high-risk groups such as close household and sexual contacts.
- Adherence to universal precautions while handling blood and body fluids in occupational settings.
- Raising public awareness of the infection and promoting safer sex and safer injecting practices (including provision of needle and syringe exchange programmes for PWIDs).
- Treating infected people to reduce their transmissibility.

Hepatitis C

- Professional and public education, including targeting PWIDs.
- Adherence to universal precautions in all settings to reduce the possibility of exposure to infected blood, which is particularly important when dialysing patients with HCV in renal dialysis units.
- Care must also be taken in domestic, commercial, and prison settings to reduce cross-contamination of infected blood, e.g. via tattooing, piercing, razors, hair clippers, toothbrushes, and acupuncture needles.
- Screening of blood donors, virus inactivation, and testing of blood donations.
- Routine antenatal screening of pregnant women is carried out in some countries.
- Reducing exposure in risk groups: in countries that have introduced the screening of blood products, most new infections are in PWIDs. Strategies to reduce new infections of HCV concentrate on:
  - stopping people from initiating injecting drug use
  - helping those who inject illicit drugs to quit injecting
  - harm minimization among those who continue to inject (e.g. needle exchange, opiate substitution treatments, and education on cleaning and not sharing drug-injecting equipment).
- Targeted testing of high-risk groups, such as PWIDs, to get infected individuals into treatment.
- Treating infected people to reduce the disease burden.

Epidemiological and molecular investigations of outbreaks

Only a small proportion of HBV and HCV outbreaks in the community and healthcare settings are likely to be detected because of the long incubation period and asymptomatic nature of acute HBV and HCV infection. Prompt recognition of outbreaks of HBV or HCV is critical to identify the source and establish effective control measures such as immunization of an at-risk group (see ➲ Chapter 12). Molecular characterization of HBV and HCV infections using sequence typing techniques aids identification of identical or related viral strains in an outbreak and provides important information for targeted control.

Surveillance

Surveillance systems provide information on trends in incidence and prevalence and identify at-risk groups to inform health policy and prevention and control strategies (see ➲ Chapter 2). The main surveillance methods for viral hepatitis are:

- laboratory reports of confirmed cases
- clinical-based notifications.

Surveillance may be supplemented by data on HBV- and HCV-related hospital admissions and outcome data such as liver transplant rates and deaths from national registers. These surveillance and supplementary data together help to describe the burden of disease from HBV and HCV.

Conclusions

Chronic HBV and HCV infections are responsible for a significant proportion of liver disease globally and have impacted considerably on national healthcare systems. Continued surveillance of these infections allows countries to define the epidemiological and virological trends of infection, to evaluate prevention and control strategies, and to assess the overall disease burden.

References

1. Nebbia G, Peppa D, Main MK (2012). Hepatitis B infection: current concepts and future challenges. *QJM*, **105**, 109–13.
2. Lemoine M, Thursz M Hepatitis C. (2014). a global issue: access to care and new therapeutic and preventive approaches in resource-constrained areas. *Semin Liver Dis*, **34**, 89–97.
3. Chen DS (2009). Hepatitis B vaccination: the key towards elimination and eradication of hepatitis B. *J Hepatol*, **50**, 805–16.
4. Romanò L, Paladini S, Zanetti AR (2012). Twenty years of universal vaccination against hepatitis B in Italy: achievements and challenges. *J Public Health Res*, **1**, 126–9.
5. Van Damme P, Kane M, Meheus A (1997). Integration of hepatitis B vaccination into national immunisation programmes. *BMJ*, **314**, 1033–6.

6. Kane MA (2003). Global control of primary hepatocellular carcinoma with hepatitis B vaccine: the contributions of research in Taiwan. *Cancer Epidemiol Biomarkers Prev*, **12**, 2–3.
7. Honegger JR, Zhou Y, Walker CM (2014). Will there be a vaccine to prevent HCV infection? *Semin Liver Dis*, **34**, 79–88.
8. Ahn J, Flamm SL (2014). Frontiers in the treatment of hepatitis C virus infection. *Gastroenterol Hepatol (N Y)*, **10**, 90–100.
9. Degasperi E, Aghemo A (2014). Sofosbuvir for the treatment of chronic hepatitis C: between current evidence and future perspectives. *Hepat Med*, **6**, 25–33.
10. Hou J, Liu Z, Gu F (2005). Epidemiology and Prevention of Hepatitis B Virus Infection. *Int J Med Sci*, **2**, 50–7.
11. McMahon BJ, Alward WL, Hall DB, *et al.* (1985). Acute hepatitis B virus infection: relation of age to the clinical expression of disease and subsequent development of the carrier state. *J Infect Dis*, **151**, 599–603.
12. Koziel M J, Siddiqui A (2005). Hepatitis B virus and hepatitis delta virus. In: Mandell LG, Bennett JE, Dolin R (eds). *Mandell, Douglas, and Bennett's principles and practice of infectious diseases*. Elsevier, New York, pp. 1428–40.
13. Mahoney FJ (1999). Update on diagnosis, management, and prevention of hepatitis B virus infection. *Clin Microbiol Rev*, **12**, 351–66.
14. Fattovich G, Giustina G, Schalm SW, *et al.* (1995). Occurrence of hepatocellular carcinoma and decompensation in western European patients with cirrhosis type B. *Hepatology*, **21**, 77–82.
15. Simmonds P, Bukh J, Combet C, *et al.* (2005). Consensus proposals for a unified system of nomenclature of hepatitis C virus genotypes. *Hepatology*, **42**, 962–73.
16. Micallef JM, Kaldor JM, Dore GJ (2006). Spontaneous viral clearance following acute hepatitis C infection: a systematic review of longitudinal studies. *J Viral Hepat*, **13**, 34–41.

Further reading

European Association for the Study of the Liver (2012). EASL clinical practice guidelines: management of chronic hepatitis B virus infection. *J Hepatol*, **57**, 167–85.

European Association for the Study of the Liver (2014). EASL clinical practice guidelines: management of hepatitis C virus infection. *J Hepatol*, **60**, 392–420.

Ramsay ME, Balogun K, Quigley C, Yung CF (2013). Surveillance for viral hepatitis in Europe. In: M'ikanatha NM, Lynfield R, Van Beneden CA, de Valk H (eds). *Infectious disease surveillance*, 2nd edn. Wiley-Blackwell, Chichester, pp. 288–303.

Thomas HC, Lok ASF, Locarnini SA, Zuckerman AJ (eds) (2013). *Viral hepatitis*, 4th edn. Wiley-Blackwell, Chichester.

Further reading

Chapter 23

Sexually transmitted infections: epidemiology and control

Pam Sonnenberg and Anne Johnson

Introduction to sexually transmitted infections

Sexually transmitted infections (STIs) are infections that have a significant probability of transmission between humans by means of sexual behaviour, including vaginal intercourse, anal sex, and oral sex. Some STIs can also be transmitted from mother to child during pregnancy, childbirth, and breastfeeding, and through blood products.

Table 23.1 shows examples of microorganisms that are primarily transmitted sexually. Many infections that are transmitted person-to-person can also be transmitted during sexual contact due to the close contact involved (e.g. respiratory or skin infections). Some organisms that are predominantly spread by other routes (e.g. faeco–oral route) may also be transmitted during specific sexual practices (e.g. *Shigella* spp., *Giardia lamblia*, and hepatitis A virus). However, they are not considered as STIs, even though they are sexually transmissible.

STIs tend to cause minimal morbidity initially and may be asymptomatic. However, they can cause long-term sequelae and death. For example, gonorrhoea and chlamydia can cause pelvic inflammatory disease and subsequent ectopic pregnancy and infertility; oncogenic subtypes of HPV may cause cervical cancer, and untreated syphilis leads to a wide range of serious systemic disease.

Table 23.1 Examples of microorganisms that are primarily transmitted sexually

Type of microorganism	Example
Bacteria	• *Chlamydia trachomatis* serovars D–K (chlamydia) • *Chlamydia trachomatis* serovars L1, L2, L3 LGV • *Haemophilus ducreyi* (chancroid) • *Klebsiella granulomatis* (granuloma inguinale) • *Neisseria gonorrhoeae* (gonorrhoea) • *Treponema pallidum* (syphilis)
Mycoplasmas	• *Mycoplasma genitalium* • *Ureaplasma urealyticum*
Arthropods	• *Phthirus pubis* (pubic lice) • *Sarcoptes scabeii* (scabies)
Protozoa	• *Trichomonas vaginalis* (trichomoniasis)
Fungi	• *Candida albicans*
Viruses	• Hepatitis B (see ➲ Chapter 22) • HSV types 1 and 2 • HIV (see ➲ Chapter 25) • HTLV-1 • HPV • *Molluscum contagiosum* (pox virus)

HIV, human immunodeficiency virus; HPV, human papillomavirus; HSV, herpes simplex virus; HTLV-1, human T-lymphotropic virus 1; LGV, lymphogranuloma venereum.

Epidemiology of sexually transmitted infections

According to the WHO global estimates in 2008, 498.9 million new cases of four curable STIs (syphilis, gonorrhoea, chlamydia, and trichomoniasis) occur annually in adults aged 15–49 years. Data on the epidemiology of STIs worldwide mainly come from surveillance (see ➲ Surveillance of sexually transmitted infections, p. 331, and Chapter 2), but both the methods and quality of data vary substantially from country to country.

The incidence and prevalence of STIs are determined by:

- patterns of sexual behaviour in the population
- efficiency of transmission of infection (including safe sex practices)
- duration of infectiousness of infected individuals
- effectiveness of control programmes
- current burden and level of infection in the population
- socio-economic environment
- social and cultural context, including stigma influencing behaviour and health-seeking.

The incidence and prevalence of STIs vary substantially worldwide. In general, prevalence is higher in resource-poor countries. In a given setting, the incidence of STIs is highest among groups most likely to be exposed to infection, i.e. those experiencing the highest rates of sexual partner change and unsafe sex. This tends to be among:

- young sexually active people (aged 15–29 years)
- unmarried people
- sex workers and their clients
- injecting drug users, especially those exchanging sex for drugs
- MSM
- single men living and working away from their families (e.g. businessmen, migrant workers, and truck drivers).

These groups are often proportionately larger in urban populations. Some may be referred to as core groups, i.e. groups experiencing particularly high rates of partner change and unsafe sex, and thus contributing a greater proportion of STI transmission than would be expected from population rates. The concept of core groups is important for control purposes, as interventions within core groups may be especially effective in reducing the transmission of STIs, **but** it is important to note that their monogamous asymptomatic partners may also be at risk.

Dynamics of STI transmission

The incidence of STIs is influenced by dynamic factors related to the behaviour of populations, ecology of organisms, and impact of control programmes within the context of the socio-economic and demographic environment (Figure 23.1).

Behaviour of populations

Sexual behaviour studies in representative populations show marked heterogeneity in sexual behaviours between individuals and demographic groups. In particular, there is great variation in the number of sexual partners reported by individuals (most people have few partners, while a few people have many). The importance of concurrent partnerships, compared with serial partnerships, is important in augmenting transmission of STIs.

Epidemiological studies have improved our understanding of variability in STI epidemiology between and within societies (see ➔ Chapter 4). Current areas of STI research include the study of 'sexual mixing'. Data on sexual mixing and sexual networks are difficult to collect, and some researchers are studying social networks to understand sexual networks and looking at new ways in which people identify sexual partners (e.g. via the Internet) (see ➔ Chapter 15).

Challenges to measuring sexual behaviour and obtaining unbiased and precise measures of individual and population behaviour patterns on this private and potentially sensitive subject area include finding ways to reduce participation bias and improving questionnaire design, content, and delivery (e.g. through computer-assisted personal interviews (CAPIs)).

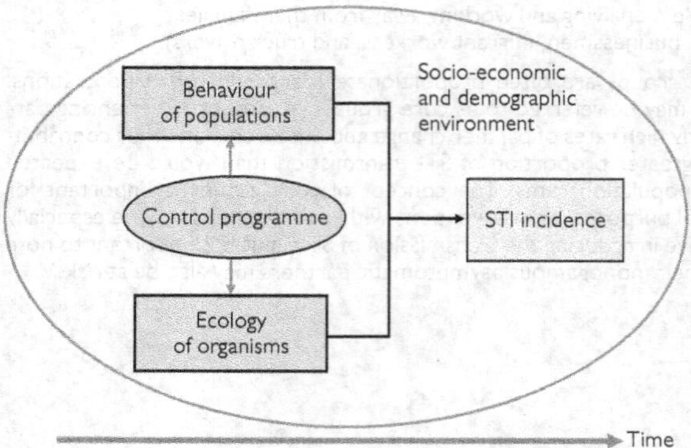

Figure 23.1 Transmission of sexually transmitted infections (STIs).

Ecology of organisms

Sexually transmitted organisms are generally fragile outside of the human body and rely on transmission through close sexual contact and their presence in body fluids, semen, cervico–vaginal secretions, and blood.

In general, successful microorganisms that are predominantly transmitted through sexual intercourse rely on the following biological characteristics for survival in human populations:

- frequently cause asymptomatic infection
- if untreated, typically have long infectious periods and rarely cause early mortality
- typically infection does not lead to protective immunity (so repeated infection is possible).

The transmission of STIs can be summarized mathematically using the standard equation for transmission of infections, expressed in terms of the basic reproduction number (R_0) (Figure 23.1).

$$R_0 = \beta CD$$

where R_0 = basic reproduction number (average number of secondary cases that result from one primary case in a susceptible population), β = probability of transmission of infection per partnership, C = mean effective rate of sexual partner change, and D = duration of infectiousness.

If $R_0 > 1$, the organism will be sustained in the population. If $R_0 < 1$, the organism will eventually reach extinction.

Efficiency of STI transmission (β) is influenced by:

- infectivity of the organism
- infectious period and phase of infection (e.g. varies in HIV and syphilis)
- sexual behaviours that increase or decrease risk (e.g. anal sex and condom use)
- biological interactions with other organisms (e.g. genital ulcers may increase infectivity in HIV-positive individuals and susceptibility in HIV-negative individuals)
- male circumcision (e.g. reduces female-to-male transmission of HIV).

Effective rate of partner change (C) is influenced by:

- mean rate (and variance) of partner acquisition
- patterns of serial or concurrent partnerships
- patterns of sexual mixing:
  - age (older men tend to have relationships with younger women)
  - sex (e.g. percentage of MSM in the population)
  - degree of heterogeneity in partner selection (i.e. assortative or disassortative mixing)
  - 'connectivity' of networks
  - 'core groups' (groups with high rates of partner change, who mix together and contribute disproportionately to STI transmission, e.g. commercial sex workers and their clients).

Duration of infectiousness (*D*) is influenced by:
- antibiotic/antiviral therapy (e.g. aciclovir for HSV and antiretroviral therapy (ART) for HIV)
- interaction with other organisms (e.g. HIV/HSV)
- case-finding/screening
- partner notification
- immune system.

Surveillance of sexually transmitted infections

Public health surveillance is the ongoing and systematic collection, analysis, and interpretation of data to help guide prevention, treatment, and care programmes (see ➲ Chapter 2).

Surveillance of STIs aims to:

- describe rates and trends of STIs in relation to geography, demography, and behaviour
- monitor behaviours that increase risk of transmitting STIs
- provide data for planning, targeting, and evaluating health promotion interventions aimed at reducing risk behaviours
- monitor the effectiveness of therapeutic control programmes
- provide comparative international data
- monitor sensitivity/resistance of organisms to antibiotic/antiviral therapies.

Surveillance of STIs may be syndromic (e.g. urethritis or genital ulcer disease) or aetiological (e.g. chlamydia). The latter relies on clinical or laboratory surveillance.

The asymptomatic or non-specific symptoms of many STIs mean accurate diagnoses rely on laboratory tests. The sensitivity and specificity of tests will depend on the specimen taken (e.g. urine or self-collected vaginal swabs) and the test used. Laboratory diagnosis of STIs is a rapidly evolving field, with many infections now diagnosed using nucleic acid amplification tests (NAATs) and the introduction of POC tests. Improved surveillance and/or diagnostic tests may lead to a spurious increase in 'incidence'.

The surveillance and control of STIs has special difficulties stemming from the importance of certain higher-risk populations, which are often marginalized and difficult to access, and issues of confidentiality associated with the sensitivities and stigma surrounding sexual matters in general.

Control strategies for sexually transmitted infections

Primary prevention includes:
- sexual health education/promotion to reduce population risk behaviours: this may be directed at individuals, at specific groups (e.g. school sex education or sex worker outreach projects), or at the general population. Programmes vary in their approaches, but use of condoms and reducing partner change rates are key components
- vaccination: vaccines against HBV and HPV are now available, with the latter being rolled out in certain countries for teenage girls
- male circumcision
- pre- and post-exposure prophylaxis (e.g. HIV).

Secondary prevention includes:
- detection and treatment programmes for symptomatic individuals (typically provided through dedicated confidential sexually transmitted disease (STD)/STI clinics), but organization of clinical care is very variable worldwide
- partner notification of exposed individuals
- population screening (e.g. antenatal screening for syphilis and national chlamydia screening programmes in young adults)
- mass treatment (occasionally used in situations of high prevalence).

Tertiary prevention comprises prevention of complications and long-term sequelae (e.g. antiviral drugs).

The various strategies to prevent or control STIs can be organized using the $R_0 = \beta C D$ formula described above, for example:
- β = measures to reduce transmissibility
  - condoms
  - microbicides
  - lower-risk sexual practices
  - antivirals
  - male circumcision.
- C = measures to reduce the rate of partner change
  - individual/population health education
  - changing social norms/sociodemographic context (the role of women, poverty, migration, etc.)
- D = measures to reduce the duration of infectiousness (D)
  - screening and treatment
  - case-finding
  - partner notification
  - health-seeking behaviour
  - service accessibility.

Evaluating the effectiveness of control programmes

In general, health promotion activities involving behavioural interventions to reduce the incidence of STIs have been poorly evaluated or rely on reported behavioural outcomes. A systematic review of the global literature focused on RCTs with (non-HIV) incidence of STIs as outcomes.[1] Forty-one trials were identified, 22 (53%) of which showed effectiveness against STIs. Effective interventions included: individual risk reduction counselling, group counselling, and skills building; HBV vaccination; HPV vaccination; partner treatment to reduce transmission; and syndromic management of STIs. RCTs of male circumcision in adults have shown reductions in STIs (HPV and possibly HSV type 2), as well as transmission of HIV. More recently, the strategy of 'treatment as prevention' for HIV (treating HIV-infected people to improve their health and reduce the risk of onward transmission) has been shown to have public health benefits.

The need to integrate prevention and treatment programmes is increasingly recognized, but further national investment in educational programmes demands the commitment of political, educational, and religious leaders.

It is often difficult to disentangle the relative contributions of behavioural and biomedical components of effective interventions, and a 'combined prevention' approach that includes both behavioural change and biomedical components is most likely to be effective. Furthermore, although no single prevention approach may be sufficient to control an infection, strategies that combine partially effective interventions may have population-level impacts.

Reference

1. Manhart L, Holmes KK (2005). Randomised controlled trials of individual-level, population-level and multilevel interventions for preventing sexually transmitted infections: What has worked? *J Infect Dis*, **191**(Suppl 1), S7–24.

Further reading

Althaus CL, Turner KME, Mercer CH, *et al.* (2014). Effectiveness and cost-effectiveness of traditional and new partner notification technologies for curable sexually transmitted infections: observational study, systematic reviews and mathematical modelling. *Health Technol Assess*; **18**, 1–100, vii–viii.

Fenton KA, Johnson AM, McManus S, Erens B (2001). Measuring sexual behaviour: methodological challenges in survey research. *Sex Transm Infect*, **77**, 84–92.

Holmes K, Mardh PA, Sparling PF, *et al.* (eds) (2008). *Sexually transmitted diseases*, 4th edn. McGraw Hill, New York.

Mercer CH, Tanton C, Prah P, *et al.* (2013). Changes in sexual attitudes and lifestyles in Britain through the life course and over time: findings from the National Surveys of Sexual Attitudes and Lifestyles (NATSAL). *Lancet*, **382**, 1781–94.

Sankar N, Pattman R, Handy P, Elawad B, Price DA (2010). *Oxford handbook of genitourinary medicine, HIV, and sexual health.* Oxford University Press, Oxford.

Wasserheit JN, Aral SO (1996). Dynamic topology of sexually transmitted disease epidemics: implications for prevention strategies. *J Infect Dis*, **174**(Suppl 2), S201–13.

Yorke JA, Heathcote HW, Nold A (1978). Dynamics and control of transmission of gonorrhoea. *Sex Transm Dis*, **5**, 51–6.

Chapter 24

Transmissible spongiform encephalopathies

Peter G. Smith

Introduction to transmissible spongiform encephalopathies

Transmissible spongiform encephalopathies (TSEs) are caused by the accumulation of abnormally folded prion protein (PrP) in the brain. The resulting neurodegeneration leads invariably to death, and there is no effective treatment. TSEs are very rare in humans; the commonests form of the disease Creutzfeldt–Jakob disease (CJD), which was first recognized in the 1920s, mainly affects elderly people, with a population incidence of around 1–2 per million per year in all populations in which specific surveillance has been undertaken.

Before 1986, interest in TSEs was primarily focused on the unusual nature of the causative agent—a transmissible infectious protein containing no DNA, with remarkable survival characteristics and resistance to autoclaving. The focus turned to their potential public health impact following a large epidemic in the UK of an apparently new TSE in cattle—bovine spongiform encephalopathy (BSE)—which was first recognized in 1986. BSE was initially considered likely to be a problem only for animal health, but cases of a new TSE affecting young adults reported in 1996, variant CJD (vCJD), were considered likely to be caused by the ingestion of beef products contaminated with the BSE agent. Because the BSE epidemic in cattle was very large and beef products are a very common food item in the UK and many other countries, there was widespread concern about the public health impact of this epidemic.

The two epidemics of BSE and vCJD illustrate how a newly emerging infectious disease could become a major global public health problem in the right circumstances. In fact, for reasons that are still not clear, the epidemic of vCJD has been much smaller than many feared initially.

This chapter focuses mainly on BSE and vCJD, but other TSEs are mentioned when they are important for understanding epidemiological features (Table 24.1).

Table 24.1 Main transmissible spongiform encephalopathies in humans

Infectious agent	• Abnormal prion protein		
Diseases caused	• CJD	• vCJD	• Kuru
Transmission	• Most cases not known • Small number are iatrogenic	• Probably contaminated beef products	• Endocannibalism
Incubation period	• Not known • Iatrogenic cases: average ~10 years	• Average ~10 years	• Average ~10 years
Main diagnostic tests	• Clinical with neuropathological confirmation		
Regions most affected	• Global	• UK • Smaller number of cases in other countries	• Papua New Guinea
Estimated global burden	• ~1–2 million/year	• ~200 cases in total	• Several thousand cases in total

CJD, Creutzfeldt–Jakob disease; vCJD, variant Creutzfeldt–Jakob disease.

The diseases

Most cases of CJD occur 'sporadically'; consistent risk factors for the disease, other than advanced age, have not been identified in case-control studies. These sporadic cases are thought likely to have arisen through endogenous mutation of PrP. About 10–15% of cases arise through inherited mutations in the *PRNP* gene that encodes PrP, with an autosomally dominant pattern of inheritance. vCJD presents with clinical features similar to CJD, but it generally affects young adults and has a longer clinical course (on average about 18 months from first symptoms to death, compared with 6 months for CJD). The two conditions are also distinguishable by their neuropathological features.

Transmission

Both CJD and vCJD are associated with transmissible agents, which are demonstrable by intracerebral injection of post-mortem-derived brain tissue from affected cases into experimental animals. CJD has been transmitted through contaminated batches of pituitary-derived human growth hormone (hGH) harvested from cadavers. Although there are no reports of transmission of CJD through blood transfusion, vCJD has been transmitted via this route.

The BSE epidemic resulted from the practice of recycling waste parts of ruminants—at the end of abattoir lines—into a high-protein product, meat and bone meal (MBM), which was used as a supplementary feed for farmed animals. The BSE agent was probably introduced into this system in the 1970s. The source of the original introduction is not known, but once it was in the system, the epidemic mushroomed, as infected animals were slaughtered and infected waste tissues were recycled into feed. This evolution was not dissimilar to the way in which the epidemic of the TSE kuru in Papua New Guinea is thought to have occurred through the practice of endocannibalism, probably initiated through someone who had died of CJD being the subject of endocannibalistic funeral rituals.

Incubation periods

The average incubation period of BSE is about 5 years. For cases of CJD arising through the use of contaminated hGH, the average period is about 10 years. Estimates of the incubation periods for kuru and vCJD, derived from mathematical modelling, are similar. However, the incubation periods are variable, and incubation periods in excess of 30 years have been described for kuru.

Control measures

The crucial control measure to curb the BSE epidemic was a ban on feeding MBM to ruminants. Initially, non-ruminants, including pigs and poultry (which seem not to be susceptible to infection with the BSE agent), were not included in the ban, but it became apparent that feed intended for these animals was leaking back to cattle. The feeding of MBM was subsequently banned for all farmed animals, and these measures were effective in controlling the epidemic and almost eliminating the disease (Figure 24.1); a small number of infected animals were still being detected in 2015, but the origin of these cases is unknown.

To reduce transmission of CJD or vCJD through contaminated surgical instruments, all such instruments that are used on someone known to have the disease should be destroyed after use. The possibility of such transmission remains through instruments used on people incubating the disease, as there are currently no diagnostic tests for infection, but such transmission has not yet been reported for vCJD.

When the BSE epidemic was first recognized, the risk of transmission to humans was assessed as 'remote'; nonetheless, some control measures were put in place to limit any risk, and bovine tissues likely to have the highest titres of the infective agent were banned from the human food chain, particularly the brain, spinal cord, and intestines. After the first evidence of transmission of BSE to humans, additional control measures were put in place, including only allowing cattle younger than 30 months into the food chain. When diagnostic tests that detect late-stage infections in brain tissue became available, these were applied to all cattle going through abattoirs, and infected animals were removed.

The absence of a diagnostic test means that measures to prevent transmission of vCJD through blood transfusion have been problematic. Some countries have not allowed people to donate blood if they spent more than 3 or 6 months in the UK between 1980 and 1996 (a compromise to avoid losing too high a proportion of blood donors). The UK has banned blood donations from anyone who has themselves been the recipient of a blood donation.

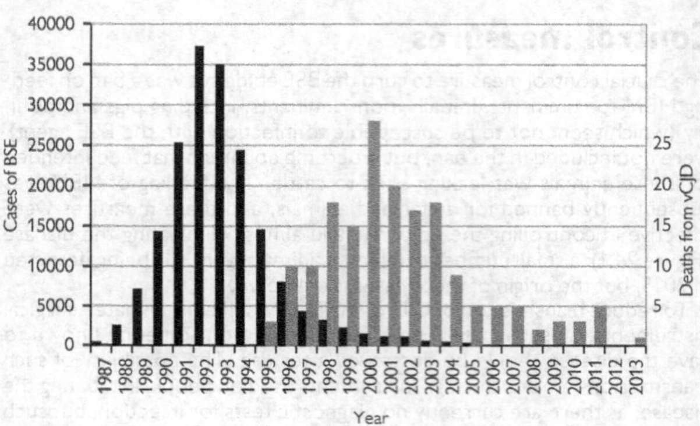

Figure 24.1 Cases of bovine spongiform encephalopathy (BSE) and deaths from variant Creutzfeldt–Jakob disease (vCJD) in the United Kingdom (UK) by year.

Source: data from The National CJD Research and Surveillance Unit (NCJDRSU), *Creutzfeldt-Jakob disease in the UK (by calendar year)*, Copyright © The University of Edinburgh 2012, available from http://www.cjd.ed.ac.uk/documents/figs.pdf; and The World Organisation for Animal Health (OIE), *Number of cases of bovine spongiform encephalopathy (BSE) reported in the United Kingdom*, Copyright © OIE 2015, available from http://www.oie.int/animal-health-in-the-world/bse-specific-data/number-of-cases-in-the-united-kingdom/.

Surveillance and the evolution of the epidemics

Good surveillance was key to recognizing the BSE epidemic, guiding the control measures, and evaluating their impact (see ➲ Chapter 2). Early recognition of the epidemic prompted epidemiological studies, which implicated MBM and informed the principal control measure. Such surveillance also enabled failings in the initial feed ban to be identified and corrective measures put in place.

Anticipating the 'remote' possibility that BSE might pass into the human population, national surveillance for CJD was set up in 1990. This led directly to the identification of vCJD in 1996, and the associated neuropathological surveillance characterized vCJD as distinctly different from CJD. Given the large number of infected cattle that entered the food chain, there were fears that the human epidemic of vCJD would be enormous. However, the epidemic of vCJD peaked in around 2000 (Figure 24.1), with very few cases in recent years. Why these particular individuals developed the disease and why the epidemic has not been much larger is unknown. Case-control studies of those with vCJD have not identified distinguishing features from controls.

A remaining question is how many people are currently incubating vCJD. Some cases of vCJD had an appendicectomy prior to developing symptoms of vCJD. Tests on these tissues found evidence of infection in the appendices several years before the onset of any symptoms of vCJD. This discovery led to two large anonymized surveys of samples of appendix tissue stored in pathology departments in the UK. In the most recent survey, 16 of 32 441 appendix samples were positive for abnormal PrP—an overall prevalence of infection in the range of about 300–800 per million population, a much higher number than the fewer than 200 cases of vCJD identified in the UK to date. Some of these individuals may be silent carriers of infection, not destined to develop disease, and whether or not they represent a risk of transmission, should they donate blood, is unknown.

Further reading

Alpers MP (2008). The epidemiology of kuru: monitoring the epidemic from its peak to its end. *Philos Trans R Soc Lond B Biol Sci*, **363**, 3707–13.

BSE Inquiry (2000). *The BSE Inquiry: the report*. Available at: http://collections.europarchive.org/tna/20090505194948/ http:/bseinquiry.gov.uk/report/index.htm (accessed 5 November 2015).

Collinge J (1999). Variant Creutzfeldt–Jakob disease. *Lancet*, **354**, 317–23.

Smith PG, Bradley R (2003). Bovine spongiform encephalopathy (BSE) and its epidemiology. *Br Med Bull*, **66**, 185–98.

Smith PG, Cousens SN, Huillard d'Aignaux, Ward HJ, Will RG (2004). The epidemiology of variant Creutzfeldt–Jakob disease. *Curr Top Microbiol Immunol*, **284**, 161–91.

Chapter 25

Human immunodeficiency virus (HIV) infection

Andrew Boulle and Leigh Johnson

Introduction to human immunodeficiency virus

The human immunodeficiency virus (HIV) destroys human immune cells, thereby severely weakening the immune system and increasing the risk of opportunistic infections (OIs), some cancers, and chronic diseases (Table 25.1). In 2014, 35 million people were estimated to be living with HIV globally; cumulatively, HIV had resulted in 39 million deaths. The estimated global prevalence of adult HIV is 0.8%, but there is extensive geographic diversity, with country-level adult prevalences ranging from <0.1% to >20% in the most severely affected countries of Southern Africa.

The two main types of HIV are further subdivided into groups and clades (or subtypes). HIV was initially a zoonotic infection from apes (HIV-1, which is responsible for most infections globally) and sooty mangabey monkeys (HIV-2). Each of the major viral groups are thought to have resulted from separate zoonotic infections in Central and West Africa, with the transmission event for the ancestral strain of the HIV-1 group M viruses that predominate today most likely occurring in the early part of the 20th century.

The course of untreated HIV-1 infection is characterized by a long initial period of mostly asymptomatic infection, which typically lasts 4–6 years, although glandular fever-like symptoms may occur during the first few weeks of infection. After several years, the infected individual starts to experience intermittent symptoms such as weight loss, diarrhoea, and oral infections. Finally, when the individual's immune system has been severely weakened by HIV, they can experience a variety of characteristic OIs, some of which are regarded as defining acquired immune deficiency syndrome (AIDS). The median time from infection to death is usually estimated at 10–12 years in the absence of treatment. For infants who are infected perinatally, disease progression and death occur much more rapidly. Individuals who are infected with HIV-2 survive for longer and are less infectious than those infected with HIV-1.

A number of laboratory tests have been used to determine the prognosis of people infected with HIV. The two laboratory measures most commonly used are viral load and $CD4^+$ T-lymphocyte cell count. $CD4^+$ T-lymphocytes are an essential part of a well-functioning immune system; an uninfected individual typically has a $CD4^+$ count >800 cells/microlitre, while an individual with AIDS would usually have a $CD4^+$ count <200 cells/microlitre. The viral load is a measure of the concentration of HIV in the body and can be thought of as determining the rate of decline in the $CD4^+$ count. Figure 25.1 shows the typical changes in viral load and $CD4^+$ count over the course of HIV infection. Viral load (often reported on a logarithmic scale) tends to be high at the time of seroconversion and then falls after the individual's immune system responds to the virus. The viral load is important not only as a prognostic marker, but also as a measure of an individual's infectiousness, as individuals with a high viral load are most likely to transmit HIV.

Table 25.1 HIV summary

Infectious agent	• HIV
	• Genus *Lentivirus* of the *Retroviridae* family, with two types (HIV-1 and HIV-2)
	• Most HIV-1 viruses are of major group M, which is further divided into subtypes A–D, F–H, J, and K
	  • Groups A–C predominate
	  • Additional groups (N–P) confined to West Africa
	• HIV-2 divided into groups A–H and further subtypes
	  • Only groups A and B are epidemic and are largely confined to West Africa

Disease	• Symptoms and opportunistic infections of increasing severity with duration of disease, characterized in four WHO-defined stages • Most advanced stage (stage IV) is termed AIDS
Incubation period	• 4–6 years until pre-AIDS symptoms • 9–10 years until AIDS
Main diagnostic tests	• Rapid or laboratory-based (e.g. ELISA) antibody tests most commonly used to test for HIV and become positive within a few weeks of infection (at seroconversion following the window period) • Antigen-based tests (for viral RNA, DNA, or proteins) are able to detect HIV infection soon after infection • A second, and sometimes third test (in low-prevalence settings), using different rapid or laboratory tests, are recommended to confirm infection
Global epidemiology	• Most of the 35 million people living with HIV in 2013 were in sub-Saharan Africa (71%) and South, South East, and East Asia (14%) • HIV prevalence exceeded 10% in nine countries (all in sub-Saharan Africa), and 1% in a further 40 countries • Global incidence thought to have peaked at 3.4 million new infections in 2001, declining to 2.1 million in 2013 • 12.9 million HIV-infected individuals on HIV treatment at end of 2013 • HIV mortality had fallen by 35% since 2005

AIDS, acquired immune deficiency syndrome; DNA, deoxyribonucleic acid; ELISA, enzyme-linked immunosorbent assay; HIV, human immunodeficiency virus; RNA, ribonucleic acid; WHO, World Health Organization.

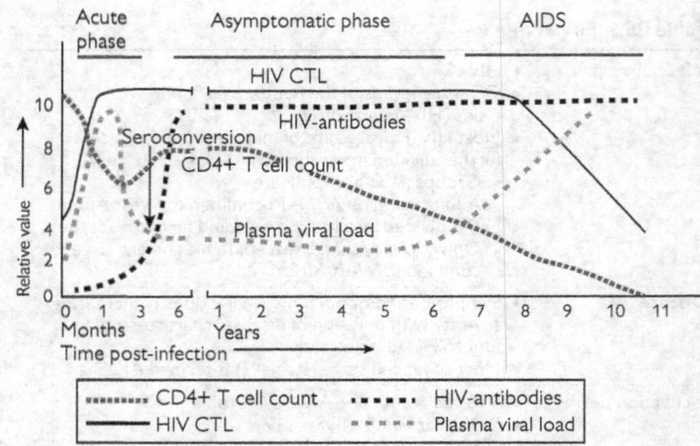

Figure 25.1 Natural history of HIV-1 infection.

HIV, human immunodeficiency virus; RNA, ribonucleic acid. HIV CTL, HIV-specific cytotoxic T-lymphocytes.

Reproduced with permission from *Laboratory Guidelines for enumerating CD4 T Lymphocytes in the context of HIV/AIDS*, World Health Organization (WHO) Regional Office for South-East Asia New Delhi, India, Copyright © WHO 2007.

Mode of transmission

The main route of transmission of HIV to adults is currently through sexual contact, with heterosexual transmission predominating in generalized epidemic settings such as Southern Africa. When AIDS was first recognized as a clinical syndrome in 1981 and in subsequent years, sexual transmission predominantly took place in men who have sex with men (MSM). The third most important route of transmission is contaminated needles shared by people who inject drugs (PWIDs), which is the predominant mode of transmission in some countries, including many in Eastern Europe and the former Soviet Union. Rarely, HIV is transmitted through blood products. Most children with HIV are infected from their mothers *in utero*, at the time of delivery, or post-partum through breastfeeding. In the absence of prevention, about a quarter of children born to HIV-infected women are infected with HIV.

Factors associated with the sexual transmission of HIV are described in detail in ➲ Chapter 23. In the context of multiple concurrent sexual partnerships, the high HIV viral load soon after HIV infection is especially important in increasing transmission to secondary contacts. A complex interplay also exists between other STIs (see ➲ Chapter 23) and HIV, with ulcerative STIs being important cofactors for HIV transmission, accelerating the epidemic spread, especially early in HIV epidemics.

Diagnosis and treatment

Most screening for HIV disease is based on rapid or laboratory-based antibody tests on blood, plasma, or serum. Current versions of laboratory-based antibody tests, such as ELISA, have sensitivities approaching 100% and specificities of >99%. Many rapid tests achieve this level of performance, but it can vary by test, operator, and field characteristics. In high-prevalence settings (prevalence >5%), it is recommended that positive results are confirmed by a second test, while a third confirmatory test may be required in settings of low prevalence.

Antigen tests that detect parts of the virus itself are increasingly used, especially in infants. They have the advantage of detecting HIV before an antibody response is detectable (the so-called window period). A common test is the PCR, which amplifies and detects a segment of RNA or DNA in infected individuals. These tests are commonly used to diagnose HIV in infants, as the presence of maternal HIV antibodies in children born to infected mothers precludes the use of antibody tests.

The past 25 years have seen rapid development of pharmacological treatment options for HIV, termed antiretroviral therapy (ART). The availability of three-drug treatment regimens from 1995 onwards heralded a new era in treating HIV, with enduring recovery and survival in those treated. The drugs target different stages of the HIV replication cycle, and tolerability and durability have improved over time with the approval of newer antiretroviral drugs. The recommended time to start treatment has been shifting earlier, in line with improved tolerability, greater appreciation of clinical benefits of treatment at higher $CD4^+$ counts, and the secondary benefits of decreased transmission of HIV. Some current guidelines recommend starting ART in symptomatic patients and those with $CD4^+$ T-lymphocyte count <350 or 500 cells/microlitre, but most guidelines now recommend the introduction of ART for all persons living with HIV, independent of the $CD4^+$ count, to reduce population transmission. Although HIV is now considered a treatable disease, there is still no known cure.

Prevention and control

Programmes to prevent HIV need to begin with **information and education campaigns** to build awareness around HIV, its consequences, how it is transmitted, and measures to prevent transmission. These campaigns may include promotion and distribution of condoms and promotion of safer sex.

Improving access to **HIV counselling and testing** (HCT) is also important in the control of HIV, as undiagnosed HIV-positive individuals are believed to contribute disproportionately to HIV transmission, and HIV diagnosis is associated with positive changes in risk behaviour. Improved **treatment of other STIs** may also be an important strategy for limiting the spread of HIV, as STIs increase the probability of HIV transmission. **Male circumcision** has been shown to reduce men's susceptibility to HIV infection by about 60% and can therefore also be considered an important HIV prevention strategy.

Prevention of mother-to-child transmission (PMTCT) of HIV involves the provision of ART to the mother and infant before and after birth and counselling on infant-feeding options (formula feeding or exclusive breastfeeding are usually promoted). Programmes for PMTCT can theoretically reduce transmission rates to <2% if all pregnant women start long-term highly active antiretroviral therapy (HAART) prior to delivery and do not breastfeed or are adherent to ART during breastfeeding.

Although ART has traditionally been seen as a treatment strategy, rather than a prevention strategy, interest in the use of **ART in prevention** has been growing, as ART reduces the concentration of HIV in the body to very low levels and thereby reduces the infectiousness of HIV-positive individuals. Antiretroviral drugs were also shown recently to be effective in prevention when used by HIV-negative individuals. **Pre-exposure prophylaxis** (PrEP) refers to oral or topical administration of ART prior to sex to reduce the risk of HIV acquisition. Use of **microbicides** (topical PrEP) may be particularly important for women who are unable to insist that their sexual partners use condoms, notwithstanding the adherence challenges for preparations which require peri-coital self-administration.

Needle exchange programmes have also been shown to be effective in preventing HIV transmission among PWIDs. **Post-exposure prophylaxis** (PEP), which involves the temporary administration of ART following exposure, is also important in reducing the risk of HIV infection in health workers who have experienced needle-stick injuries and victims of sexual assault.

Although there are substantial challenges in the development of an HIV **vaccine**, one candidate vaccine has so far been shown to be modestly effective, reducing the risk of HIV transmission by 31%. Ongoing work is aimed at confirming and improving on this through new approaches.

While the above described prevention programmes are crucial in reducing the risk of HIV at an individual level, it is also important that interventions be developed in relation to **social determinants** of HIV risk. Factors, such as gender inequality, migration, livelihood challenges, substance abuse, and stigma around HIV/AIDS, fuel the growth of the epidemic, and many country-level HIV prevention programmes seek to address these as part of a comprehensive response to the epidemic.

Surveillance

Surveillance of HIV differs substantially between countries. In most high-income countries, case reporting of new HIV diagnoses is the main source of estimates (see ➲ Chapter 2).

In countries with a high prevalence of HIV, nationally representative household surveys are usually considered the gold standard to estimate the prevalence and are further able to estimate other indicators such as HIV treatment coverage and treatment success. Surveys of HIV prevalence in pregnant women provide useful additional information regarding HIV prevalence trends in developing countries, but they may be biased, because they represent mainly young sexually active women who are not using contraception.

In many developing countries, the focus of surveillance has gradually shifted from measuring HIV prevalence to measuring the incidence of HIV, as the latter better reflects the success (or failure) of recent control programmes. However, the incidence of HIV is difficult to measure directly, and a number of approaches have been proposed, including the conduct of longitudinal studies in sentinel populations, improved laboratory methods to detect recently acquired HIV in survey samples, and the use of mathematical models fitted to data from prevalence surveys.

Further reading

Abdool Karim SS, Abdool Karim Q (eds) (2010). *HIV/AIDS in South Africa*, 2nd edn. Cambridge University Press, Cape Town.

Bertozzi SM, Laga M, Bautista-Arredondo S, *et al.* (2008). Making HIV prevention programmes work. *Lancet*, **372**, 831–44.

Joint United Nations Programme on HIV/AIDS (UNAIDS) (2014). *GAP report*. UNAIDS, Geneva.

Maartens G, Celum C, Lewin SR (2014). HIV infection: epidemiology, pathogenesis, treatment, and prevention. *Lancet*, **384**, 258–71.

Sharp PM, Hahn BH (2011). Origins of HIV and the AIDS pandemic. *Cold Spring Harbor Perspectives in Medicine*, **1**, a006841.

United Nations, World Health Organization (2015). *Guideline on when to start antiretroviral therapy and on pre-exposure prophylaxis for HIV*. World Health Organization, Geneva.

Vermund SH (2014). Global HIV epidemiology: a guide for strategies in prevention and care. *Curr HIV/AIDS Rep*, **11**, 93–8.

Chapter 26

Parasitic infestations

Mauricio L. Barreto and Phil J. Cooper

Introduction to parasitic infestations

Parasites are important causes of disease and death in humans. A parasite is an organism that lives at the expense of its host; the three main types are protozoa, helminths, and ectoparasites. The protozoa and helminths that cause 'parasitic diseases' are usually endoparasites, while ectoparasites live on the surface of the host.

This chapter focuses on helminth infections of greatest public health importance: soil-transmitted helminth (STH) infections and schistosomiasis.

Soil-transmitted helminths (intestinal helminths)

Introduction to soil-transmitted helminths

The four main STHs of global public health relevance are *Ascaris lumbricoides* (819 million estimated to be infected worldwide), *Trichuris trichiura* (465 million), and the hookworms *Necator americanus* and *Ancylostoma duodenale* (439 million) (Table 26.1). *Strongyloides stercoralis* is less common but can cause severe disseminated infection in immunocompromised individuals (30–100 million). Other STHs with a global distribution are *Enterobius vermicularis, Toxocara canis*, and *Toxocara cati* (which cause visceral and ocular larva migrans).

Mode of transmission of soil-transmitted helminths

Transmission of *A. lumbricoides* and *T. trichiura* is faeco–oral, whereas hookworms and *S. stercoralis* transmit through skin contact with infective larvae. Adult STHs live in the human intestine (the hookworm *A. lumbricoide* and *S. stercoralis* parasitize the small intestine; *T. trichiura* the large intestine, especially the caecum) where females produce thousands of eggs a day (or larvae for *S. stercoralis*), which are expelled in faeces. The eggs require a period of 2–3 weeks in the environment to mature and become infective, except for *S. stercoralis* where the larvae may lead to auto-infection.

Clinical presentation of soil-transmitted helminths

Infections caused by STHs are generally asymptomatic, with the risk of clinical disease increasing with heavier parasite burdens. Clinical manifestations are generally non-specific, varying from mild (including abdominal discomfort and poor appetite) to severe (including intestinal obstruction (*A. lumbricoides*), anaemia that is occasionally severe (hookworm), and colitis and dysentery (*T. trichiura*)). *S. stercoralis* is generally asymptomatic but may cause severe disseminated disease in immunocompromised patients with sepsis, multi-organ failure, and significant mortality.

Diagnosis of soil-transmitted helminths

Diagnosis is made by the detection of eggs or larvae in faeces. One common detection method is the direct smear where a small quantity of faeces suspended in saline is examined on a microscope slide. Other common, more sensitive methods include egg concentration techniques (e.g. the Kato–Katz faecal thick smear and the McMaster method). Serology is superior to microscopy for *S. stercoralis*, but poor specificity is a problem with standard serological assays in endemic populations. Molecular methods, such as PCR-based assays, have much better sensitivity but are expensive. The sensitivity of standard microscopic methods can be improved by multiple sampling to up to three stool samples. In non-endemic populations, peripheral blood eosinophilia is highly suggestive of a helminth infection.

Table 26.1 Characteristics of soil-transmitted helminths

Infectious agent	Disease caused	Reservoir	Incubation period	Main diagnostic tests	Regions/countries most affected	Estimated global burden (cases)
Ascaris lumbricoides	• Ascariasis (common roundworm infection)	• Eggs in soil and infected humans act as reservoirs	• 4–8 weeks	• Stool examination	• Worldwide • Greatest frequency in tropical and subtropical regions and areas with inadequate sanitation	• Estimated 807–1,221 million people
Trichuris trichiura	• Trichiuriasis (whipworm infection)	• Eggs in soil or infected humans act as reservoirs	• 15–30 days	• Stool examination	• Worldwide • Greatest frequency in tropical and subtropical regions and areas with inadequate sanitation	• Estimated 604–795 million people
Ancylostoma duodenale/ Necator americanus	• Ancylostomiasis (hookworm infection)	• Humans	• Varies between a few weeks to many months	• Stool examination	• Worldwide in areas with warm, moist, climates	• 576–740 million people
Strongyloides stercoralis	• Strongyloidiasis (threadworm infection)	• Humans • Cats, dogs, and monkeys have been infected	• 2–4 weeks	• Stool examination	• Most common in tropical or subtropical climates	• 30–100 million people infected
Enterobius vermicularis	• Enterobiasis (pinworm infection)	• Humans	• 1–2 months	• Search for eggs in perianal skin with transparent tape that is examined with microscope	• Worldwide	• 4–28% of children

Toxocara canis/T. cati	• Visceral and ocular larva migrans	• Dogs, foxes, and cats	• 1 week to months	• Serological test using PCR or finding larvae in biopsy or autopsy specimens	• Worldwide	• 2–80% of children
Schistosoma haematobium	• Schistosomiasis haematobium • Urinary schistosomiais	• Humans and other mammals • Freshwater *Bulinus* spp. snails as intermediate hosts	• 14–84 days for acute form	• Urine examination or tissue biopsies for eggs	• Africa • Middle East	• 112 million infected
Schistosoma mansoni	• Schistosomiasis mansoni • Intestinal schistosomiais	• Humans and other mammals • Freshwater *Biomphalaria* spp. snails as intermediate hosts	• 14–84 days for acute form	• Stool examination or tissue biopsies for eggs	• South America • Caribbean • Africa	• 80 million infected
Schistosoma japonicum	• Schistosomiasis japonicum • Asian intestinal schistosomiais	• Humans and other mammals. • Amphibious freshwater *Oncomelania* spp. snails as intermediate hosts	• 14–84 days for acute form	• Stool examination or tissue biopsies for eggs	• China • Southeast Asia	

PCR, polymerase chain reaction

Treatment of soil-transmitted helminths

The drugs most widely used to treat STH infections are benzimidazoles (e.g. mebendazole and albendazole). The standard dose is 400 mg albendazole or 500 mg mebendazole as single oral doses. The efficacy of benzimidazole drugs varies according to the parasite; a single dose cures >90% of infections with *A. lumbricoides*. Hookworm cure rates vary; albendazole is preferable to mebendazole, and, in some settings, cure rates >90% can be achieved only with three doses over consecutive days. Three doses of 400 mg albendazole, given over consecutive days, are recommended against *T. trichiura*. Greater cure rates may be achieved by the addition of a single dose of ivermectin (200 micrograms/kg). The treatment of choice for strongyloidiasis is a single oral dose of ivermectin 200 micrograms/kg, which has >90% efficacy. Albendazole is an effective alternative. Disseminated disease requires daily treatments with ivermectin for prolonged periods.

Prevention and control of soil-transmitted helminths

There is currently no effective vaccine against STHs. In endemic communities, the distribution of worms displays an overdispersed distribution, with a few individuals (usually children) harbouring a large proportion of all worms and acting as the main reservoir of infections. Control of the disease in endemic areas has relied on periodic (annual or semi-annual) mass treatments of schoolchildren with benzimidazole to reduce transmission and the risk of morbidity by reducing parasitic burdens. Infections with STHs thrive in conditions of poverty where access to sanitation is limited and faecal contamination of the environment is widespread.

A growing awareness of the limitations of chemotherapy strategies has led to renewed emphasis on education and good hygiene (i.e. using soap to wash hands after defecation) and improvements in access to clean water and sanitation, together known as WASH (water, sanitation, and hygiene) strategies.

Schistosomiasis (intestinal and genitourinary)

Introduction to schistosomiasis

The three schistosome species of public health relevance are *Schistosoma haematobium*, which occurs mainly in Africa; *S. mansoni*, which occurs in the Middle East, South America, and Africa; and *S. japonicum*, which occurs in parts of China and the Philippines. An estimated 200 million people are infected worldwide.

Mode of transmission of schistosomiasis

The adult male and female worms live within the veins of abdominal and pelvic organs within their human host where they mate and produce fertilized eggs. The eggs are either shed into the environment through faeces or urine or are retained in host tissues where they cause disease. Eggs that reach fresh water hatch, releasing free-living ciliated miracidia that infect a suitable snail host. In the snail, the parasite undergoes asexual replication, eventually shedding thousands of cercariae that infect humans through exposed skin.

Clinical presentation of schistosomiasis

Acute schistosomiasis (Katayama syndrome) occurs most often in travellers or immigrants to endemic regions when infected for the first time. It presents weeks to months after infection, with sudden onset of fever, malaise, myalgia, headache, eosinophilia, fatigue, and abdominal pain, which generally resolves within 2–10 weeks of onset.

Chronic schistosomiasis is a slowly progressive condition caused by retention of schistosome eggs in intestines and liver for *S. mansoni and S. japonicum* and the bladder and urogenital system for *S. haematobium*. In the case of *S. mansoni* and *S. japonicum*, a chronic intestinal form of the disease may develop over many years, with periportal fibrosis (Symmer's pipe-stem fibrosis) and portal hypertension. Clinical features include upper abdominal discomfort, with palpable nodular and hard hepatomegaly, often with splenomegaly. The clinical picture can become severe, with ascites and haematemesis from oesophageal varices. Pulmonary hypertension caused by granulomatous pulmonary arteritis can also occur in patients with advanced hepatic fibrosis disease.

Spinal schistosomiasis is an atypical, but severe, form in which adult females become located in atypical sites, and the eggs embolize in the spinal cord, which may be associated with rapidly progressive neurologic deficits.

The most characteristic symptom for urogenital schistosomiasis (*S. haematobium*) is haematuria. As with severe intestinal schistosomiasis, severe urogenital schistosomiasis occurs more often in individuals with the highest burden of infection and is a consequence of poor immunoregulation of antischistosome egg responses, leading to chronic fibrosis of the urinary tract, which presents as obstructive uropathy (hydroureter and hydronephrosis).

Infection with *S. haematobium* is associated with a high frequency of squamous cell carcinoma of the bladder. It may affect female fertility and cause inflammatory lesions in the female genital tract, affecting the ovaries, Fallopian tubes, cervix, vagina, and vulva. Recent studies have shown a higher risk of HIV infection (see ➔ Chapter 25) among women with genital schistosomiasis.

Diagnosis of schistosomiasis

The standard diagnostic method for schistosomiasis, which is not very sensitive, is the microscopic detection of parasite eggs in urine (*S. haematobium*) and faeces (*S. japonicum* and *S. mansoni*) or in tissue biopsies and rectal snips. Microscopic examination of polycarbonate filters for eggs in the urine and the Kato–Katz faecal examination for eggs in stool are the most commonly used methods. Molecular techniques and serological assays are also used but have limitations. More recently, sensitive and specific POC diagnostics tests have been developed, and the availability of these in endemic areas may greatly aid treatment and control strategies.

Treatment of schistosomiasis

Praziquantel, which is safe and effective against all *Schistosoma* spp., with relatively few adverse events, is the drug of choice. Effective doses are 40 mg/kg for *S. haematobium* and *S. mansoni*, and 60 mg/kg for *S. japonicum*; 40 mg/kg can safely be used in pregnancy after the first trimester. Praziquantel is available generally only as large tablets, and paediatric formulations are not readily available. Oxamniquine—a tetrahydroquinolone compound—is effective only against *S. mansoni* and has limited availability. Currently, no vaccine is available for the treatment and control of schistosomiasis.

Prevention and control of schistosomiasis

Mass drug administration of praziquantel has been implemented for control of schistosomiasis worldwide. As with STH infections, education to improve hygiene habits and safe disposal of faeces are key to sustainable and effective control strategies.

Improved sanitation aims to reduce soil and water contamination. To be effective against schistosomiasis, sanitation must cover a high percentage of households, with the associated economic costs rendering this not an easy task in resource-limited settings, particularly in rural areas and urban shanties.

Conclusions

Infections with STHs and schistosomiasis are common with significant morbidity, mainly on the physical fitness of endemic populations, and mortality. Diagnosis relies on relatively insensitive microscopic identification of the parasite, but more sensitive POC tests are in development. Treatment is limited to few safe and effective drugs, and drug resistance has yet to become a problem. Recent efforts to control these infections in endemic areas have involved mass drug administration for STH infections or schistosomiasis (or both where they are co-endemic). Such programmes reduce parasite burdens and morbidity, but should be accompanied, where possible, by education on hygiene and improvements in sanitation and access to clean water.

Further reading

Barreto ML, Genser B, Strina A, *et al.* (2010). Impact of a citywide sanitation program in Northeast Brazil on intestinal parasites infection in young children. *Environ Health Perspect*, **118**, 1637–42.

Bethony J, Brooker S, Albonico M, *et al.* (2006). Soil-transmitted helminth infections: ascariasis, trichuriasis, and hookworm. *Lancet*, **367**, 1521–32.

Colley DG, Bustinduy AL, Secor WE, King CH (2013). Human schistosomiasis. *Lancet*, **383**, 2253–64.

Greaves D, Coggle S, Pollard C, Aliyu SH, Moore EM (2013). *Strongyloides stercoralis* infection. *BMJ*, **347**, f4610.

Hotez PJ, Bundy DAP, Beegle K, *et al.* (2006). Helminth infections: soil-transmitted helminth infections and schistosomiasis. In: Jamison DT, Breman JG, Measham AR, *et al.* (eds). *Manson's tropical diseases*. World Bank, Washington, DC.

Jia TW, Melville S, Utzinger J, King CH, Zhou XN (2012). Soil-transmitted helminth reinfection after drug treatment: a systematic review and meta-analysis. *PLoS Negl Trop Dis*, **6**, e1621.

Chapter 27

Congenital infections

Lakshmi Ganapathi and Tanvi Sharma

Introduction to congenital infections

Congenital infections are infections that affect the unborn fetus or newborn infant. These infections are either transmitted directly to the fetus from infected mothers via the placenta (transplacental transmission) or acquired by the newborn via the birth canal during delivery. They are therefore also known as vertically transmitted infections or mother-to-child transmitted infections. The global burden of congenital infections has been hard to estimate, given the lack of high-quality surveillance data, particularly in low- and middle-income countries. In general, the burden of vaccine-preventable congenital infections, such as rubella, is highest in regions or countries where vaccines are not available or uptake is low. Table 27.1 provides examples of congenital infections, the disease-causing pathogen, diagnostic techniques, and areas of disease burden worldwide.

Table 27.1 Examples of congenital infections and associated disease-causing pathogens, diagnostic techniques, and areas of disease burden worldwide

Infectious agent	Disease caused	Reservoir	Incubation period	Main diagnostic tests	Regions most affected
CMV	• Congenital CMV infection	• Humans • In case of perinatal infection, reservoirs include breast milk, maternal secretions, and transfused blood products	• Up to 90% of newborn babies infected congenitally are asymptomatic at birth; remaining 10% exhibit symptoms at birth • As many as 15% of asymptomatic infants can experience progressive hearing loss • Hearing loss may also manifest later in childhood	• Urine/saliva shell vial assay • Urine/saliva viral culture • Urine/saliva CMV DNA PCR	• Global birth prevalence of congenital CMV infection is estimated at 0.6–6.1%, although there is a paucity of studies from developing countries to determine true prevalence • In developed countries, birth prevalence is 0.2–2%

Treponema pallidum	• Congenital syphilis	• Humans are only known reservoir	• Early congenital syphilis presents with clinical manifestations before age of 2 years
			• Late congenial syphilis presents with clinical manifestations after age of 2 years
				• In clinical settings:
				  • Direct visualization of *T. pallidum* by dark field microscopy or fluorescence antibody staining of infected body fluids, lesions, placenta, or umbilical cord
					• Congenital syphilis complicates about 1 million pregnancies per year worldwide
					• Regions affected include:
					  • sub-Saharan Africa
					  • South and South East Asia
					  • Latin America and the Caribbean

(Continued)

Table 27.1 *(Contd.)*

Infectious agent	Disease caused	Reservoir	Incubation period	Main diagnostic tests	Regions most affected
			• About 40% of infants of untreated mothers develop late congenital syphilis	• Demonstration of *T. pallidum* by special stains or histopathological examination • Demonstration of serology typical of syphilis from venous blood • Point-of-care testing kits are commercially available and can be used in settings where laboratory testing is not available	• Congenital syphilis in the USA occurs primarily in infants whose mothers were untreated or demonstrated inadequate serological response to treatment
Rubella virus	• Congenital rubella syndrome	• Humans are only known reservoir	• Most infants with congenital rubella syndrome are asymptomatic at birth but develop clinical manifestations over next 5 years	• Viral isolation from nasopharyngeal secretions • Serological confirmation: • Demonstration of rubella-specific IgM antibody or infant IgG rubella antibody levels that persists at higher levels and for a longer time than expected from passive transfer of maternal antibody	• Regions where vaccine coverage is the lowest, including countries in Africa and South East Asia • In the USA, congenital rubella is rare because of routine vaccinations and rubella serology being checked in mothers during pregnancy

HSV I and II	• Intrauterine HSV (rare), perinatal and post-natal HSV	• Humans	• Intrauterine HSV is rare, and manifestations primarily occur in the neonatal period • Disseminated disease often presents in first week of life	• Isolation by viral cell culture • DFA and EIA of HSV antigens in skin and mucous membrane lesions • Detection of HSV DNA by PCR in the CSF	• Regions affected include sub-Saharan Africa • In general, prevalence is higher in developing countries • Estimated 1500 cases of neonatal HSV in the USA annually
Toxoplasma gondii	• Congenital toxoplasmosis	• Cats	• Newborns infected in second and third trimesters present predominantly with subclinical infection in neonatal period; severe manifestations can also occur during this period • Mild or severe disease can also present in first few months of life • Sequelae or relapse of undiagnosed infection can occur later in infancy, childhood, or adolescence	• Screening maternal and newborn serology and subsequent confirmation in reference laboratory • Newborn serology to be screened include toxoplasma-specific IgM antibody; when this is equivocal, toxoplasma-specific IgM and IgA may also be obtained	• South America • Some countries of the Middle East
Hepatitis B virus	• Congenital hepatitis B infection	• Humans	• Affected newborns remain asymptomatic, although small number of infants may have acute hepatitis by age 2 months	• Detection of hepatitis B viral DNA in blood, persistence of hepatitis B surface antigen	• Asia and Pacific regions • Sub-Saharan Africa

CMV, cytomegalovirus; DFA, direct immunofluorescence assays; DNA, deoxyribonucleic acid; EIA, enzyme immunoassays; HSV, herpes simplex virus; Ig, immunoglobulin; PCR, polymerase chain reaction; USA, United States of America.

Diagnosis

One challenge is to decide when the diagnosis of a congenital infection should be pursued, as the clinical symptoms and signs of vertically transmitted infections vary between pathogens.

Several infections that are transmitted from mother to child cause subtle symptoms in mothers—such as a transient fever and influenza-like symptoms—and may not be noticed. Careful investigation of a maternal history of exposure (such as to cat litter in the case of toxoplasmosis), maternal immunization status, a history of mononucleosis-like illness, lymphadenopathy, and rash during pregnancy may elicit useful information. When ultrasounds are performed routinely during pregnancy, signs of a congenital infection in the fetus can include intrauterine growth restriction, fetal microcephaly, hydrocephalus, intracranial calcifications, fetal hepatomegaly, and intrahepatic calcifications. A constellation of findings may be observed in newborn babies; several congenital pathogens and associated findings are described in Table 27.2.

Laboratory abnormalities, such as thrombocytopenia, anaemia, and elevated levels of liver enzymes, may also provide early signals of a congenital infection in a newborn child. Definitive diagnosis is established by performing pathogen-specific tests in the mother and newborn (Table 27.1). In general, every effort should be made to recover the causative organism from the newborn. Serology may be helpful, e.g. in the case of paired sera in mothers to document seroconversion during pregnancy. On the other hand, passively acquired antibody from mothers may complicate interpretation of serological tests in newborns and infants. Nevertheless, post-natal serial titres from the infant that show an increased titre at age 2–4 months or persistently high titres at age 6–8 months can be helpful in establishing the diagnosis. Exceptions for which serial titres are not helpful include CMV antibody, which may also be acquired peri- or post-natally, and HIV (see ➲ Chapter 25). In addition, IgM-associated antibodies in the mother and newborn child are unreliable and thus not recommended for diagnosis, except in the case of rubella-specific and toxoplasmosis-specific IgM. Of note, toxoplasmosis-specific IgM is a screening test to determine the need for further review or reference laboratory testing.

Table 27.2 Tests to diagnose congenital infections

Finding(s)	Possible congenital infection
Microcephaly	• CMV • Rubella • Toxoplasmosis • HSV
Anaemia with hydrops	• Syphilis • CMV • Toxoplasmosis
Jaundice with or without thrombocytopenia	• CMV • Toxoplasmosis • Rubella
Hepatosplenomegaly	• CMV • Rubella • Toxoplasmosis • HSV • Syphilis
Progressive hearing loss	• Rubella • CMV • Toxoplasmosis • Syphilis
Purpura (usually present on first day of life)	• CMV • Toxoplasmosis • Syphilis • Rubella • HSV
Ocular findings	• CMV • Toxoplasmosis • Rubella • HSV • Syphilis
Congenital heart disease	• Rubella
Cerebral calcifications	• Toxoplasmosis (widely distributed) • CMV and HSV (periventricular)
Hydrocephalus	• Toxoplasmosis • CMV • Syphilis
Pseudoparalysis	• Syphilis

CMV, cytomegalovirus; HSV, herpes simplex virus.

Treatment

Several examples of treatment of congenital infections are provided in Table 27.3. Treatment also includes management of sequelae of congenital infections such as hearing loss, neurodevelopmental delays, and congenital heart disease.

Table 27.3 Pathogen-specific treatment of congenital infections

Congenital infection	Prevention	Treatment	
		Mothers	Newborns
CMV	• Education on hygienic measures (for example, in day-care centres)	• None	• Ganciclovir for prevention of progression of hearing loss
Syphilis	• Education on prevention of STIs	• Penicillin	• Penicillin
Rubella	• Rubella vaccination	• Supportive care	• Supportive care
Toxoplasmosis	• Education on avoidance of exposure to cat litter/ faeces during pregnancy • Avoidance of undercooked meat • Screening of seronegative pregnant women following exposure and initiation of treatment	• Pyrimethamine and sulfadiazine	• Pyrimethamine and sulfadiazine
HSV	• Education on prevention of STIs • Valaciclovir prophylaxis in pregnant women • Consideration of Caesarean section delivery in women with open lesions during labour	• Aciclovir	• Aciclovir
Hepatitis B	• Education on prevention of STIs • Avoidance of intravenous drug use • Safe blood transfusions • Hepatitis B vaccination series • Hepatitis B vaccine and immunoglobulin for newborns of carrier mothers	• Supportive care • Antiviral therapy in chronic hepatitis B on case-by-case basis under supervision of specialist	• Supportive care

CMV, cytomegalovirus; HSV, herpes simplex virus; STI, sexually transmitted infection.

Prevention

Several strategies may be used to prevent congenital infections; some of these are highlighted in Table 27.3. Immunizations prior to pregnancy are very efficient in preventing infections such as rubella, hepatitis B, and varicella.

In cases where early intervention, including treatment of the infected mother, prevents transmission to the fetus, screening programmes can identify maternal infections that may otherwise be unrecognized. For example, congenital syphilis can be prevented by early antibiotic treatment in pregnancy; mother-to-child transmission of HIV can be prevented by ART during pregnancy, and hepatitis B infection in the newborn child can be prevented by vaccination in the mother or by hepatitis B Ig and vaccine given at birth to newborn babies of mothers who carry hepatitis B.

Unfortunately, in the case of certain congenital infections, such as toxoplasmosis, screening and treatment of exposed mothers can be difficult. *Toxoplasma gondii*-seronegative women, who may be exposed at any time during pregnancy, need to be screened monthly, and treatment should be initiated if they seroconvert. Such a strategy is often challenged by difficulties determining the interval between visits, adherence to the screening programme, logistics of procedures such as sampling, and prescription.

For infections, such as syphilis and HIV, in which early antimicrobial therapy is highly effective, testing pregnant women at the point of their earliest antenatal care is crucial. In addition, education and dissemination of knowledge on basic preventive strategies, such as avoidance of cat litter during pregnancy, vaccinations, and prevention of STIs (e.g. hepatitis B, HIV, and syphilis) in childbearing women and the larger population, are equally important.

Surveillance of mother-to-child transmissible infections is particularly important to estimate the true burden of such infections in pregnant women and newborn babies. Surveillance is also necessary to evaluate the efficiency and efficacy of prevention programmes. Surveillance strategies include the creation of case registers in the community, at national levels, monitoring the extent of antenatal testing and uptake of vaccinations, and international collaborative surveillance networks (see ➲ Chapter 2).

Further reading

Ford-Jones EL (1999). An approach to the diagnosis of congenital infections. *Paediatr Child Health*, **4**, 109–12.

Forsgren M (2009). Prevention of congenital and perinatal infections. *Euro Surveill*, **14**, 2–4.

Kamb ML, Newman LM, Riley PL, *et al*. (2010). A road map for the global elimination of congenital syphilis. *Obstet Gynecol Int*, **2010**, 312798.

Lanzieri TM, Dollard SC, Bialek SR, Grosse SD (2014). Systematic review of the birth prevalence of congenital cytomegalovirus infection in developing countries. *Int J Infect Dis*, **22**, 44–8.

Manicklal S, Emery VC, Lazzarotto T, Boppana, SB, Gupta RK (2013). The 'silent' global burden of congenital cytomegalovirus infection. *Clin Microbiol Rev*, **26**, 86–102.

Index

S